Fundamentals of Nursing

Fundamentals

PRENTICE-HALL, Inc.
ENGLEWOOD CLIFFS, NEW JERSEY

# of Nursing

Malinda Murray
University of Pennsylvania School of Nursing

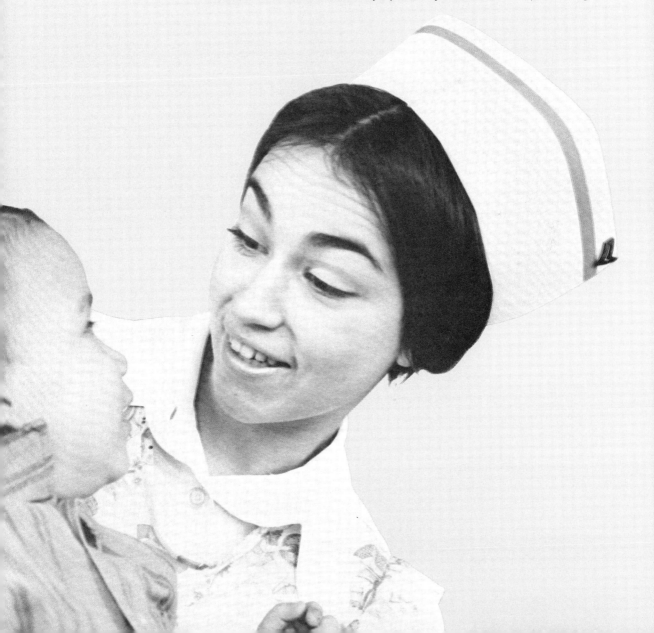

To Bill, with love

Library of Congress Cataloging in Publication Data

Murray, Malinda.
   Fundamentals of nursing.

   Includes bibliographies and index.
   1. Nursing. I. Title. [DNLM: 1. Nursing care.
WY100 M982f]
RT41.M87   610.73   75-33107
ISBN 0-13-341354-3

Printed in the United States of America

10 9 8 7 6 5 4

PRENTICE-HALL INTERNATIONAL, INC., London
PRENTICE-HALL OF AUSTRALIA, PTY. LTD., Sydney
PRENTICE-HALL OF CANADA, LTD., Toronto
PRENTICE-HALL OF INDIA PRIVATE LIMITED, New Delhi
PRENTICE-HALL OF JAPAN, INC., Tokyo

Photo credits:

*Cover photo, title page, Parts One, Two, Four, Five, and Seven—
Robert Goldstein; Part Three—Joel Gordon; Part Six—United
Hospital Fund of New York.*

Contents

5 Assessment   68

6 Planning, implementation, and evaluation   114

7 Record keeping and charting   133

Part Three   Psychosocial and interpersonal concerns of the nurse

8 Psychosocial and emotional needs of the patient   153

9   Nursing throughout the life cycle   179

10   Communication aspects of nursing   204

11   Teaching-learning aspects of nursing   232

Part Four   The therapeutic environment

12   Patients' rights in the health care system   247

Preface

This book is intended for beginning students in nursing—whether enrolled in a baccalaureate degree, associate degree, or diploma program. All these students need to develop the fundamental intellectual, interpersonal, and psychomotor abilities necessary for providing effective nursing care in a variety of situations. Today, nurses are increasingly accountable for their own actions. In addition to interdependence with the health team, the nurse must also be prepared for independent thought and action toward the goal of improved health care.

My experience with nursing students has convinced me that usually they are more highly motivated, goal-directed, and sensitive to human needs than their peers whose career plans are not so clearly defined. Provided with appropriate learning opportunities, encouragement, and a sound knowledge base, most nursing students clearly demonstrate a strong commitment to improved health care for patients, families, and communities with whom they come in contact. With the proper tools, nursing students are capable of making tremendous contributions to individuals and to society as a whole.

The most important tool for a nursing student to master is the nursing process itself. Assessment, planning, intervention, and evaluation are invariably the steps that must be taken in order to interact effectively with people who can benefit from contact with a nurse. Other skills, such as communication and various types of technical dexterity, are vital components in the repertoire of the successful nurse as she applies the nursing process to each situation in which she becomes involved. Four chapters in this book explain the nursing process in detail. Other chapters illustrate the nursing process as it is related to specific health needs and dysfunctions.

Hopefully, each student's growing recognition of her own valuable personal qualities will provide her with insight into how a professional nursing role must be built on self-acceptance as a unique worthwhile human being, as well as how to use this understanding and acceptance in her dealings with patients and families. The case studies included in the text are intended to help in this development of the student's realization of the scope and depth of nursing responsibilities and her own special abilities in fulfilling them. The case studies are designed to provoke careful thought and concerned creativity as the reader considers the nursing implications in each episode.

As graduate nurses, students will be expected to provide care to people in all physical, socioeconomic, and cultural circumstances and in many different settings. Therefore, most nursing curricula provide clinical experiences for students in various agencies and with different age groups. An effort has been made in this text to avoid an approach that is totally hospital-oriented, although many of the examples are directed to the care of hospitalized patients, because most clinical experiences for beginning students in most nursing programs are still in hospitals.

Recently, some nursing publications have begun to substitute the term "client" for "patient," arguing that "patient" carries the connotation of illness, whereas the nurse is also concerned with maintaining and promoting health. I agree wholeheartedly that the nurse supports the healthy person as well as the ill one. However, "client" is a rather general term referring to a person in need of an unspecified type of assistance. Thus, I believe that "patient" is a more appropriate term when implying a health need. It does not necessarily imply illness. Therefore, the term "patient" was deliberately selected in this text to refer to a person with health needs of any kind.

Because many current grammatical conventions for equalizing or eliminating pronoun gender (he or she, he/she, s/he) are awkward and distracting to the reader, I have chosen instead to designate the nurse as "she" and the patient, in most instances, as "he." This is because most nursing students and practicing nurses at this time are female, although I am glad to note that each year more men are choosing nursing as a career.

Acknowledgments

I would like to express my heartfelt thanks to all of my students, teachers, and colleagues who have profoundly influenced my ideas about nursing and the education of nurses. In preparing this book, I am grateful to the excellent team of research assistants, professional writers and editors, artists, photo researchers, market specialists, and production personnel who have contributed their special expertise to its development. A special word of appreciation is due to Claudia Wilson for her outstanding editorial contributions and unfailing sense of humor, which is a definite asset in publishing as well as in nursing. I also wish to thank my parents, LaBlanche and Henry Murray; my husband, William Edgell; and my friends both inside and outside the nursing profession for their support and enthusiasm throughout the writing of this book.

M. M.

Philadelphia, Pennsylvania

Malinda Murray (B.S.N., Emory University, M.Ed., Teachers College, Columbia University) was previously course coordinator and instructor in nursing fundamentals and in medical-surgical nursing at Skidmore College where she was also a member of the staff of a five-year project in curriculum development and evaluation. She is presently an Assistant Professor and Curriculum Coordinator of the Generic Baccalaureate Program, at the University of Pennsylvania School of Nursing.

Fundamentals of Nursing

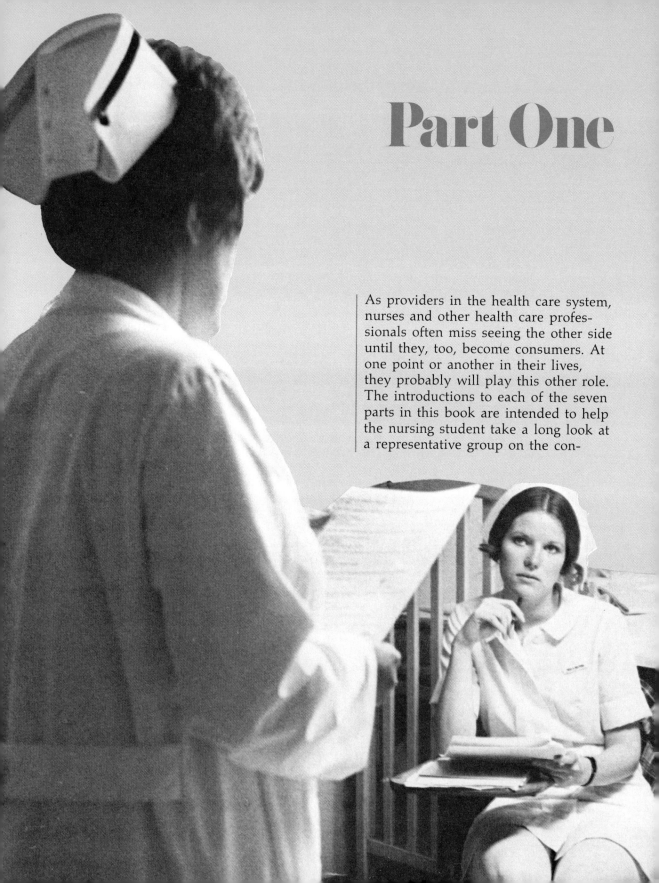

Part One

As providers in the health care system, nurses and other health care professionals often miss seeing the other side until they, too, become consumers. At one point or another in their lives, they probably will play this other role. The introductions to each of the seven parts in this book are intended to help the nursing student take a long look at a representative group on the con-

Introduction

sumer side of the health care fence. Hopefully, this will help increase the student's understanding of some of the situations faced by patients and their families.

• • •

There is nothing very extraordinary about the Harrison family, nothing dramatic that sets them apart from the Joneses, the Smiths, and the Does. Yet, the Harrisons are unique. They have their own particular problems and will certainly seek or need help to resolve them. Some of this help will be found in the health care system.

Richard Harrison, as the Census Bureau would say, is the head of the household. He is 47, and works as a foreman in a small factory that pro-

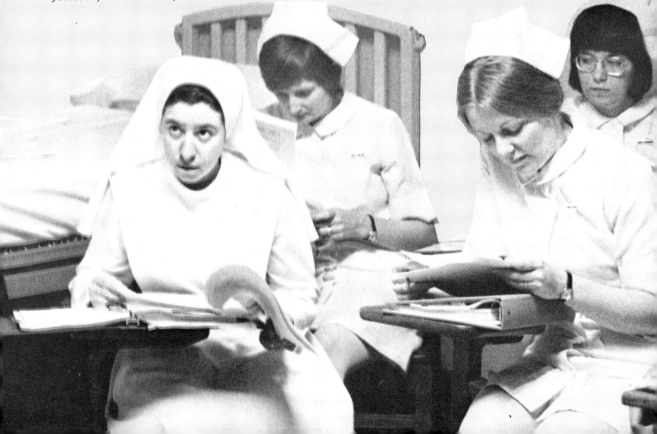

duces television parts. Richard is very handy with tools and has always been fascinated by gadgets. He does a lot of the electrical work around his own house and for friends, using the skills he learned in vocational high school and on his job. He is a stickler for detail and has a great deal of manual dexterity.

Richard, who began working right after high school as an electrician's assistant, earns about $14,000 a year. About $2,000 of this comes from overtime work at night or on weekends. In addition to his salary, he receives a number of employee benefits. These include medical insurance, which covers 65 percent of all in-hospital bills and some drug prescriptions. He also has a small pension and an allowance for disability.

Richard's factory is located in an old part of town. Most of the buildings there, including the factory, are over 50 years old. Lack of adequate public transportation in the area means that Richard must drive to work.

Richard is usually a congenial fellow. He enjoys good company, hearty meals, an occasional drink, and an occasional card game. It seems he has been enjoying the hearty meals a little too much lately and has been putting on weight for the past few years. So far, he has shrugged off his wife's suggestions that he get more physical exercise.

Anita, his wife, is 39 and very active physically and socially. After finishing high school, she worked for a year as a file clerk for an insurance company before marrying. She and Richard have three children, the first of whom was born when she was 20. The others arrived when she was 22 and 26.

Anita is a meticulous housekeeper and is considered an excellent cook by her family. She has a busy life and is very involved in volunteer work. Most of her activities are connected with her church. Although her life is busy, she feels she would like to go back to office work, now that her children are getting older.

Linda, the Harrisons' 19-year-old daughter, is a sophomore at the local community college, where she is majoring in child care. An ambitious young woman, she is the first in her family to attend college. In order to help pay for her tuition, she is working part time in the nursery school of a neighborhood recreation center. About 6 months ago, she started dating a co-worker at the center, a young man whose father is an alcoholic.

Paul, the Harrisons' oldest son, is 17 and a junior in high school. He likes automobiles, and he and his friends spend a great deal of time repairing old cars. Paul works as a service station attendant after school and on Saturday mornings. As a student, Paul is rather easygoing and not very interested in his academic courses. His attitude is reflected in his grades, which are mostly C's and D's. Paul is not sure what he wants to do later on, but he talks about being a sports car racer. College does not figure in his plans, but Anita and Richard are urging him to improve his grades and at least finish high school.

The youngest Harrison child, Steve, is 13 and in the eighth grade. He is a cheerful, friendly boy with lots of friends and many interests. His grades are mostly B's, with A's in science and math, his favorite subjects. He says he wants to study medicine eventually.

Steve is very good at sports and participates in one team sport or another almost every afternoon at the local YMCA. He always has a scratch or bruise to prove it, but has never had any serious injury. Steve looks up to his older brother and sister. He admires his sister's ambition and independence and his brother's casual attitude. He would like to tag along with Paul sometimes, but he is still considered the baby of the family, much to his dismay.

The Harrisons live on the outskirts of a large midwestern city. When they bought their house 15 years ago, the area was a well-kept residential neighborhood. Since then, however, some of their neighbors have moved away in order to escape the factory-generated smog and the noise of a nearby airport. Many of the neighborhood stores have closed and moved to more profitable areas. Groceries and other essentials are no longer available within walking distance.

The Harrison family is closely knit, although the children are now asserting their independence more and more. This sometimes takes the form of rebellion against parental advice, but the family is usually able to talk out its disagreements. To date, the Harrisons have had no major medical problems.

There are other family members with whom the Harrisons maintain close ties. These include Charlotte Harrison, Richard's older sister. She owns and manages a small, successful florist shop and has three people working for her. At 53, Charlotte has never been married. She was engaged at one time, but her fiancé was killed during World War II. Charlotte is devoted to the Harrison children and has dinner with the family every Sunday.

Charlotte lives alone in a one-bedroom apartment in the suburbs, about 20 minutes away from the Harrisons. She loves to travel and has vacationed abroad frequently. She has been to some 20 foreign countries and has seen many attractions "off the beaten path." By now, she has even become pretty well conditioned against "tourista" and other typical travelers' ills. She is also active in community affairs. Among other activities, she has helped to coordinate the annual blood bank drive for many years.

Charlotte and Richard lost both parents within the last 10 years. Their mother died of cancer in her early sixties and their father died of heart failure in his late fifties. An older sister died of undetermined causes while still a child.

Estelle Tanner, Anita's mother, is a 71-year-old widow. Her husband died last year at the age of 78 after a long, debilitating illness. Estelle nursed him at home. She has never worked outside the home. She raised five children, whose births spanned a period of 15 years. Estelle lives in a small, three-bedroom house in a small town about 300 miles from the Harrisons. Although she has lived in the same area all her life, she no longer knows well many of the people in the town.

Many of her old friends have passed away. Recently, she has considered taking in a boarder, not only to supplement her small pension but also to provide companionship. She sees the Harrisons about once every two months and speaks to them on the phone every week.

What are the projected health care needs for this family as a unit? for individual members?

What are the family's probable strengths in the area of health maintenance? What are their liabilities?

From what sources would the family most likely obtain health services?

In what settings is the family likely to come into contact with a nurse?

1 What is nursing practice?

What is health? What is illness?

"If you have your health, you have everything," people say to one another, and generally they understand what is meant.

For nursing and other health sciences, however, the concepts of **health** and **illness** are central to the work of delivering "health care." For them, a more definitive and complete understanding of health is needed.

The definition of health proposed by the World Health Organization (WHO) has been accepted by many professionals. It does not, however, tell us precisely what is meant by the term "health." WHO states:

Health is a state of complete physical, mental, and social well-being, and not merely the absence of disease or infirmity.[1]

One critic of this definition claims that one vague concept (health) is defined in terms of the absence of another even more imprecise concept (disease).[2] Another problem arises in the ambiguity of the term "well-being." Does this imply that health is a state of complete happiness or euphoria? (If so, most of the world is unhealthy.) A woman in labor may feel pain and discomfort, not a sense of well-being—but would we say that she is sick? And if health is the complete absence of any disease, what about people who function fully but who are handicapped, or people with myopia who wear glasses? What about the temporary grief and depression associated with real-life crises?

No known definitions of health and illness answer every objection and exception, of course. Nurses, along with other involved workers and researchers, continue to work at defining exactly what is meant by health, illness, and all states in between.

[1]World Health Organization. 1947. Constitution of the World Health Organization. *Chronicle of the World Health Organization* 1.
[2]Marie Jahoda. 1958. *Current concepts of positive mental health*, pp. 10–15, 73. New York: Basic Books.

Upon completing this chapter, the reader should be able to:

1. Define health in various ways.

2. Understand the subjectivity of the health-illness continuum that individuals experience.

3. Identify the human factors that influence the development of a nurse-patient relationship.

4. Explain the position of the nurse in relation to the health team and its members.

5. Define the concept of primary care and its implications for nursing.

6. Describe the relationship between health team members and their shared goal of enhancing the patient's health and welfare.

People experience
health and illness in
about as many different
ways as there are
cultures and
individuals.

The following are some current attempts at defining health:

Wellness [i.e., health] is a status in which an individual of a given sex and at a given stage of growth and development is capable of meeting the minimum physical, physiological, and social requirements for appropriate functioning in the given sex category and at the given growth and developmental level.[3]

Most people seem to perceive health in terms of their own ability to function according to their own perception of what is normal.[4]

Somatic [physical] health is, sociologically defined, the state of optimum capacity for the effective performance of valued tasks.[5]

And the *American Heritage Dictionary of the English Language* states:

Health is the state of an organism with respect to function, disease, and abnormality at a given time.

The health-illness continuum

From these examples, it is obvious that no clear, comprehensive definition has yet been found. Many attempts to explain health and illness are "either-or" propositions—that is, an individual must be *either* healthy *or* ill. In real life outside the definitions, however, we know that people can be both ill and well at the same time. We can see that there are healthy elements in otherwise ill people, as well as elements of sickness in otherwise well persons. Likewise, the potential for one state is present in the existence of the other.

Factors influencing our attitudes toward health and illness

People experience health and illness in about as many different ways as there are cultures and individuals. In order to know that he is "ill," an individual must have some standard against which to measure current (or past) physical or mental changes. A person measures these changes against his (and his society's) concept of what his physical and mental state usually is or should be. For example, a person with anemia may not always experience the symptoms of fatigue as unusual or indicative of an "illness."

[3]Betty Jo Hadley. Current concepts of wellness and illness: Their relevance for nursing. *Image*, p. 24.
[4]Carter L. Marshall. 1972. *Dynamics of health and disease*, p. 2. New York: Appleton-Century-Crofts.
[5]Talcott Parsons. 1958. Definitions of health and illness in light of American values and social structure. In *Patients, physicians, and illness*, ed. E. Gartly Jaco, pp. 167–68. New York: Free Press.

("Everyone's always complaining about being tired, so I didn't think anything of it," one anemic patient stated.) And in many underdeveloped countries, where malaria, tuberculosis, and intestinal diseases are common, most people consider themselves "sick" only if they are unable to work.[6]

Even the belief that one should try to maintain a certain level of health and the ways health should be kept up are influenced by societal values. Also important are age, education, social class, religious beliefs, and current physical condition. Thus, one study showed that poorer people in the United States were concerned about health only when it interfered with daily activity and independence. This would suggest that lack of concern with health may relate to the economic value placed on health in comparison with other expenditures.[7]

In the study from which the following examples were taken, clinic patients and third-year medical students were asked how they would define being "healthy" or "physically fit":

> She or he doesn't get dizzy spells, or pain in the arms like I do. Such people wouldn't get other things I've had—the pressure in my chest, for instance. (Housewife with arteriosclerotic heart disease)

> Most people consider they are in good health when they are unaware of any disease process being present. I would define it as the absence of any predisposition to disease, no pain, fatigue, or loss of appetite; a total absence of somatic complaints. (Medical student)[8]

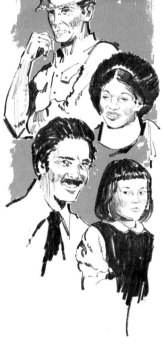

"Illness" does not mean the same thing to all people.

The clinic patient with a chronic disease describes health as the absence of the particular symptoms that she has experienced. The medical student defines health solely in **somatic** terms, and the description lacks a personal referent. (The medical students, on the average, were 20 years younger than the clinic patients and presumably in good health.)

Although, at some time or other, "illness" confronts everyone, it does not mean the same thing to all people. In fact, no two individuals, even with the same diagnosis, will see their illnesses in exactly the same way. The same illness may be associated with punishment and shame for one person and relief plus needed family support for another. There is some indication that a higher educational level may increase awareness of symptoms. It has also been observed that physical and emotional states can determine how and what is perceived. Fear, for example, produces thinking that is slow, narrow in scope, and rigid in form. It tends to reduce

[6]L. M. Hanks, Jr., and Jane R. Hanks. 1955. Diphtheria immunization in a Thai community. In *Health, culture and community*, ed. Benjamin D. Paul, p. 156. New York: Russell Sage.

[7]H. Ashley Weeks, Marjorie Davis, and Howard Freeman. 1958. Apathy of families toward medical care. In *Patients, physicians, and illness*, ed. E. Gartly Jaco, pp. 159–65. New York: Free Press.

[8]Barbara Baumann. 1961. Diversities in conceptions of health and physical fitness. *Journal of Health and Human Behavior* 2. In *Social interaction and patient care*, ed. James K. Skipper, Jr., and Robert C. Leonard, p. 209. Philadelphia: Lippincott.

Nursing is putting "the patient in the best condition for nature to act."

—*Florence Nightingale*

the alternatives an individual can choose to handle a particular situation. When fear is tied to illness-perception, the resulting behavior can prove bizarre, or at least unreasonable. One nurse, acutely aware of possible anesthetic and surgical risks, refused to undergo a simple surgical procedure. She chose instead to cope with nagging, chronic medical complaints.

For nursing, then, any workable concept of health must include social, psychological, and cultural factors as well as medical and physical aspects. Moreover, the nurse giving care must understand that she, too, is part of this pattern of culture and values. She must be aware of her own individual prejudices and fears, expectations, and reactions to illness. She can recognize this, and when caring for patients, she can make a conscious effort to see values and wishes concerning health through their eyes.

What is nursing practice?

As with the concepts of health and illness, there are many definitions of **nursing practice.** There is the historical dictum of Florence Nightingale that nursing is putting "the patient in the best condition for nature to act."[9] There are also modern ideas of nursing as "diagnosing and treating human responses to actual or potential health problems."[10]

Basic to many of the definitions, however, is the concept of nursing as an activity which helps the individual to help himself in achieving or maintaining health. In other words, nursing involves complementing the patient's own abilities. "The unique function of the nurse," nursing theoretician Virginia Henderson says in "The Nature of Nursing," is to "assist the individual, sick or well, in the performance of those activities contributing to health or its recovery (or to peaceful death) that he would perform unaided if he had the necessary strength, will or knowledge."[11]

In order to do this, the nurse must, as much as possible, "get inside the patient's skin." She must try to see where his responses originate and realize that she herself could feel, and perhaps has felt, some similar reactions. Human beings are often able to understand extremes of feeling in other human beings, and those in professional nursing develop this quality to a high degree. After sharing another person's emotional burden,

[9]Florence Nightingale. 1859. *Notes on nursing: What it is and what it is not,* p. 79. Facsimile edition, 1946. Philadelphia: Lippincott.

[10]The New York State education law, amendment to article 139, sec. 6902, defining the practice of nursing effective March 15, 1972, continues as follows: ". . . through such services as case finding, health teaching, health counseling, and provision of care supportive to or restorative of life and well-being, and executing medical regimens prescribed by a licensed or otherwise legally authorized physician or dentist. A nursing regimen shall be consistent with and shall not vary from any existing medical regimen."

[11]Virginia Henderson. 1964. The nature of nursing. *American Journal of Nursing* 64. In *Nursing fundamentals,* ed. Mary E. Meyers, p. 8. Dubuque, Iowa: Brown.

she is then in a better position to help him bear, lessen, cope, or deal with the particular situation.

An official definition of nursing, from the 1973 American Nurses' Association's *Standards of Nursing Practice,* states that "nursing practice is a direct service, goal directed and adaptable to the needs of the individual, family and community during health and illness." In addition, the practitioner of nursing "bears the primary responsibility and accountability for the nursing care clients/patients receive."

The following standards of nursing practice, as formulated by the American Nurses' Association (ANA), apply to nursing in any setting. They provide a means for determining the quality of nursing care that is given:

1. The collection of data about the health status of the client/patient is systematic and continuous. The data are accessible, communicated, and recorded. (*Rationale: Comprehensive care requires complete and ongoing collection of data in order to determine nursing needs. All health status data about the client/patient must be available for all members of the health care team.*)
2. Nursing diagnoses are derived from health status data. (*Rationale: The health status is the basis for determining nursing care needs.*)
3. The plan of nursing care includes goals derived from the nursing diagnosis. (*Rationale: The determination of the results to be achieved is an essential part of planning care.*)
4. The plan of nursing care includes priorities and the prescribed nursing approaches or measures to achieve the goals derived from the nursing diagnoses. (*Rationale: Nursing actions are planned to promote, maintain, and restore client/patient well-being.*)
5. Nursing actions provide for client/patient participation in health promotion, maintenance, and restoration. (*Rationale: The client/patient and family are continually involved in nursing care.*)
6. Nursing actions assist the client/patient to maximize his health capabilities. (*Rationale: Nursing actions are designed to promote, maintain, and restore health.*)
7. Client/patient progress or lack of progress toward goal achievement is determined by the client/patient and the nurse. (*Rationale: The quality of nursing care depends upon comprehensive and intelligent determination of nursing's impact upon the health status of the client/patient. The client/patient plays an essential part in this determination.*)
8. Client/patient progress or lack of progress toward goal achievement directs reassessment, reordering of priorities, new goal setting, and revision of the plan of nursing care. (*Rationale: The nursing process remains the same, but the input of new information may dictate new or revised approaches.*)[12]

---

[12] American Nurses' Association. 1973. *Standards of nursing practice.* Kansas City, Mo.

> "Nursing practice is a direct service, goal directed and adaptable to the needs of the individual, family and community during health and illness."
>
> *—American Nurses' Association's Standards of Nursing Practice*

The focus of nursing practice

The individual patient

In the previous paragraphs we have discussed at least some of the factors that go into a person's reaction to illness. We have also outlined current standards of nursing practice. Now let us see what happens when this unique individual, the patient, with his own prejudices, fears, and vulnerabilities, encounters the health care system that is supposed to help him:

"Here, sir, take this medication."
"But what's it for?"
"I'm sorry, but you'll have to ask your doctor tomorrow."

"Here's your dinner, sir."
"But it's only 5:30. I usually don't eat this early."
"Sorry, sir, here's your dinner."

"Time to go for X-ray studies."
"What for?"
"For a bone study. Didn't you know?"
"Why no, what's wrong with my bones?"

In actual patient care situations, many conflicts may arise between an individual patient's needs and the desire of the institution for order and efficiency. There may also be differences between nursing theory and actual nursing practice. Nurses will see examples of impersonal and often fragmented methods of giving care and the effect that these have on the patient. Often the effects include anger, fear, intimidation, withdrawal, or acceptance. Nurses then realize, perhaps acutely, the importance of focusing their care and interest on the *individual* patient and what he considers important. By caring for only one patient, family, or small group of patients at a time, nursing students can see the whole person (the patient) within his total environment (to be discussed further in chapter 15). They will also become acquainted with the consequences of caring for people as "the gall bladder in room 650."

The family

Illness in an individual is like a pebble thrown into a still pond. The waves and ripples from even a small stone are far reaching. Even with a so-called "minor" illness, other people, families, and friends of the ill person are often deeply affected. Other people are related to the sick person, whether by blood or by concern. They too need personalized care in order to recover a sense of balance and help the patient recover or accept his illness.

Illness in an individual is like a pebble thrown into a still pond.

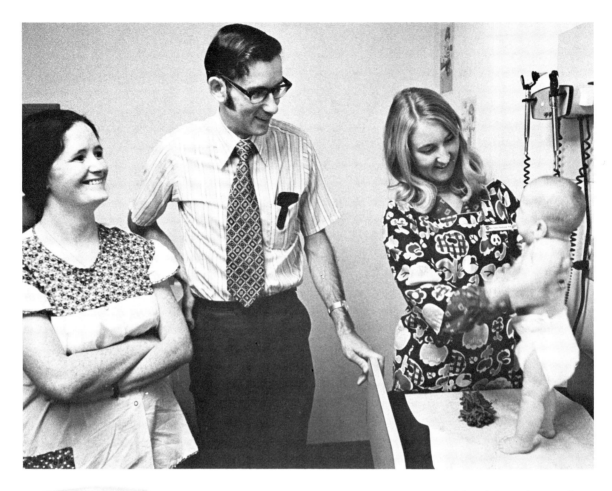

The community

Individuals are also part of a larger community. In some fields of nursing, including public health, mental health nursing, and teaching, this larger population is the major focus of nursing practice. Even in expanded settings, however, nursing's aim is still to give continuous good care to every individual.

The nurse is also part of a specialized community. This is the community of nurses and other health providers. Nurses can play key roles in initiating and implementing ways of improving and humanizing specific aspects of care. These include hospital admission procedures, which are notoriously impersonal and anxiety-producing for the patient and his family. Also important are methods of communicating to patients their rights upon admission and about routine hospital procedures. Nurses are also involved in educational programs for preoperative and clinic patients. At all employment levels, nurses are in a unique position to provide leadership in many areas of patient care. They work through nursing care groups within hospitals, local nursing organizations, consumer rights committees, and meaningful continuing education courses.

The whole family, as well as the whole patient, must be treated.

[Photo by Dan Bernstein, courtesy of the *American Journal of Nursing*]

11

Acceptance of patients'
behavior depends on
an emotional
self-awareness and
self-acceptance on the
part of the nurse.

Factors influencing the nurse-patient relationship

Periodically, nursing journals feature articles written by nurses who experience nursing and hospitalization from the "other side"—as patients or members of a patient's family. Only then do they really know the way a patient or his family feels and reacts. The disappointment, shock, and fear they experience in the hospital situation is obviously surprising to them. They feel alienated, resentful, isolated, and "problematic" to the very nursing staffs they have, in other situations, been part of.

One nurse recalled her feelings as she was impersonally shifted from her role as wife to that of "visitor" when her husband was hospitalized for a heart attack:

> I was a relative—that enemy who is told nothing, kept as far from the patient as possible, and by all means, kept from the doctors. That much I remembered. Relatives complain. They ask questions. They pounce from behind doors to demand tea or vases for their miserable flowers.[13]

Another nurse, whose child was dying in a hospital, spoke of the experiences she and her husband had with hospital personnel:

> People were unfailingly kind and sympathetic, but conversation was always general, almost social in nature, and no one seemed able to talk with us about what was uppermost in our minds. Namely, how could we bear this tragedy? How could we and his brother and sisters attempt any sort of normal living again? We requested an autopsy, but we were never offered the results. We were tormented by wondering if earlier medical care might have made any difference, whether keeping John in bed might have prevented the lethal complications, whether certain physiological differences had contributed to his vulnerability. But these questions, and others, went unanswered.[14]

This author hoped to help nurses realize the importance of expressing understanding, sensitivity, and compassion toward people in similar situations. She concluded her article this way:

> Attempts on the part of the nurse to show empathy, to understand, and to communicate more understandingly with families who suffer the death of a child, would not only help them in accepting and coping with their immediate anguish, but would probably make the long adjustment easier to endure.[15]

And when hospitalized patients, in one study on pain, were asked what

[13]Ethel H. Naugle. 1971. Knock and wait. *American Journal of Nursing* 71:312.
[14]Joyce Guimond. 1974. We knew our child was dying. *American Journal of Nursing* 74:249.
[15]Ibid.

doctors and nurses could do to help patients in pain, these were their responses:

> Don't make judgments when you don't know and haven't hurt.
>
> Don't ignore patients in pain and give them the brushoff—we aren't a bunch of neurotics.
>
> See patients as individuals and not textbook pictures.
>
> What is more important than talking to patients about pain?
>
> Be prompt. Try to understand. Make more of an effort.[16]

Nursing attitudes and patient care

Just about every nursing student experiences anxiety about whether her care of patients will ever be the care of a "good" nurse. And all dread the ever-present possibility of being told by the instructor that "you just don't have what it takes to be a good nurse." But just what does it take? Is it a mystical composite of unattainable, unlearnable qualities? If these qualities are not inborn, can they ever be learned well enough, and soon enough, to help current patients?

What follows is an exploration of some of the factors that influence the kind of relationship a nurse will have with a patient. Included are suggestions on how nursing students can begin building on the qualities they already possess to develop excellence in nursing.

Acceptance

The quality of acceptance in nursing does not necessarily mean approval of the patient's attitudes, values, or behavior. Rather, it is a developing attitude by which the nurse is able to work with the patient as he really is. The nurse accepts his negative as well as his positive qualities, without judging them to be "bad" or "good." At some level she may judge the patient's behavior according to her own personal standards. In her work as a nurse, however, her motive is to understand the person constructively, rather than to judge him. This constructive understanding, not moral judgment, will allow the patient to recognize and express his feelings. Eventually it will help him to find his own answers to the conflicts he expresses.

Acceptance of patients' behavior depends on an emotional self-awareness and self-acceptance on the part of the nurse. In addition, she must

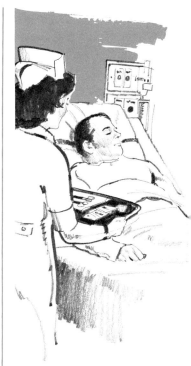

"See patients as individuals and not textbook pictures."

[16]Laurel Archer Copp. 1974. The spectrum of suffering. *American Journal of Nursing* 74:493.

have a knowledge of human personality, patterns of behavior, and factors influencing potential for change.

In a study of 105 hospital surgical patients, all of the patients indicated a need for acceptance by the nurse. Factors contributing to their feelings of acceptance varied, however. The following conclusions were made about their responses:

1. Patients felt accepted if the nurse created an environment in which the patient could comfortably express his feelings.
2. Patients felt accepted if they "didn't have to keep up a front" and could share their feelings. (One postoperative patient said: "It was ridiculous the way I acted. I didn't know why I was so scared when I arrived, but it helped to know that it was all right to cry.")
3. Patients felt accepted if time was taken by the nurse to ascertain how they "really felt about things."
4. Patients felt accepted if the nurse demonstrated nonjudgmental attitudes toward them. (These attitudes were expressed by the nurse more through her tone and manner of conversing than by any direct statements.)[17]

How is acceptance demonstrated by the nurse? To show acceptance, the nurse must start with a real desire to help the patient (caring). She then comes to accept him as a person and communicates this acceptance to him.

Some of the ways that the patients said a nurse could show acceptance and caring include:

1. Demonstrating spontaneity in friendly relations and attention to social amenities
2. Thoughtfulness to details
3. Paying attention to personal preferences
4. Respecting the patient's modesty
5. Stopping to see if the patient needs anything, even though his call light may not be on

Sensitivity

Sensitivity is nothing new. We are already sensitive to certain things. That is, we "pay attention to," we "respond to" people and situations around us that we consider important. Among these are red lights, storm warnings, and the people close to us. The key to expanding our sensitivities

---

[17]Laurel Archer Copp and John Dixon Copp. 1960. Look to the pattern of relationships. *American Journal of Nursing* 60:1284.

to include patients lies in learning to do explicitly and frequently what we naturally do implicitly and only occasionally.[18]

To acquire sensitivity, an individual must first accept the other person's perception of reality. Even though this perception may be different from his own, he must come to recognize it as valid for the other person. Then he must focus on the other person and what he is really saying. This means temporarily postponing his own immediate needs in order to be available to the other person and his wishes. It means learning to listen carefully and objectively and learning to watch the other person's behavior for the meaning it expresses.

Sensitivity can be learned by simply looking at things receptively. This means observing and noting observations and reactions to experiences, whether real or vicarious (as through literature), and by sharing other people's experiences. It also means not becoming involved with whether the other person's behavior measures up to one's own expectations or "correct" behavior. Being sensitive need not mean that an individual must give up his own perceptions. He must be willing, however, to recognize the reality and validity of others' views of what life is all about.

Empathy

The concept of **empathy** has been explored by authorities in many fields—philosophy, psychiatry, religion, and sociology. Basically, empathy involves the feelings of identification that people can develop when interacting with other persons. It has also been described as openness and understanding between two persons, a feeling of entering into the feeling of another person.[19] And finally, it has been characterized as "stepping into another person's shoes and stepping easily out of them."[20]

Anyone who takes on the role of helper is faced with some degree of empathetic involvement since the nature of helping demands subjective involvement with others. The phases of developing a "relatedness" relationship with another person begin with an initial encounter and lead to the development of a rapport (a relationship of mutual trust).

It has been said that the ability to empathize is the distinguishing characteristic of the committed nurse.[21] "She must learn to feel in herself something of his [the patient's] unaccustomed feelings, his strange new fears, his silently pleading hopes"[22]—to realize what it is to be this person.

[18] Arthur W. Combs, Donald L. Avila, and William W. Purkey. 1971. *Helping relationships: Basic concepts for the helping professions*, p. 187. Boston: Allyn & Bacon.

[19] Martin Buber. 1937. *I and thou.* New York: Scribner's.

[20] N. Blackman et al. 1958. The development of empathy in male schizophrenics. *Psychiatric Quarterly* 32:546.

[21] Sister Madeleine Clemence. 1966. Existentialism: A philosophy of commitment. *American Journal of Nursing* 66:500–05.

[22] Copp and Copp, p. 1284.

Even after mastering
and becoming
proficient with many
technical skills, the
good nurse retains her
empathy for patients
and their problems.

Even after mastering and becoming proficient with many technical skills, the good nurse retains her empathy for patients and their problems.

Since the degree of empathy seems to be determined by the bounds of individuals' similarities, empathy may not always occur as a natural process. The ability to comprehend the behavior of another is generally limited by one's personal background. Many nursing students, for example, have very little in common with their patients in the way of age, social class, and past experiences. These differences may interfere with the process of communication and identification, unless the student can objectify her own perceptions. She must understand the patient's perceptions and realize that people, regardless of culture, have basically similar needs, even though these needs may differ in strength, intensity, and manner of expression.[23]

Among aids for the student in developing empathy are experiences that will deepen her life perspective. These include literature (behavioral sciences, poetry, fiction) and continued contact with individuals from varying backgrounds. Recognition and clarification by the student, through discussion groups, of the similarities and differences between herself and her patients is also important. Role-playing, in which students reconstruct or imagine interactions with patients who are quite different from themselves, is also helpful.

Trust

Patients and nurses of quite dissimilar backgrounds can often close their obvious cultural gaps somewhat through "trust." No matter how much empathy, warmth, and sensitivity the nurse expresses toward a patient, it is not likely that the patient will express himself fully if he believes the nurse to be untrustworthy.

A person whose attitude of trust is weak is "one who expects bad from every new situation and to whom the kindness and dependability of people must be demonstrated."[24] Trust is defined as "a contentment and confidence which stems from a deep assumption that life is pleasant and will not become unmanageable."[25] Some synonyms for trust are faith, confidence, reliance, and dependence. Two of its opposites are mistrust and suspicion.

In general, a person who trusts has the following characteristics:

1. A comfortableness with an increasing awareness of himself, his goals, and his motivations

[23]Joyce Travelbee. 1971. *Interpersonal aspects of nursing,* 2d ed., p. 205. Philadelphia: Davis.
[24]A. Baldwin. 1955. *Behavior and development in childhood,* p. 547. New York: Dryden.
[25]Ibid.

2. An ability to share this awareness with appropriate people
3. An acceptance of others who deviate from his own ways of thinking, feeling, and acting without intense needs to change them
4. An acceptance of new experiences
5. An ability to demonstrate a consistency between words and actions that lasts over time
6. An ability to delay gratification[26]

People who mistrust generally demonstrate the opposite personality characteristics.

These are not mutually exclusive categories, however. Both the patient and the nurse will exhibit elements of trust and mistrust. Each person's attitude probably lies somewhere on a line between extremes.[27]

The existence of trust in any given individual depends to a large extent on his life experiences up to that point, particularly early life experiences. Infants constantly test the trustworthiness of their external and internal world. They measure to what degree their frustrations, hunger, and discomforts are being alleviated. If they receive love and understanding consistently, infants are helped to develop a basic sense of trust. If not, they may develop tendencies more toward suspicion and loneliness. In addition, an individual's later experiences continue to contribute to the further development, clarification, and evaluation of modes of self-trust and ability to trust others.

Trust is an essential element of nursing. When the patient trusts, he can reveal more of his true feelings. The nurse can then make more accurate observations and decisions about his nursing care. As a result, the patient can move more productively toward health.

> Trust is an essential element of nursing.

The need for personal satisfaction

The growth of these characteristics in the nurse not only helps the patient, but also provides greater satisfaction for the nurse. A nurse who is motivated primarily by a sense of duty will never be as happy or creative in her work as a nurse who experiences a sense of joy. The latter relates to patients with an anticipation of challenge and interpersonal rewards for herself as well as for the patient and his family. The traditional aura of "dedication" surrounding the nurse does not stop her from fulfilling some of her own needs in a constructive fashion through the satisfaction of providing high-quality nursing care.

---

[26]Mary Durand Thomas. 1970. Trust in the nurse-patient relationship. In *Behavioral concepts and nursing intervention,* ed. Carolyn E. Carlson, p. 118. Philadelphia: Lippincott.
[27]Ibid.

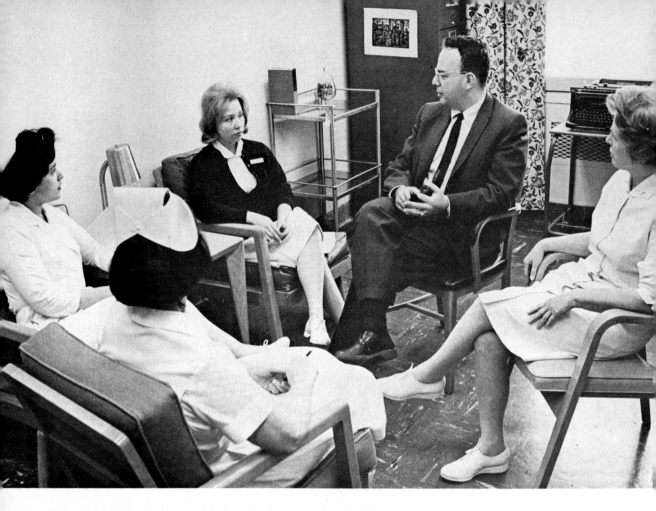

The modern health care team includes doctors, nurses, occupational therapists, nutritionists, and representatives of other helping professions.

[Courtesy of the National Institutes of Health Clinical Center]

The nurse as a member of the health care team

Not too many years ago, the doctor and the nurse, along with the local apothecary (druggist), were the only members of the "health team." Today, however, growing health care institutions are specialized and multifaceted. The number of health workers within the system of medical care has grown tremendously. In the course of one short hospital stay, a patient may be seen and evaluated not only by doctors and nurses but also by social workers, dietitians, inhalation therapists, chaplains, X-ray technicians, psychiatrists, physical therapists, physicians' assistants, and by students of every health science.

The most important members of the health team are the *patient* and his *family*, who must be active participants in the patient's care rather than mere beneficiaries of the planning of others. The professional membership of the team includes the *doctor*, who, together with the nurse and others, determines the plan of care and methods of treatment. The *professional nurse* makes additional decisions and judgments about the nursing care needs of the patient and cooperates with the doctor to implement the medical care plan. The *licensed practical* (or vocational) *nurse* assists the professional nurse and carries out various nursing procedures. Helping them are *aides, orderlies,* and *technicians.* They perform no professional function but are involved with much of the direct nursing care. They work under the supervision of the professional nurse. The health care team often includes members of other helping professions (*clergy, social work, physical and occupational therapy, speech therapy, dentistry, pharmacy,* and *clinical psychology*). There are also clerical and administrative managers, community workers, and aides within the other professions.

Independent, interdependent, and dependent nursing functions

Within the broad range of professional nursing responsibilities there are independent as well as interdependent and dependent functions. Independent functions involve actions which the nurse initiates herself. Dependent functions are those she performs on someone else's orders. Interdependent functions are those which she decides upon in collaboration with other members of the health care team. For example, a nurse functions independently when teaching a patient or family members how to give a medication. She acts interdependently when she decides to administer a medication the doctor has indicated is for "prn" (whenever necessary) use. She performs a dependent function when she administers a medication prescribed by a physician. In order to be most effective, members of the health team can never function completely independently of each other. They are all interdependent.

Primary care nursing

Nursing has currently been experimenting with expansion of its traditional services and roles to meet the multiple health needs of people. It is also acting to provide meaningful growth within the nursing profession. **Primary care** is the name given to the first contact a patient has with the health system. In the past, this contact has almost always been with a physician.

The expanded nursing role in primary care includes taking health histories, doing physical examinations, and caring for the well child (the pediatric nurse practitioner). Nurses are also working in communities in an expanded public health and medical supervisory role. One nurse, who is also a registered inhalation therapist, operates a solo practice in respiratory nursing. Another, in a rural county in New Mexico, provides primary care to a community that suddenly found itself without a physician.[28] Other

Primary care is the name given to the first contact a patient has with the health system.

[28]Carol Brierly. 1973. Thanks to Martha Schweback. *Prism.*

nurses have set up independent practices in nursing, either as solo practitioners[29] or in a group.[30]

The concept of "primary care nursing" has also evolved within the hospital. This has resulted from an attempt to lessen the confusion a patient feels when confronted by so many workers, as mentioned previously, all of whom claim to be "his" doctor, "his" nurse, or whatever. Through primary nursing, the patient is assigned on admission to a nurse on his unit. She will remain his primary nurse throughout his stay on that unit or until discharge. The primary nurse is a staff nurse (or the head nurse) who is totally responsible for the care of three or four patients. She meets with each patient and decides what nursing care is needed. Staff members who work with the patient when the primary nurse is off duty follow her initial plan and make appropriate changes on behalf of the primary nurse. At discharge, the primary nurse initiates referrals and nursing follow-up, if needed, to the public health nurse.

This method of care not only contributes to the patient's welfare but furthers the development of a nurse's professional growth. It encourages her to make independent assessments and decisions and provides accountability for care to the patient, the physician, and the head nurse. Finally, it concentrates on actual nursing care at every level of competence.

In nursing units that have not implemented the practice of primary nursing, no one person is usually held responsible for the nursing care. A patient may get lost in the shuffle. Sometimes he is discharged without adequate follow-up. He may be unsure of just exactly what his condition is and what he can do about it. Many times the patient is not even sure of just what was done to him in the hospital!

Unique vs. shared responsibilities in health care

All health professionals have certain shared interests and responsibilities in promoting and providing health care. For example, both the nurse and the physical therapist attempt to enable the patient to independently perform the activities of daily living. Both the social worker and the public health nurse want to insure adequate nutrition for foster home families and their young charges.

But each has a unique contribution to make. The surgeon determines the extent of activity a patient will be allowed postoperatively. The nurse attempts to help the patient integrate these new limitations into his own life in a satisfactory way. The internist may decide that a patient's hypertension can be controlled with diet and medication. The nurse and the dietitian help the patient with the specifics and details of just what a

---

[29]M. Lucille Kinlein. 1972. Independent nurse practitioner. *Nursing Outlook* 20:22–24.
[30]American Nurses' Association. 1974. Nurse teams hang out their shingles. *American Journal of Nursing* 74:10.

low-salt diet means, what the medications are, and how to take them. Each profession must be aware of its own special interests. They should not, however, become so preoccupied with professional territoriality that they lose sight of their commonly held goal—to defend and enhance the patient's welfare and health.

SUMMARY

Health means many things. It is a sense of complete well-being and the absence of disease. It is also the ability to meet the minimum requirements of functioning within society and performing valued tasks in a "normal" fashion. For the individual, the existence or absence of health is usually not determined by laboratory tests or medical pronouncements but by the expectations created within his particular society. It means that the person who is "sick" has demonstrated changes (physical, mental, or both) that are deemed unacceptable, abnormal, and unhealthy by that society.

The person who becomes a nurse is also part of a cultural "school" of health attitude-teaching. Family, friends, experiences, nursing curriculum, childhood training, and future expectations all go into determining many of the attitudes the student holds about health and illness. Experiences with patients will help the nursing student recognize many of the complex, irrational, and rational values held by other people concerning health. Understanding their values can be helpful in clarifying and evaluating individual concepts of health and disease.

Experience tells us that each person's health status is somewhere on a line between extremes of good health and sickness. Clinical experience at the bedside will demonstrate the many types of reactions to illness that the human organism is capable of. We can see elements of sickness in otherwise healthy people, and elements of health in sick persons.

The nurse sees healthy potential in every "sick" person and can intervene in positive ways to assist the person to help himself return to complete health. In addition, she can help family members adjust to illness situations. She recognizes the need for well individuals to continue in healthy patterns and can encourage this growth.

She does this by establishing a rapport with the patient based on mutual trust. She builds the relationship by getting to know him, his values, and the meaning sickness holds for him. She must also accept and identify with his feelings. She can then constructively and sensitively complement the patient's own efforts toward health or coping with illness.

The nurse becomes proficient in technical skills through practice. Likewise, her ability to accept and assist the *total* person is a combination of natural and learned abilities. These are developed through self-knowledge, self-acceptance, flexibility, a fine attunement to others, and an understanding that all people have basically the same needs and drives.

Both health care and nursing have changed rapidly over recent years. Medical care has become increasingly complex. Nursing, in many ways, has filled gaps in the delivery of that care. Nursing and medicine are still interdependent. Each has a unique contribution to make, along with several other involved professions, to improved patient care. Primary nursing is an example of one of nursing's innovations.

Since the focus of nursing practice is the individual, the family, and the larger community, nurses are in a unique position to provide leadership and direction for communities and groups concerned with health issues. The nurse is also part of the community of nursing. She can participate in organizations to improve the quality of nursing care and encourage professional growth. She can also help change many of the mechanisms of the all too often inadequate health care delivery system.

STUDY QUESTIONS

1. What are your definitions of health and illness? How do they compare with the definitions given in this chapter?
2. Name five factors that influence a person's beliefs about health.
3. Explain the reasons for each of the ANA's standards of nursing practice.
4. How does a nurse show acceptance? sensitivity? empathy? trust?
5. What is the difference between independent, interdependent, and dependent nursing functions? Give examples.
6. How does your concept of nursing practice compare with the ideas in this chapter?

SELECTED BIBLIOGRAPHY

American Nurses' Association. 1969. Establishing standards for nursing practice. *American Journal of Nursing* 69:1458–63.
———. 1973. *Standards of nursing practice.* Kansas City, Mo.
Baumann, Barbara. 1961. Diversities in conceptions of health and physical fitness. *Journal of Health and Human Behavior* 2:39–46.
Henderson, Virginia. 1964. The nature of nursing. *American Journal of Nursing* 64.
———. 1969. Excellence in nursing. *American Journal of Nursing* 69:2133–37.
Jamann, JoAnn Shafer. 1971. Providing for the maintenance of health. In *Advanced concepts in clinical nursing,* ed. Kay Corman Kintzel, pp. 1–20. Philadelphia: Lippincott.
Manthey, Marie. 1973. Primary nursing is alive and well in the hospital. *American Journal of Nursing* 73:83–87.
Skipper, James K., Jr., and Leonard, Robert C. 1965. Doctor, nurse and patient: Role and status relationships. *Social interaction and patient care,* pp. 325–40. Philadelphia: Lippincott.
Travelbee, Joyce. 1971. The nature of nursing. *Interpersonal aspects of nursing,* 2d ed., pp. 7–22. Philadelphia: Davis.
Wu, Ruth. 1973. *Behavior and illness.* Englewood Cliffs, N.J.: Prentice-Hall.

2   Who is the nurse?

Behind the title of RN that officially identifies a nurse is a complex pattern of qualities that fit less readily into a simple description. Behind all the traditional concepts with which nurses have been associated—caring, compassion, selflessness, and dedication—are individual people. These are people with specific cultural values, backgrounds, education, job expectations, life experiences, and attitudes. These factors, all so variable, make it difficult and unfair to give nurses a collective description.

The nurse as a person

Despite individual and unique characteristics, nurses do share two things in common: each is a person and each practices in the same profession. Moreover, these two factors are not separable but must be interrelated for successful nursing. It would be both unrealistic and counterproductive for people to "turn off" their nonprofessional selves and "turn on" their nursing selves at will.

In fact, the key to developing a nursing self is to learn how to integrate effective personal reactions with a mastery of intellectual and technical skills. The special knowledge gained in nursing school must be supplemented by an ability to understand and accept people—both oneself and others. Awareness and acceptance of one's own assets, strengths, frailties, and sensitivities must be developed before one can be receptive to those qualities in others. These are often the human characteristics that one must deal with in patients and families. Under stress of illness various qualities emerge and become aggravated and magnified. Patients faced with physical stress must also contend with a variety of social, cultural, and psychological demands. These may include physical disfigurement or disability, disruption of family life, acceptance or rejection of the illness, and the need to make a multitude of other adjustments. The ability of a patient to deal with these problems largely determines his emotional state, and his emotional state is intricately tied to his physical state. The nondefinable "will to live" or "will to die" *can* be a determinant in a person's prognosis.

Upon completing this chapter, the reader should be able to:

1. Identify the various qualities nurses use in order to be receptive to patients' needs.

2. Recognize the influence the nurse's cultural background, expectations, and value system have on her receptiveness to the needs of patients.

3. Explain the relationship between the various nursing roles and settings where nursing is practiced and the weakening stereotype of the "typical" nurse.

4. Trace the impact of current activist trends on nursing as a profession.

5. Describe the influence that the nursing profession's desire for self-determination, responsibility and accountability, increased autonomy, and economic security have had on professional standards.

Thus, the nurse's ability to deal with the patient's emotional stress is as important a therapeutic tool as the ability to deal with the patient's physical stress. The nurse must learn to listen and to listen again. She must look for unspoken signs and masked reactions, for these indicators are often clues to potential problems. As the health care provider who is often closest to and most frequently in contact with the patient, the nurse is in a unique position to pick up these clues. The nurse's receptiveness to the patient's emotional needs is influenced by her own experiences, cultural background, values, and expectations.

Cultural background

In our culture, the role of nurse is usually viewed as that of a nurturant mother. This has posed difficulties for young women entering nursing. They must overcome the social barrier of assuming supportive maternal roles toward adults old enough to be their parents. It has also helped to foster nursing as a female occupation and discouraged all but the most determined men from entering the field.

Other cultural restraints affect the expectations that patients and administrators have of nurses. To deal with these expectations, nurses often have to rely on behavior and techniques that have been socially and culturally acceptable for their profession. Generally, these include passivity and obedience to authority. The nurse, for example, may find that forceful and independent action will be condemned in some instances, but condoned, or even expected, in others. And a particular attitude or conviction may be considered perfectly acceptable when held by a physician but unacceptable when held by a nurse.

Attitudes about life and death, so integral a part of nursing, are also grounded in one's cultural background. It is usually hard to divorce them from one's attitudes toward stressful professional situations. It is easy to state, but hard to achieve, nonjudgmental attitudes toward patients' wishes in such areas as mercy killing, abortion, and Russian roulette gambles with illness. This is especially true if these attitudes conflict with basic beliefs of the nurse.

Then, too, there are patients who may serve to remind a nurse of a personal vulnerability. The dying older patient or terminally ill child will often evoke associations with family and self. The way a nurse relates to patients and situations will certainly be influenced by her personal biases and experiences, often totally unrelated to the patient himself.

Expectations of self and others

Much has been written about the process of becoming a nurse, of the transition from aspirant to practitioner. How the actual experience measures up to expectations will often have a strong influence on a nurse's future attitudes toward the profession. Unlike learners in other professions, the nursing student does not have the opportunity to become acquainted with the norms of the occupation or to master the tools of the trade solely within a closed classroom situation. There is little time to shift from self to nurse, to become comfortable with nursing skills. Much of the learning takes place at the patient's bedside. Expectations of self, of others, and of the profession itself are quickly put to the test.

Faced with the reality of patient care, hospital administration, and the political aspects of a work situation, the nurse learns to adapt and adjust. Original expectations of a helping, understanding, comforting, nurturing person are tempered by the developing need to deal with the often conflicting experiences of life and death, with different patients and situations. The nurse must be able to move quickly from one approach and stance to another. She must be able to express appropriate behavior with the dying patient, on the one hand, and the recuperating patient, on the other. Detachment, though theoretically contrary to the ideals of nursing, is an attitude that many nurses develop in spite of themselves. This detachment serves as a defense against the risks and potential discomfort of emotional involvement with suffering patients and families.

Yet, to accept such reactions is to accept one's own humanness and therefore to make one much more tolerant of the moods and problems of patients and co-workers. Expectations of self and others must become more flexible in the nursing environment as the nurse learns to revise, rethink, and integrate them with her basic values.

Value systems

Underlying nurses' attitudes toward their work are the values they hold as they grow in their profession. Extensive studies of the self-image of the nurse show that most nurses share specific attitudes and values about their field. It is significant that most place high value on the need to help others and the need to work and be with others. It is clear from these studies that nurses do not place a high value on financial success, wide open mobility, or leadership achievement. They are more oriented toward a desire to be needed and to serve the ideals of helping others.[1]

The "typical" nurse

Just who is this "typical" nurse whose values, attitudes, and background we are discussing? It may be a kindly middle-aged woman, but it may just as easily be a young woman who recently was valedictorian of

[1]Hans O. Mauksch. 1963. Becoming a nurse: A selective view. *The Annals of the American Academy of Political and Social Science* 346. In *Social interaction and patient care,* ed. James K. Skipper, Jr., and Robert C. Leonard, p. 336. Philadelphia: Lippincott.

her high school class. It may be an ex-military man who has seen 20 years of service, a grandmother who is reactivating old interests, or a young person who has broken out of the ghetto.

The nursing profession no longer appeals to a limited group. It is attracting a cross section of the population in terms of race, age, sex, ethnic background, and life experience. One of the more significant demographic changes in this formerly 99 percent female profession is the influx of increasing numbers of men. Older people, looking for "second careers," are entering nursing programs, and even the composition of the younger group is changing. Formerly, the field frequently attracted those with somewhat limited aspirations. The more ambitious often went to medical school or specialized in pure science. With increased opportunities for specialization, diversity, and challenge, ambitious and medically curious people now often opt for nursing.

The opening of the field to such a variety of people has contributed to the expansion of the boundaries of nursing. The corpsman may bring a sophisticated experience in emergency care; the "ghetto dropout," an increasing understanding of and interest in drug and alcohol-related problems. The increase in the number of older people has resulted in a new emphasis on long-term patient care.

Increasing numbers of men are now joining the nursing profession.
[Photograph by Joel Gordon]

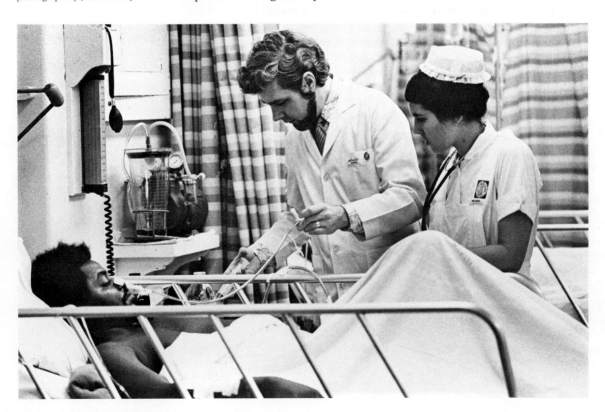

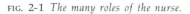

FIG. 2-1 *The many roles of the nurse.*

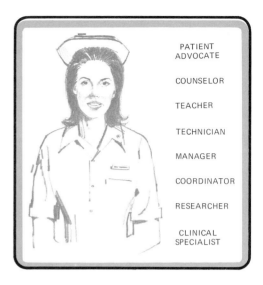

PATIENT
ADVOCATE

COUNSELOR

TEACHER

TECHNICIAN

MANAGER

COORDINATOR

RESEARCHER

CLINICAL
SPECIALIST

The nurse as a professional

As the field of nursing grows, diversifies, and expands, nurses are wearing more and more hats simultaneously. Now, they must shift back and forth from the role of technician to counselor, from teacher to manager, and many others. Because the nurse fulfills so many roles concurrently, any division of roles is artificial. For the sake of clarity, they can be separated in discussion.

The traditional concept of the nurse as supportive protector, care-giver, and health-promoter remains the primary *raison d'être* for the nursing profession. Within the terms of this broad generalization, however, nurses are now working in a variety of settings. They are found in hospitals, other health agencies, schools, industries, homes, community agencies, and doctors' offices. All of these situations provide different degrees of autonomy and different relations to patients and other members of the health team. They have widely varying priorities and demands. Still, all incorporate aspects of the following roles.

Patient advocate

To interpret, explain, defend, and protect the patient's rights and opportunities within the health care system is one of the most vital roles the nurse can and should play. At all times, the primary consideration of the nurse is the welfare of the patient. To this end, she intervenes and speaks in his behalf whenever he is unable for any reason to represent himself and his interests adequately. Such patients include those who are medically unsophisticated or uninformed, unaware of health resources, unable to communicate, mentally ill, senile, or in severe pain.

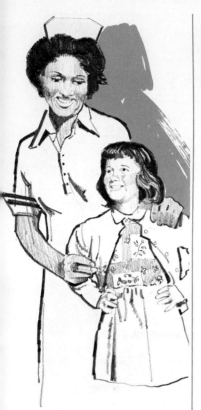

Because of the different vantage points and perspectives that physicians and nurses have, the same patient is often seen in two quite distinct lights by each professional. The nurse emphasizes the patient-centered objectives and social factors, while the doctor sees the disease-oriented objectives and biological prognostic factors.[2] The value of the nurse as patient advocate in patient-doctor relations is often that of interpreter, making for a more effective relationship between patient and doctor.

The patient-advocate role of the nurse may also be exercised in patient-family relations in order to protect the patient from undue emotional demands. Under stress, familial crises are often aggravated. The nurse can help them deal with these crises in a way that will relieve some of the stress placed on the patient.

Counselor

The nurse tries to create a therapeutic environment by offering emotional counseling, support, reassurance, and understanding. In one nurse's words, the most important contribution a nurse can make is not always in what she says, but in her ability to be there and to understand, to have the courage to listen and not run away. This type of emotional counseling is invaluable for patients as a way of lowering their tension level during the tension-producing illness.

The nurse's concern for the patient includes providing effective and appropriate counseling so that patients and their families will know how to obtain essential health care services.

Emotional counseling is invaluable for patients. . . .

Teacher

The close contact that the nurse has with the patient (and often with his family) enables her to promote his well-being through instruction in the basic principles of health maintenance. Such instruction is in addition to the particular skills and techniques that may be required in the treatment of specific health problems. Teaching may involve explaining at the patient's level the reasons for and importance of certain clinical procedures or the sequence of the healing process. Such explanations will usually do wonders to reassure the patient and his family. They thereby prevent complications or recurrences, in addition to promoting rehabilitation.

Technician

The role of the nurse includes a high degree of technical competence with responsibility for carrying out many diagnostic, treatment, and com-

[2] Barbara Bates. 1970. Doctor and nurse: Changing roles and relations. *New England Journal of Medicine* 283:129–30.

fort procedures. These include safe and prudent administration of medicines, preparation of patients for diagnostic procedures, surgery, and other
kinds of care, and monitoring the condition of the patients. As technicians,
nurses must also function as interpreters of treatment and procedures and
be the executors of emergency care.

While background and education equip a nurse for a technician role,
nursing has also urged its members to be more person-oriented than their
disease-oriented physician counterparts. Thus, nurses are always called
upon to recognize the many factors that influence human health and illness.
They must also be prepared to deal with the problems that these factors
may create.

Manager

Everyone involved in providing health services eventually converges
on the patient care unit. As a result, the managerial function of the nurse
in an inpatient setting is to delegate prerogatives and priorities. The
primary concern of the nurse-manager is to create as calm an environment
as possible for the patient. This often involves duties other than direct
patient care.

Coordinator

Efforts to meet the patient's needs can be grouped into functional
subgroups—diagnostic and therapeutic functions, comfort functions,
housekeeping functions, and allied health functions. All of these must be
coordinated. This responsibility, which often overlaps with that of manager,
is aimed at establishing and maintaining as beneficial an environment as
possible for the patient. It may be achieved by assuring that there is a
continuity of function among all those involved in the patient's care.

Clinical specialist

The clinical specialist is a nurse who has achieved a greater depth of
knowledge and skill in one particular area than the average nurse and who
can function as an autonomous unit. These specialties include pediatrics,
geriatrics, or obstetrics. In her specialty, the nurse participates in the
diagnostic process, in the planning of patient care, and in the selection
of resources.

Researcher

The growing complexities and expanding bodies of knowledge inherent
in the health field today demand that practitioners continue to educate
themselves. A nurse's technical knowledge may become outdated shortly

The primary concern of
the nurse-manager is to
create as calm an
environment as
possible for the patient.

after graduation from nursing school unless she seeks out information as a continuing professional responsibility. In addition to her own inquiries, the professional nurse may be called upon to participate in research projects initiated by fellow nurses or by other members of the health team. And even if she is not engaged in such projects herself, the effective nurse must be able to read and understand the results of the research efforts of others in order to offer the most up-to-date care to her patients.

Professionalism in nursing

Just as the scope of nursing practice is expanding and changing, so are the attitudes *of* nurses *about* nursing being rethought and redefined. These new attitudes, which indicate a growing sophistication about the profession, are primarily geared to achieving improved position and status for the nurse. Ultimately, their aim is improved care for the patient.

Nurses now want a say in what they do, how they do it, and, most of all, in how their patients are treated. Fewer and fewer nurses are content to silently accept salaries, working conditions, and hiring practices imposed on them by administrators and other nonnursing professionals. They are demanding an active role in determining the conditions of their practice. Their demands are being strengthened by an increasing willingness of nurses to join together to be heard.

Not only are nurses speaking more frequently as a collective unit, but they are becoming more insistent, even militant, about ensuring that their profession be practiced as they think it should be. This growing militancy has only infrequently erupted in strikes, mass resignations, or even picket lines. The fact that such actions have occurred at all, however, is indicative of the major changes taking place in nursing ranks.

For years, the nursing profession has been so bound by its tradition of service orientation that demands for better working conditions, better salaries, and increased control have seemed inappropriate and almost heretical. Many of these attitudes can be traced to three ideologies that have been identified with nursing: **Nightingalism, employeeism,** and **professional collectivism.**[3] Nightingalism can be interpreted as a selfless ideal that precludes concern with economic and job conditions. Employeeism refers to the belief, held by employees, that the employer has the employees' best interests at heart and will therefore be just and fair in bestowing benefits. This attitude developed during the Depression when nurses were grateful for hospital employment. It has lasted well beyond the period when such gratitude for employment was appropriate. Profes-

[3]Norma K. Grand. 1971. Nightingalism, employeeism, and professional collectivism. *Nursing Forum* 10:290–93.

sional collectivism is the feeling held by nurses that the profession's high standards of service are the responsibility of all practitioners.

These attitudes of passivity and obedience have worked against the attainment of increased status and professional gains for nurses. Only gradually are nurses and society beginning to realize and accept the fact that better working conditions will help attract more and better people to the nursing profession. This, in turn, will result in better patient care, both quantitatively and qualitatively.

These attitudes have not been changed overnight or because of any single incident. Rather, they have been gradually influenced by many of the ideas and trends that are influencing the entire society—consumerism, women's liberation, equality, and activism.

Because of the large number of women in nursing, the nurse-doctor and nurse-administrator relationships have reflected the traditional male-female relationship of dependence and subservience. Increased consciousness of women's roles and the influx of men into nursing have forced some of these sex-role expectations to change. Gradually, nursing personnel are becoming more independent and more assertive.

Consumerism has forced health care personnel to reevaluate the position of the patient. Nurses have gained professionally as a result. It is finally being accepted that nurses can better serve the patients if they themselves are happy and satisfied with their conditions of employment.

Just as nurses are changing their own self-image, so others are taking a long look at nursing and seeing it as a profession rather than as a vocation. Attainment of professional standing has meant a new focus on the aims and objectives of nursing. Nurses are characterized by a drive for self-regulation, self-determination, autonomy, and economic security. In order to better understand what is happening in the push for increased professional status, we should examine each of these characteristics in detail.

Self-regulation

One of the aims of today's nurses is to control the conditions of their practice rather than to have them controlled by outsiders. Licensure, accreditation of schools, and definition of what is and is not appropriate nursing responsibility are only a few of the spheres that have moved under nursing control in recent years. The National League for Nursing, with a membership of 15,000 individuals and 1,800 education and service agencies, is responsible for the accreditation of all nursing programs throughout the United States. These include basic nursing education programs (baccalaureate, associate degree, diploma, and practical nursing programs), graduate nursing programs, and continuing education programs. In addition, the League provides testing services and maintains research programs in the area of nursing education.

Nurses are increasingly called upon to carry out more complex patient care involving major independent decision making.

On the state and national levels, the nursing profession has achieved increasing degrees of self-regulation. Nursing leaders are working to change licensure laws and **nurse practice acts** so that they will more accurately reflect changes in health practice and social needs. Areas under particular scrutiny are those that deal with requirements for licensure and licensure renewal, standards for continuing education, and state board membership.

The principle of total self-regulation in nursing is not accepted unconditionally, however. Some within the profession believe that the participation of other disciplines and consumers in decision making can enrich the deliberations of a professional board and enhance mutual understanding.

Self-determination

Nurses are also striving to determine their own choices, their role on the health care team, and their future professional destiny. In the past, nurses as a group have not consistently attempted to exercise control. Many times they have refused opportunities to do so. They have rarely participated meaningfully in decision making about the delivery of health care to people.[4]

Such a passive and obedient attitude, one that was bred in many nursing schools, is being replaced by independence and a desire to become involved in determination of issues. Both nurses and administrators are beginning to accept the premise that nurses themselves are best able to understand the demands of their profession and are therefore entitled to help plot its future direction. Representation by nurses on planning and implementation boards is becoming more frequent as nurses assert themselves and turn increasingly to collective bargaining and other methods of forceful action.

Even though the primary focus of collective bargaining has been economic, nurses have used it as a tool for negotiating professional issues. For example, they have pressed for inclusion on interdisciplinary patient care committees, development of orientation programs for nurses, paid educational leave for attendance at seminars and workshops, and establishment of nursing care committees.

Responsibility and accountability

Nurses are increasingly called upon to carry out more complex patient care involving major independent decision making. As a result, the burden of responsibility for their actions is shifting from those who oversee nurses to the nurses themselves. They must be accountable for their actions to

[4]Ingeborg G. Mauksch. 1971. Attainment of control over professional practice. *Nursing Forum* 10:235.

the administration and, above all, to the patients they serve. This increased accountability is the price that professionals must pay for increased freedom to practice.

However, nurses must achieve a balance between their responsibility to safeguard the public and legitimate concern for their own welfare. For example, nurses are being increasingly asked to practice in those "gray areas" of health care that are neither strictly allowable nor disallowable nursing functions. They are now demanding that they be given legal sanction and an aura of respectability to carry out these functions.

Increasing autonomy

Work-related autonomy for the professional can be defined as the freedom to practice in accordance with his training. One of the questions nursing is asking in its quest for autonomy is whether it is possible for an occupation whose members are primarily employees to practice autonomy within the framework of an institutional employment setting. As an employed professional, the nurse finds aspects of her work are influenced by hospital policy. Other professionals in the hierarchy can claim authority to determine and provide some of the services for the patient. These constraints on the nurse's autonomy are being counteracted by the passage of legislation and the establishment of specific regulations that allow nurses to perform clearly defined patient care functions. As nurses move into roles requiring greater independence, such as that of clinical specialist, their autonomy increases.

Economic security

Economic aims are the most tangible and socially understandable needs sought by the nursing profession. The economic picture for nurses has changed radically in the past two decades, with salaries doubling and tripling. However, with nursing's history of low wages and poor conditions, nurses now want to ensure that their gains will continue to grow in line with cost-of-living increases and with gains won by other workers. Thus, economic security has become a top priority for nursing associations.

While most nurses welcome higher salaries and better working conditions, many reject attaining them through such methods as collective action and collective bargaining. The principle of collective bargaining, in which employer and employee come together to achieve settlements on working conditions, has long been considered taboo in nursing. It has faced years of rejection or only partial acceptance by nursing organizations. The American Nurses' Association required years of careful consideration before it accepted the concept of collective bargaining as a tool. Even then, it did not give approval to strikes as a means of achieving gains until 1968. Strikes by nurses were considered detrimental to patient care.

As nurses move into roles requiring greater independence, their autonomy increases.

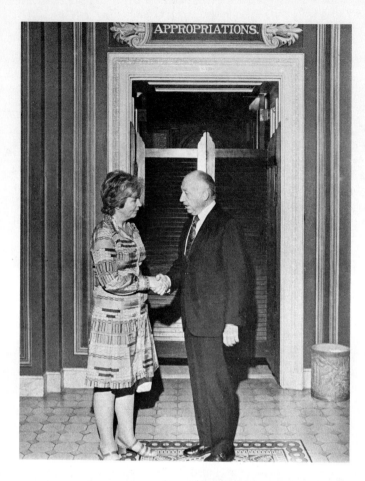

Professional nursing organizations are now lobbying for better health care services. Here, a representative of the American Nurses' Association talks with Senator Jacob Javits of New York.
[Courtesy of the *American Journal of Nursing*]

Legislation passed in 1974 finally removed one of the last legal restraints against strikes by nurses. With this new legislation, which amends the Taft-Hartley Labor-Management Relations Act, nurses in nonprofit hospitals are entitled to engage in collective bargaining activity. This new legislation should give all nurses more latitude in their efforts to attain equitable pay. In the long run, this and other provisions favoring nurses' bargaining positions could do much to give nursing the professional status most of its members have sought.

Professional organizations

Behind the drive for increased professionalism in nursing has been the build-up of professional organizations at the national and local levels to represent nurses in both generalized and specialized areas.

The American Nurses' Association was the forerunner and is still the leader of professional nurses' organizations in this country. It is now involved in influencing and giving direction to nursing education programs and trying to organize nurses. It is also lobbying for legislative and economic gains and providing guidelines for the achievement of some of the goals and objectives just discussed.

Because of nurses' resistance to act collectively (fewer than 30 percent of all nurses belong to the ANA),[5] the ANA's effectiveness in influencing actual conditions of practice and salary has been limited. However, some leaders in the nursing field are beginning to see a growing spirit of unification among nurses.[6] This unity has been hastened by a growing awareness of common concerns about patient advocacy, standards of practice, continuing education, certification, and accountability.

Indicators of such a move are the establishment of splinter groups representing nursing specialties. These include nurses in obstetrics/gynecology, emergency care, and pediatrics. An umbrella group, the Federation of Specialty Organizations, has been organized to represent these groups. Other developments prompted by nurses' explorations into constructive action groups geared to their specific needs are the formulation of organizations to represent black nurses, student nurses, practical nurses, and other subgroupings in the nursing field. State and local level nursing groups are becoming more involved in specific activities directly concerned with their membership. These activities have included representation as the collective bargaining agent in negotiations with hospital administrators. As nurses awaken more to their own potential and to a positive self-image, their demand for and interest in increasing the effectiveness of specialized groups and local associations will likely grow.

SUMMARY

There are a multitude of forces at work today influencing the nursing profession, its goals and objectives, and the attitudes and self-image of its practitioners. Nurses are being challenged by society, by administrators, by consumer-patients, by co-workers, and by themselves. Part of this change is expressed in a new respect for the demands of the profession. These demands now include not only increasing clinical expertise but also person-to-person effectiveness in human relationships. Nursing education is emphasizing the need to expand the practitioner's knowledge of the physical and psychological needs of self and of patients, both at the initial learning stage and thereafter on a continuing basis.

How is the nursing profession reacting to all these challenges and dynamic forces? It is searching and feeling its way through new definitions of roles, new expectations, and new goals. In this search, nursing is asserting itself as a powerful profession.

[5]Ada Jacox. 1971. Collective action and control of practice by professionals. *Nursing Forum* 10:254.
[6]Rosemary Amason Bowman and Rebecca Clark Culpepper. 1974. Power: Rx for change. *American Journal of Nursing* 74:1055.

Nurses are being challenged by society, by administrators, by consumer-patients, by co-workers, and by themselves.

STUDY QUESTIONS

1. Name four roles fulfilled by the nurse. Give examples of the way she functions in each of these roles.
2. Define Nightingalism, employeeism, and professional collectivism.
3. What are nurse practice acts?
4. What are the functions of the National League for Nursing? the American Nurses' Association?
5. What do you think are legitimate and ethical ways in which nurses can improve their status?
6. What factors in your background influenced you to become a nursing student?

SELECTED BIBLIOGRAPHY

Corwin, Ronald G. 1961. The professional employee: A study of conflict in nursing roles. *American Journal of Sociology* 66:604–15.

Kelly, Lucie Young. 1974. Nursing practice acts. *American Journal of Nursing* 74:1310–19.

Lewis, John A. 1960. Reflections on self. *American Journal of Nursing* 60:828–30.

Mauksch, Hans O. 1963. Becoming a nurse: A selective view. *The Annals of the American Academy of Political and Social Science* 346:88–98.

———. 1972. Nursing: Churning for change? In *Handbook of medical sociology,* 2d ed., ed. Freeman, Levine, and Reeder, pp. 206–30. Englewood Cliffs, N.J.: Prentice-Hall.

Mereness, Dorothy. 1970. Recent trends in expanding roles of the nurse. *Nursing Outlook* 18:30–33.

Tagliacozzo, Daisy L. 1962. The nurse from the patient's point of view. Address to a regional conference of the department of hospital nursing, National League for Nursing, St. Louis, Mo. Reprinted in *Social interaction and patient care,* ed. James K. Skipper, Jr., and Robert C. Leonard, pp. 219–27. Philadelphia: Lippincott, 1965.

3 Health care settings and agencies

Why do we need health care services?

The health of the people has always been a concern of American society. With public funds the early colonists built almshouses for the poor. Physicians and midwives were employed by the larger cities. Thanks to private contributions, the country's first hospital—Pennsylvania Hospital in Philadelphia—was begun in 1786. The first local health department had been established by the end of the eighteenth century.[1]

Yet today, for a variety of reasons, the United States is low on the list in terms of the quality of health care available to the average person. Although we are among the richest and most technologically advanced nations, our infant mortality rate is fifteenth in the world.[2] Efforts are constantly being made by medical and political groups to change this picture and bring better health care to larger numbers of people. In 1965, two famous amendments to the Social Security Act were passed. These were Title XVIII **(Medicare)** and Title XIX **(Medicaid).** Medicare provides a federally administered program of health insurance for the aged. This includes hospital insurance financed through social security taxes and a voluntary program of supplementary benefits financed by matching contributions. Medicaid provides a program of grants to states for medical assistance.

Diagnosis and treatment of illness

Vast changes have taken place in the practice of medicine in the past 20 years. Thanks to new techniques and instruments of ever-increasing refinement, we are now gaining more insight into the mysteries of cell structure. Researchers are unraveling the complex biochemical processes which maintain life and which are disturbed in disease.

Upon completing this chapter, the reader should be able to:

1. Define the general goals of the health care system: promote health, cure illness, rehabilitate patients after acute illnesses, and prevent further disease.

2. Discuss the role of modern technology in diagnosing and treating illness and its impact on the preventive aspect of illness.

3. Name and give examples of the four types of agencies and organizations in the United States whose purpose is to provide health care.

4. Discuss nontraditional settings such as community agencies, outpatient clinics, and independent nursing practice as appropriate sites for the practice of nursing.

[1]Carter L. Marshall. 1972. *Dynamics of health and disease,* p. 341. New York: Appleton-Century-Crofts.
[2]Doris Cook Sutterley and Gloria Ferraro Donnelly. 1973. *Perspectives in human development: Nursing throughout the life cycle,* p. 6. Philadelphia: Lippincott.

Some of these advances in diagnosis and treatment are:

1. The control of many infections and parasitic diseases
2. The production of potent synthetic drugs
3. The use of cortisone and allied steroids
4. The exploitation of radioactive isotopes
5. Renal and cardiac transplantation

As diseases once common and serious grow rare, other conditions gain attention. The heavy load of infectious disease has been lightened, but the vast numbers of genetic disorders are now being discovered. Also, longer life expectancy has brought the two great problems of cancer and cardiovascular disease into the immediate foreground.

Prevention of illness

An increasing number of Americans now lead long lives and develop chronic diseases. This explains why the interest of many health care workers has shifted to prevention of disease rather than treatment alone. For example, cardiovascular disease, the nation's number one killer, is the result of a gradual building process that can sometimes be slowed or arrested when a person is young. By the time he reaches old age, the destructive processes have done irreparable damage. As a result, specialists in coronary disease have been urging for years the importance of proper diet, exercise, and not smoking.

A major development in preventive medicine is the growing number of screening programs for certain diseases. Mass screening for tuberculosis using chest X-rays has been a familiar feature on the health care scene for some time. More recently, routine screening has been used to detect diabetes, cervical and prostatic cancer, metabolic disorders in infants, and psychiatric disturbances. Many other screening tests are being developed in the nation's laboratories.

Health agencies today are stressing the importance of preventive medicine and urging cooperation from the public. But many people still hesitate to see a doctor unless they feel they are ill. In cases where a person belongs to a prepaid group, such as a Health Maintenance Organization (see p. 44), preventive health care has been more successful.

Restoration to optimum health (rehabilitation)

Before the twentieth century, relatively few disabled persons survived. Today, life expectancy has increased from 48 to 72 years.[3] Infant mortality

[3]Kathryn L. Riffle. 1973. Rehabilitation: The evolution of a social concept. *Nursing Clinics of North America* 8:669.

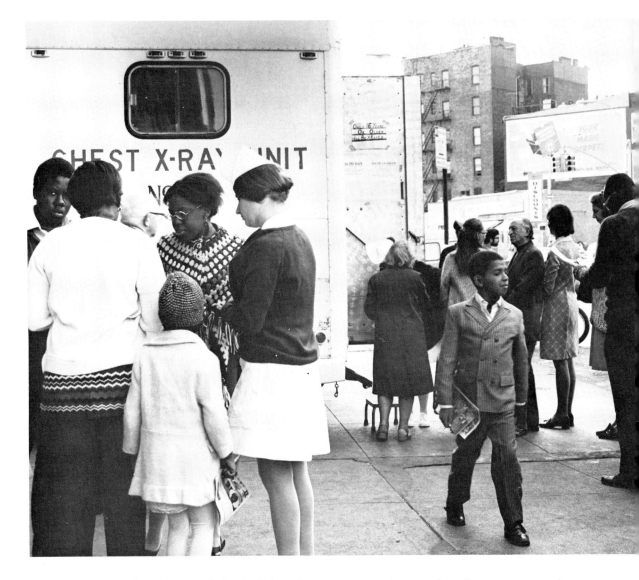

has decreased, and children with birth defects have a greater chance of survival. The growing elderly population adds daily to the lists of the chronically ill. Thus **rehabilitation** has become a major concern of professional health care providers.

In the early days of this country, rehabilitation was mainly in the hands of voluntary organizations. They developed standard programs of activities for the disabled, such as rug weaving or chair caning. At that time, physical disability was looked upon as a form of social deviance. Today that stigma has largely disappeared. State and local governments provide not only vocational rehabilitation but various medical and psychosocial services.

Rehabilitation and nursing have been linked for many years. Today, teachers of nursing are making earnest attempts to integrate rehabilitative concepts into nursing curricula.

Screening programs play a vital role in health maintenance and prevention of disease.

[Photo by Irene Bayer from Monkmeyer Press Photo Service]

39

Health care settings

There are four main types of health organizations which make up the American health care system. These are:

1. Official or public agencies
2. Voluntary, or nonprofit, agencies
3. Hospitals and nursing homes
4. Health-related organizations[4]

Health care in the United States is provided by many different agencies and organizations. These agencies are able to provide the consumer with far more services than he would be able to obtain simply by consulting a private practitioner.

Like other government organizations, official agencies depend upon tax funds and operate within relatively clear legal limits. Most federal agencies have only an indirect effect on local communities. A few, however, offer services on the local level. Most important of these agencies is the Department of Health, Education and Welfare. Its wide-ranging activities include research, demonstration projects, and financial grants-in-aid to states and institutions. Other federal agencies of considerable significance at the local level are the Veterans' Administration and the Rehabilitation Services Administration.

Each state has its own system of health care organizations. Usually there are several state departments involved in providing health services, and their activities often overlap. Basically, the most important organization on the state level is the department of health. This department provides various programs and services, such as mobile personnel and equipment for dental care, diagnostic X-rays, and other health services.

On the local level, city and county health departments are primarily concerned with the following activities:

1. The recording and analysis of vital statistics
2. The control of communicable diseases
3. The maintenance and supervision of environmental sanitation
4. Public health laboratory services
5. Maternal and child health services
6. Health education[5]

Nongovernment, or voluntary, agencies are supported by donations from the public. They include such well-known organizations as the

[4]Sol Levine and Paul E. White. 1972. The community of health organizations. In *Handbook of medical sociology*, 2d ed., ed. Freeman et al., p. 359. Englewood Cliffs, N.J.: Prentice-Hall.
[5]Ibid., p. 361.

American Cancer Society, the American Heart Association, and the Visiting Nurse Association. These agencies vary widely in services and activities. Many sponsor research and provide financial aid to patients and their families. They also maintain educational programs for the community.

Hospitals

Hospitals are the major medical treatment centers of the community. Some are official and some voluntary. Some concentrate on specific diseases, and others are general.

General hospitals. From ancient times until late in the nineteenth century, hospitals mainly cared for the sick poor. Only in the last few decades have hospitals treated a wide variety of patients from all social and economic classes. In the United States, the establishment of large general hospitals has been the result of the growth of urban areas. The concentration of professionals in the cities has resulted in the development of teaching and research facilities there. Most such hospitals are now associated with medical schools and universities. They are concerned with teaching and research as well as with patient care.[6]

While the total number of hospitals has increased in the past 15 years, patient stays are shorter. The number of hospitals providing long-term care has decreased. In part, this fact reflects a profound change in the treatment of certain diseases such as tuberculosis and mental illness. It also suggests a lack of interest in facilities for the chronically ill, bedridden patient.

Specialized hospitals. The number of hospitals which limit themselves to care of specific problems—eyes, obstetrics, pediatrics, mental illness—has also declined in recent years. Unless they are near a general hospital, such institutions are sometimes unable to provide all the services necessary for complete patient care. However, they still play a very important role in concentrating expertise and facilities in specific areas. For example, cancer is usually best treated at large, research-oriented cancer institutions.

Some specialized hospitals are losing prominence because of changes in the overall health care picture. The number of maternity hospitals has decreased largely as a result of a decline in the birth rate. And the care of psychiatric patients is now being provided by the urban general hospital rather than left to the specialized, often-isolated asylum.

Nursing homes

Nursing homes are currently known by a variety of names—"rest homes," "convalescent homes," "sanitoriums." According to the American

---

[6]John H. Knowles. 1973. The hospital. *Scientific American* 229:131.

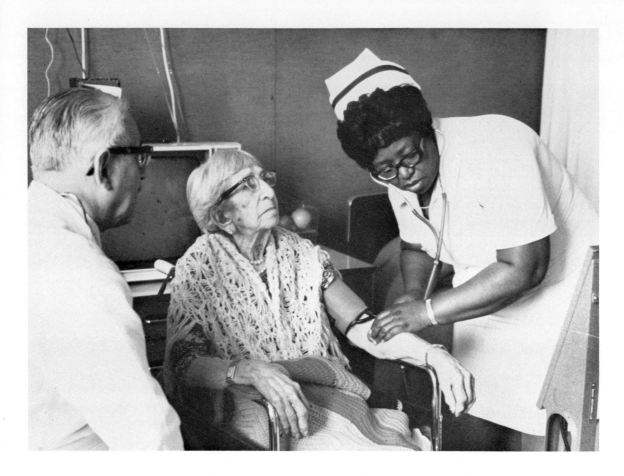

Nursing homes provide care for the aged and infirm, as well as for those with chronic illnesses.
[Photo courtesy United Hospital Fund]

Nursing Home Association, a nursing home is a licensed home for those whose illnesses or injuries do not require hospitalization. It is a home in which the residents are usually aged, infirm, or chronically ill and where special personal attention and sympathetic care are provided.[7]

The increase in the number of nursing homes in this country can be attributed to three factors:

1. The growing number of aged persons with chronic diseases
2. The social changes that have produced families who are unable or unwilling to care for their aged, infirm members at home
3. The advent of Medicare and Medicaid, which cover payments for care in certain types of nursing homes[8]

Nursing in nursing homes is basically the same as nursing in other situations. The nurse takes care of the bedridden and the ambulatory residents. Service may include the entire gamut of health care—prevention, diagnosis, treatment, and rehabilitation.

[7]Allen Podell. 1973. The role of the private nursing home. *Nursing Homes* 22:25–26.
[8]Marshall, p. 358.

Community agencies

Public health nursing. The life of a public health nurse differs in many respects from that of the hospital-based nurse. Because she sees many healthy family members while visiting a sick one, she often tends to be oriented more toward prevention than cure.

Education is a particularly important function of the public health nurse, who is in a good position to influence people to improve their health care. Among the areas in which she is most likely to provide instruction are:

1. *Home safety.* The nurse can identify potential and actual safety hazards of all types.
2. *Personal and environmental hygiene.* It is the nurse's job to set an example and to offer advice in this area.
3. *Nutrition.* Elderly patients, in particular, need investigation and help.
4. *Mental health.* The public health nurse is in an ideal position to observe early signs of stress that may have serious consequences.
5. *Use of health and social services.* The nurse should have all necessary referral information.[9]

Neighborhood health centers. Authorized by Congress in 1966, **neighborhood health centers** are located in areas where not enough traditional types of health manpower are available. They are found in rural areas as well as in the inner city. These centers offer a broad scope of comprehensive health services tailored to fit specific community needs. Hospitals or other health care institutions are used for services not available at the center. Neighborhood residents are trained to work at the center and help define problems and shape services to meet the needs of the people. Fees are based on ability to pay, with the government making up the difference. These centers have helped many who would ordinarily not go to private physicians to receive adequate health care. The emphasis is usually on care of the entire family.

The type of care provided varies somewhat according to location. It is not always limited to strictly medical care. At the Family Health Services in rural West Virginia, for example, health workers have found themselves fixing roofs, repairing radiators, rounding up warm clothing, and hauling wood. In a poverty area of Manhattan, the staff deals with heroin addicts and with lead-poisoned infants who have eaten paint chips from the peeling walls of apartments. Patients are checked routinely for venereal disease and tuberculosis.[10]

[9]Hugh Ruddick-Bracken. 1973. The district nurse as health educator. *Nursing Times* 69:1188.
[10]Neighborhood health centers—bringing more care to needy. 1973. *U.S. News & World Report* 71:62–64.

Education is a particularly important function of the public health nurse . . . .

Health maintenance organizations. The **health maintenance organization (HMO)** concept established a system of private, comprehensive, prepaid health care programs as an alternative to conventional health care arrangements. The HMO is the newest entry on the American health scene. As of 1973, more than fifty HMOs were in various stages of development throughout the United States.

All HMOs share three common features:

1. They offer an organized system, in contrast to the present system, which is oriented to individual service.
2. They serve groups who voluntarily agree to seek most of their medical care from the HMO.
3. They determine the price of services in advance, agreeing by contract to provide all the medical care enrollees will require.[11]

Although HMOs have not been around for very long, a number of predictions have been offered about their potential effect on the American health care scene. One public health nurse suggests that HMOs will make school and occupational health nurses obsolete. They will also take the place of health departments, emergency rooms, and intensive care, coronary care, and kidney dialysis units.[12]

In HMO demonstration projects, the professional nurse has assumed considerably greater responsibility for delivery of primary health care services. Candidates for these nursing positions have been carefully screened. Nurses in HMOs must have demonstrated the ability to work independently, to plan and schedule actively, and to work well in a team situation.[13]

Schools, industry, etc. The school nurse has many functions. She is a health specialist, teacher, counselor, mental health worker, and a participant in community health planning. The school nurse must understand school organization and be familiar with the normal growth and development of children. She must also be very knowledgeable about clinical deviations and their significance.

A series of radically changing needs demands new approaches from school nurses. In 1969, the National Council for School Nurses published a monograph entitled "Solutions to Critical Health Needs." This included discussions of smoking, alcohol and drug abuse, venereal disease, teen-age

---

[11]Paul M. Elwood, Jr. 1973. Concept organization and strategies of HMOs. *Journal of Nursing Administration* 3:29.

[12]Joan E. Mulligan. 1973. There's an HMO in your future: Is your future in the HMO? *Journal of Nursing Administration* 3:36, 38.

[13]Betty M. Callow. 1973. An R.N.'s view of the health maintenance organization. *Journal of Nursing Administration* 3:40.

pregnancy, family life, education, and mental health.[14] Previously such subjects were seldom presented as of interest to the nurse.

A nurse who is interested chiefly in prevention of illness and promotion of health may find a satisfying job in the field of occupational health. As the employee of an industrial concern, her objectives are:

1. To protect the worker from any health risk on the job
2. To contribute toward his physical and mental adjustment to the job
3. To help establish and maintain his physical and mental well-being[15]

The individual occupational health nurse may be part of a health team, or she may work alone in a small company. One of her satisfactions is being able to see patients over a long period rather than during times of illness alone.

Outpatient clinics

Outpatient clinics represent another attempt to fill the gap in medical service to rural and ghetto areas. Many large hospitals have established and staffed clinics in outlying areas where it is difficult for the residents to travel to the main hospital. If the patient cannot be given the treatment he needs at the clinic, he is referred to the main hospital.

The nurse's functions in an outpatient clinic are likely to be centered on ambulatory rather than acute care. Often she has more autonomy in patient care than the hospital nurse, who is usually more closely supervised.

A nurse who spent 8 years working in an outpatient clinic noted that

I became more assertive in my nursing intervention and in taking the initiative for patients. I learned to assume more of the care sharing in a less threatening fashion to some physicians. I was in the latter years a more independent practitioner than in the beginning.[16]

Another type of outpatient clinic which has sprung up in the last decade is the "free clinic." These clinics are mainly geared to serve young people who either do not trust or cannot afford standard medical treatment. These clinics are staffed by professionals and funded by groups ranging from the Salvation Army to the Black Panther Party. They offer medical, gynecological, and dermatological care, as well as counseling in nutrition, legal and personal problems, birth control, pregnancy, and venereal disease. Routine tests and medications are usually free of charge.

[14]Irma B. Fricke. 1972. School nursing for the 70s. *The Journal of School Health* 42:203.
[15]Betty Jarman. 1973. Occupational health nursing. *Nursing Mirror* 136:21.
[16]Barbara Noonan. 1972. Eight years in a medical nurse clinic. *American Journal of Nursing* 72:1130.

Physicians' offices

The nurse who works in a physician's office has a valuable opportunity for health teaching, counseling, and follow-up care. She can greatly expand the "receptionist" role that has often been filled by office nurses in real life and in television dramas.

Independent nursing practice

Today, growing dissatisfaction with professional limitations is causing an increasing number of nurses to strike out on their own. Many are frustrated by administrative tasks that take them away from direct patient care. They often resent the "handmaiden" attitude that many physicians and hospital administrators have toward nurses.

One result of this movement toward independence has been an increase in nursing specialization. The first formalized program for **nurse-practitioners,** or **clinical nurse specialists,** was established in 1965 at the University of Colorado School of Nursing. It was used for the training of pediatric nurses. Since then, many other programs have been established. Among the specialties covered are pediatric, family, medical, and maternal-child care. Some programs require on-the-job training. Others involve a full four-year master's degree course. The specialists trained in these programs work in a variety of settings and assume varying degrees of independence.[17]

Laws restricting the activities of the independent nurse-practitioner vary widely from one state to another. A major problem is certification. The mechanisms for this do not exist so far. The problem is currently under consideration by the American Nurses' Association.

SUMMARY

The concept that people have a right to medical care reaches far back into history. In the early days, health care was primarily an after-the-fact function of attending people who were already diseased or disabled. Hospitals were unpleasant places, and only people who were too poor to hire their own physician resorted to them.

Today, the goal of health care is not only to promote health or to cure the immediate illness, but to rehabilitate the patient after the acute phase. The prevention of future illness is also a major objective. Unfortunately, the reality remains a far cry from the ideal in almost every country, including the United States.

In the early part of this century, infectious diseases were the greatest

[17] Alice M. Robinson. 1973. The nurse-practitioner: Expanding your limits. *RN* 36:29.

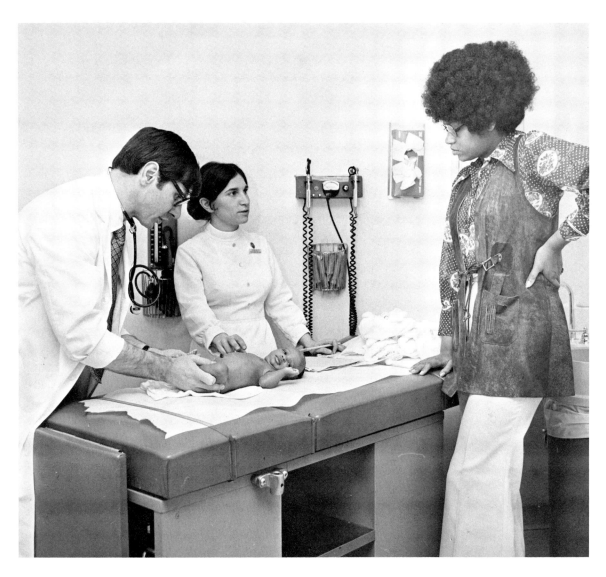

worldwide health problem. With the introduction of antibiotics, medicine has been able to turn its attention more to the chronic diseases. These include cancer, cardiovascular disease, diabetes, and arthritis, among others. As diagnosis and treatment have been increasingly refined, prevention has assumed greater importance. Today, there are a large number of screening centers where people can go for tests that early disclose the existence of potential medical problems. And for those who suffer permanent disabilities or chronic illnesses, rehabilitation services are widely available.

The United States is overlaid by a complex network of agencies and organizations whose purpose is the delivery of health care. Some are run

Independent nurse practitioners are now providing care in such fields as pediatric and maternal-child nursing.
[Photo courtesy the March of Dimes]

by the federal, state, or local government, others by voluntary agencies. An important agency in the system is the general hospital, which has taken on an increasing variety of responsibilities in the past half-decade. Today, many urban hospitals are affiliated with medical and nursing schools. Their functions include teaching and research in addition to patient care.

Effective treatment of disease has increased life expectancy. One result has been the growth in the number of nursing homes. Basically, a nursing home is a place where the aged, infirm, or chronically ill can receive special care.

Community agencies offer somewhat different settings for the practice of nursing. For example:

1. *Public health nursing.* The public health nurse finds herself as much in contact with well people as with sick ones. In consequence, she has many opportunities to teach preventive medicine.
2. *Neighborhood health centers.* These government-supported centers are located in rural or inner-city areas where medical care is scarce.
3. *Health maintenance organizations.* These are private, prepaid health care programs that encourage the preventive approach to health care.
4. *Schools and industry.* The school nurse's concern is with the health and well-being of the school child, while the occupational health nurse cares for the employees of a company. Ambulatory care and preventive medicine are prominent in the responsibilities of both.

The outpatient clinic represents another attempt to bring health care to more people. Most outpatient clinics are run by large area hospitals, although some are privately financed.

A growing phenomenon in the nursing profession is the trend toward specialization and independent practice. This stems largely from the nurse's desire to increase the clinical responsibility she feels she was trained to undertake.

STUDY QUESTIONS

1. Define Medicare and Medicaid.
2. What are the four major types of health care organizations in the United States? What is the role of each in the health care system?
3. What is a health maintenance organization?
4. Identify and state the function of several health care agencies located in your community. How do these agencies relate to one another?

SELECTED BIBLIOGRAPHY

Ellwood, Paul M., Jr. 1973. Concept organization and strategies of HMOs. *Journal of Nursing Administration* 3:29–34.

Knowles, John H. 1973. The hospital. *Scientific American* 229:128–37.

Levine, Sol, and White, Paul E. 1972. The community of health organizations. In *Handbook of medical sociology,* 2d ed., ed. Freeman et al., pp. 359–85. Englewood Cliffs, N.J.: Prentice-Hall.

Marshall, Carter L. 1972. *Dynamics of health and disease,* pp. 338–72. New York: Appleton-Century-Crofts.

Robinson, Alice M. 1973. The nurse-practitioner: Expanding your limits. *RN* 36:27–34.

Part Two

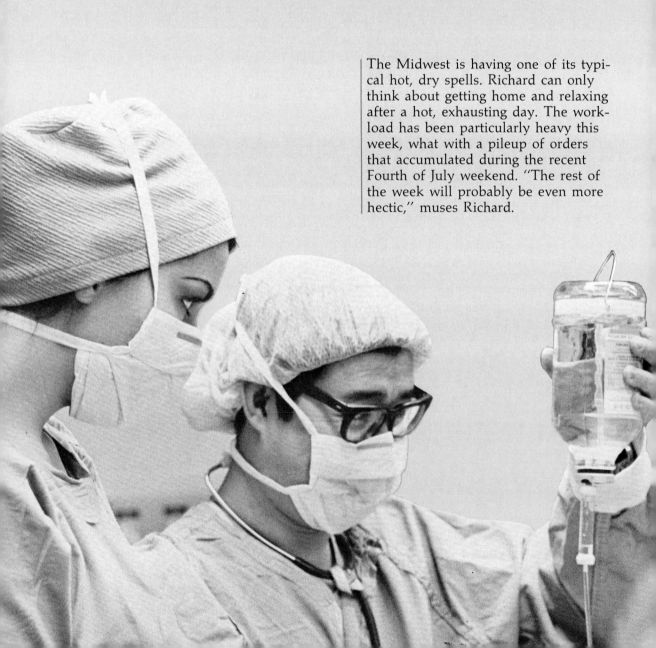

The Midwest is having one of its typical hot, dry spells. Richard can only think about getting home and relaxing after a hot, exhausting day. The workload has been particularly heavy this week, what with a pileup of orders that accumulated during the recent Fourth of July weekend. "The rest of the week will probably be even more hectic," muses Richard.

The nursing process

His thoughts shift from work to home and the prospect of a relaxing hour or two in the garden before dinner. Anita will be at choir rehearsal until about 8, and the kids are on a two-day visit to Charlotte's rented cottage on a nearby lake.

Suddenly, there is a loud explosion. The factory seems to shake from its very foundation. Richard's office is plunged into darkness. He opens the door and his office fills with smoke. Gasping and choking, with eyes tearing, he gropes his way down the smoke-filled hall, and then remembers nothing.

Although the fire-fighting squad arrives quickly, the flames from the exploding boiler are spreading even more quickly. Walls are ablaze in some sections of the factory and acrid smoke is everywhere.

The firemen pull several unconscious men out of the smoking building, including Richard. His shirt is singed, and to prevent further burning, the firemen quickly rip off Richard's clothing and wrap him in a blanket. A 20-mile ambulance ride to the county hospital gives the ambulance team a short time

to try to revive Richard and to monitor his vital signs. He is still unconscious when the ambulance reaches the hospital emergency room. Emergency measures are continued in order to revive him, stabilize his vital signs, and treat his burned right hand and arm. The emergency room is chaotic, with some dozen victims of the fire requiring various types of emergency care, observation, and assessment.

When Richard regains consciousness about a half-hour later, he is dazed and in pain. Looking around from his vantage point on a stretcher, he becomes panicky. "What happened? Was I in an accident? My wife, my children. Are they all right?" he asks frantically. By the time a nurse reassures Richard and explains what has happened, several minutes have elapsed and his anxiety level is extremely high.

It is late in the evening by the time Anita is notified of the accident. By now, Richard's burns have been treated and he is resting fairly comfortably in a four-bed room. The health care team has decided to keep him overnight for observation.

"I don't know why I have to stay in

this place until tomorrow," he mutters with annoyance. "I'll be late for work this way, and this room is so noisy, what with all the comings and goings, that I'll never get any sleep." Annoyance turns to anxiety and frustration when Richard learns that his first-degree burns will require daily dressings. On top of this, the movements of his right hand and arm are bound to be somewhat limited for the next few weeks. Work, says the doctor, is out of the question for the next few days. So is driving for the next week.

"Richard will never stay quietly in bed," Anita tells the nurse in the corridor. "We specifically postponed our summer vacation for two weeks because he has so much work to do right now." She then realizes that, with the factory in shambles, the job of setting up temporary quarters elsewhere will demand even more of Richard's time and thoughts.

Richard's boss calls to inquire about Richard's condition and to reassure him that everything will be brought under control at the factory. This is little comfort to Richard, who feels exhausted and terribly sore from all the smoke inhalation. His right side hurts from the burns, and his mind is still reeling from the events of the afternoon.

Anita leaves him for a fitful night's sleep. She promises to arrive early the next morning to pick up Richard and to receive instructions from the nurse on how to change his burn dressings.

Richard's family doctor is notified by the attending physician. He agrees to come over to the hospital first thing in the morning to have a look at Richard. He offers some information to the emergency room team about Richard's medical background, giving details that Richard and Anita had been unable to supply because of their anxiety or because of lack of information.

After he has been home for several days, Richard finds that his burns are draining more profusely. He calls the hospital and is told to come to the clinic that afternoon.

How would nurses in the emergency room and on the patient unit go about assessing Richard?

How would they develop a plan of care?

What kinds of plans should be made for discharge and follow-up care? How should these plans be developed?

What kind of information should be included in the record? Why?

How can a nurse evaluate care that is planned and implemented during a patient's overnight stay in the hospital?

4 Introduction to the nursing process

What is the nursing process?

The **nursing process** is a specific method for organizing nursing actions. It is similar to the scientific method but with less strict control of variables. Although it involves a series of orderly and disciplined steps, the nursing process is not static. It changes constantly in accordance with different situations.

Essentially, the nursing process is a combination of intellectual and physical activities. It is a systematic means of analyzing the patient's problems, determining how to solve them, carrying out a plan of action, and then evaluating its effectiveness.

Ideally, the nursing process combines the attitude of sharing oneself with the patient in knowledgeable service to him. Neither quality alone is enough. Kindness and consideration are essential, but they cannot substitute for sound scientific knowledge. On the other hand, someone who is abrupt or impersonal with patients is not following the nursing process, no matter what her scientific or technical expertise.

The term "nursing process" has entered the language only in the last decade or so. The existence of such a process has been a fact for many years, however. What is new is that professionals have recently been attempting to identify nursing problems specifically and outline the steps necessary to resolve them. They now see the need for a systematic method of problem solving. This is a method that good nurses had always used but which had not previously been specifically defined and outlined.

Some nurses objected to the term "nursing process" when they first encountered it in the literature. "This is what we've been doing all along—why put a scientific name to it?" they asked. True, a good nurse always knew what she was doing and why. But it was usually not possible to evaluate her actions scientifically because her goals and methods had not been clearly defined.

A nurse uses the nursing process when she deliberately analyzes the patient's health problems and decides how she will act to meet these

Upon completing this chapter, the reader should be able to:

1. Demonstrate that the nursing process as a systematic approach to nursing establishes the scientific basis of nursing as a profession.

2. Explain the relationship between the "scientific method," problem solving, and the nursing process.

3. Recognize that the nursing process requires integration of interpersonal skills, scientific knowledge, and physical actions.

4. Define the four steps of the nursing process: assessment, planning, implementation, and evaluation.

5. Define the three major skills and their related subskills in the execution of the nursing process: intellectual, technical, and interpersonal.

A professional nurse is characterized chiefly by her ability to make decisions about nursing care.

problems. She continues the process by outlining a course of action, putting it into effect, and then evaluating how effective it has been. This progression is essentially what is called for by the scientific method. It was first developed by philosopher-scientists such as Sir Francis Bacon and Sir Isaac Newton and their followers. The scientific method can be stated as follows:

1. Recognize and define the problem
2. Collect data from observation and experimentation
3. Formulate and implement a solution
4. Evaluate the solution

The scientific method and the nursing process are almost identical in form, but they are different in purpose. While the scientist is looking for new knowledge, the nurse is usually looking for answers to an immediate problem in a particular setting. Also, while many scientists deal with facts, a nurse deals with people. The way in which she views her job has a great effect on what she does, feels, and says in her encounters with the patient. Ideally, the nurse and patient help each other by establishing an "I-you" relationship. The goal of this relationship is to relieve the patient as much as possible.

Twenty years ago Lydia Hall used four prepositions to define levels of nursing. She labeled them nursing *at* the patient, *to* the patient, *for* the patient, and *with* the patient.[1] Of these four levels, the last, "nursing *with* the patient," is the most important. The goal of all nursing action is to involve the patient in his own care. This means planning care with the patient as well as implementing it.

Another definition was offered in 1967 by a committee for curriculum development in the western states. They defined the nursing process as "that which goes on between a patient and nurse in a given setting: it incorporates the behaviors of patient and nurse and the resulting interaction. The steps in the process are: perception, communication, interpretation, intervention, and evaluation."[2]

Lois Knowles points out that a professional nurse is characterized chiefly by her ability to make decisions about nursing care. Her visible activities must be the end product of a conscious process which reflects her education and experience. The Knowles model of nursing hinges on "the five D's": discover, delve, decide and plan nursing approaches, do, discriminate.[3]

[1] As quoted by Helen Yura and Mary B. Walsh. 1973. *The nursing process: Assessing, planning, implementing, evaluating,* 2d ed., p. 20. New York: Appleton-Century-Crofts.
[2] Ibid., p. 21.
[3] Ibid.

Why use the nursing process?

The intelligent use of the nursing process helps one avoid the extremes. Patients are not benefited by a nurse who is only a technician, who works in an automated, "cookbook" fashion. In other words, they are not benefited by a nurse who thinks only in terms of a specific duty and carries it out, oblivious of the total picture. On the other hand, if a nurse is not working in a planned way, she may be wasting a lot of time and energy.

When nursing care is given in a disorganized or instinctive (even though sincere and compassionate) fashion, the patient is likely to become puzzled and uncooperative. The nurse in turn may become frustrated or resentful because the patient seems "ungrateful."

The framework of a nursing plan is based on information about why a person needs care and judgments made about what kind of care he needs. Although this plan may undergo revision with time, the essential structure will remain as a guide. The nursing plan begins the mostly practical phase of the nursing process in which the patient is helped to care for himself (or his family for him). Formulating this plan depends to a large extent on the technique of problem solving.

Problem solving

Two kinds of reasoning are used in **problem solving.** (See p. 62 for a further discussion of problem solving.) The first is **inductive** reasoning, which is the development of knowledge and the formulation of generalizations or principles. The second is **deductive,** which requires drawing inferences from general principles or applying knowledge already at hand.

It is not necessary for every nursing action to be backed up by carefully reasoned scientific principles. Science does not claim to hold all the explanations for why things are as they are. Certain nursing practices are commonly accepted simply because experience shows they work. But in most cases, the nurse will provide the best care when she systematically uses scientific problem solving, rather than relying on clinical experience alone.

Some problems can be attacked with ease; others require much time and effort. Frequently, several problems will converge at the same time. In many cases, one phase of problem solving will occur with another phase, or one step will take longer than another. The problem-solving process does not necessarily evolve in a neat and orderly fashion.

All nurses are not equipped with the same inborn abilities to deal with people or to solve problems. However, the necessary techniques can and must be learned. They will enable each nurse to respond to the continuing challenge of dealing with other people.

Patients are not benefited by a nurse who is only a technician, who works in an automated, "cookbook" fashion.

What are the steps in the nursing process?

The division of the nursing process into four steps is somewhat arbitrary. In reality, one phase flows into the next. But the separation serves a function. When a nurse knows in which phase a particular action belongs, she is better able to analyze it. For teaching purposes, the separation makes it possible to have nursing actions follow the same prescribed pattern. The details will, of course, change according to each situation.

It is important to exhaust the possibilities of each stage before moving on to the next. Of course, the limits of time, safety, and other circumstances must be considered. One is easily tempted to jump to hasty conclusions and plan without enough data. This is particularly true of students who are eager to help the patient as quickly as possible.

"The ability to withhold judgment until needed data are accumulated and ordered is acquired more slowly, but learning is enhanced as students recognize their maturation in this area," one nurse educator has observed.[4] She acknowledged, however, that students who want to use the techniques of observation and communication can become frustrated when the means of doing so are not readily available.

"Just once I'd like to go to bed knowing that tomorrow I can get up without something still waiting to be finished," she reports overhearing a student remark.[5] Yet, this ongoingness is one of the elements of the nursing process that ties it most closely to the outside world.

The nursing process is not an enforced, rigid discipline. It is a set of principles that has evolved from observation of what works. It should be flexible enough to allow for some movement back and forth between the steps. For example, a nurse will often plan a patient's therapy based on an initial diagnosis. When previously unknown factors in the patient's condition are discovered, she must move back to phase one, assessment.

The framework agreed upon by nearly all teachers of nursing is outlined below, although their terms for each step vary. (The steps in the nursing process will be discussed in detail in chapters 5 and 6.)

Assessment

Assessment means the ability to make judgments and decisions and then communicate them to others. Assessment is the act of reviewing a situation in order to identify a patient's problem. To assess wisely, the nurse must be able to comprehend the patient's needs. She must be able to communicate with the patient and translate her assessment into terms that relate to his specific condition.

[4]Joyce Finch. 1969. Systems analysis: A logical approach to professional nursing care. *Nursing Forum* 8:186.
[5]Ibid., pp. 188–89.

FIG. 4-1 *The steps in the nursing process.*

**1
ASSESSMENT**

• Gathering data
 — Taking a history
   (interviewing)
 — Conducting a physical
   examination
• Making a nursing diagnosis

**2
PLANNING**

• Formulating a plan
 — Writing nursing orders
• Revising the plan
• Collaborating with the patient

**3
IMPLEMENTATION**

• Coordinating care
 — With other health
   team members
 — With relatives and
   friends of the patient

**4
EVALUATION**

• Looking for patient reactions
• Checking efficiency and
  effectiveness of care
• Making necessary changes
  (modification)

Gathering data

During the assessment phase, the nurse gathers data about the patient from all available resources. This information includes the patient's normal functioning, his present status, and the tentative goals for his future. One or more approaches may be required to make this assessment. For example, the nurse may determine the patient's ability to exchange oxygen and carbon dioxide through the respiratory system. She might also simply observe his daily activities, such as his sleeping habits.

Another line of observation involves a general "head-to-toe" report of the patient's condition. Are his spirits generally good? Does he seem tired often? What is the condition of his lower leg muscles?

A problem may be stated in a general or a specific manner. Nursing authorities have unanimously identified certain nursing problems as guides. For example, regulation of oxygen supply is a problem common to many patients. There are also specific problems related to this general one. The nurse must be aware of the relationship between these general principles and specific problems.

The value of observation has been recognized throughout the history of modern nursing. Florence Nightingale wrote, "For it may safely be said,

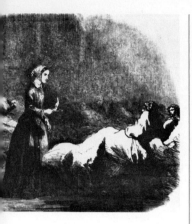

"For it may safely be said, not that the habit of ready and correct observation will by itself make us useful nurses, but that without it we shall be useless with all our devotion."

—*Florence Nightingale*

[Picture Collection, New York Public Library]

not that the habit of ready and correct observation will by itself make us useful nurses, but that without it we shall be useless with all our devotion." [6]

The nursing diagnosis

While the nurse has always been held in high regard for her skills as an observer, she has been held in some suspicion as a diagnostician. Part of the problem is in the definition of the word **diagnosis.** It does not have the same meaning when applied to the nurse's function as when it refers to the physician's. The difference lies in purpose. A doctor is concerned with identifying the cause of illness so that he can treat the underlying disease process. Although the nurse usually uses the same techniques—examining, asking questions, and observing—her goal is to identify the patient's symptoms or reactions to his situation.

For example, a physician may diagnose the victim of a stroke as a diabetic. The nurse's diagnosis might include the fact that the patient is weak and mentally confused. Her diagnosis provides the basis for **nursing orders,** which are communicated to the staff and revised as necessary. Her therapeutic plan includes both the nursing and medical diagnoses, which complement each other to work in the best interests of the patient.

Record keeping

Particularly at this point in the nursing process, it is important to keep careful records. We are all limited in our abilities to observe accurately, remember, and report. In addition, past experience often colors what we "see." Good record keeping lessens the chance of overlooking significant clues as well as misinterpreting their importance. It also eliminates the necessity of repeating information to different members of the staff.

Numerous predetermined forms have been created for this purpose. No one format is ideal; the main point is to allow for the recording of all pertinent information.

Planning

This phase of the nursing process involves drawing up a careful blueprint for carrying out the goals determined in the assessment phase. **Planning** means weighing priorities and designing methods for the resolution of problems. It also involves continually validating the information at hand. Planning demands care and deliberation—goals cannot be set arbitrarily or hastily.

[6] As quoted in Irene L. Beland. 1970. *Clinical nursing: Pathophysiological and psychosocial approaches,* 2d ed., p. 15. New York: Macmillan.

Formulating a plan

As an illustration of the components of planning, consider the patient who lacks oxygen because of internal bleeding. After collecting the necessary data, the nurse formulates possible methods for solving the problem or preventing it from getting worse. Her continuing evaluation of the situation is based on knowledge of principles related to blood pressure, respiration, pulse rate, and other factors. The soundness of her judgment rests on her ability to know how and when to initiate a nursing action and when to call a physician.

Based on her perception of patient needs and her scientific knowledge, the nurse plans not only what to do but how to do it. At the same time she determines nursing priorities, including the sequence of activities and who will perform them. Some people call this process **nursing intervention;** other terms include nursing therapy, nursing action, and nursing care.

In making her plans, the nurse uses not only the information she has recorded but the collective knowledge and experience of all members of the health care team. She also takes into account any current scientific information related to the problem. For example, an aide may observe that a patient lies on his back without changing position for three hours at a time. Combining this information with her own observations, the nurse may make plans based on the need to "maintain skin integrity and prevent decubitus ulcers." This plan would be guided by the scientific information that one hour of continuous pressure can lead to the breakdown of tissue.

Revising the plan

The nursing plan is also subject to revision based on the nurse's own reevaluation of her data. She must confirm her observations by questioning the patient directly. She must make sure that the two of them view his problem in the same light and agree on the same solutions. Failing this, she must insure that the patient is at least aware of differences in their points of view.

Reevaluation is based on the recognition of both immediate and long-range goals. It must take into account the sometimes shifting balance between the two. Short-range goals often serve the useful function of giving both nurse and patient a sense of progress. For example, the partially paralyzed patient who becomes able to feed himself can look more hopefully to the day when he will regain use of his legs.

Implementation

This is the stage of the nursing process where thoughts become words, and plans become actions. A plan of care is of no use to anybody unless it is translated into action. For example, in the case of the patient with potential decubitus ulcers, **implementation** might consist of turning him every hour. In this way all four of his body surfaces will be utilized in succession.

Coordinating care

In this patient's case, as in others, implementation would include coordinating the activities of paramedical personnel as well as those of the other people involved with the patient. Depending on where he is being cared for, the numbers and the professional status of the people will vary. But whether the patient is in his home or in a large community hospital, he will probably have friends and relatives who will be asking questions. The nurse must be imaginative and compassionate in including them in the process of patient care.

Coordinating the activities of others is not always an easy task. Patience and understanding of human nature are essential. However, coordinating many different activities and maintaining a sense of purpose may be one of the nurse's major professional challenges as well as an important source of satisfaction.

The challenge lies partly in organizing the efforts of health care personnel with a wide range of abilities, training, attitudes, and personality traits. The nurse must be familiar with the human composition of her team and make maximum use of their talents as they relate to the needs of the patient. This difficult task is another major source of professional reward. It is satisfying to know one's capabilities and to observe their effects on the patient.

Evaluation

This part of the nursing process takes place both during administration of care and afterwards. The major factors to be considered are how the nurse's actions brought about changes in the patient's condition, and how well the original therapeutic goals were fulfilled.

Evaluating a solution is as important as planning it. However, like other steps in the problem-solving sequence, **evaluation** does not necessarily occur as an isolated activity. It is usually continuous, and it may be both formal and informal.

Returning to the patient with potential decubitus ulcers, evaluation criteria might include "absence of redness and breaks in the skin." Of course, the nurse would not wait until the patient was approaching discharge to evaluate the effectiveness of her plan. If the patient's skin actually began to break, she would immediately review her approach. This review should take into account that each patient is different. What works for one may not work for another. It is not only the patient's medical diagnosis that dictates nursing care but his needs as an individual.

While evaluating, the nurse will be asking herself a number of questions:

1. How did I expect the patient to react?
2. Could I have done anything to achieve the same goals more efficiently and effectively?
3. What changes could or should be made?

Constant self-evaluation makes it possible to plan more precisely not only for the patient currently under treatment but for the next one. In effect, the nurse is going through what might be termed a fifth stage of the nursing process, **modification.**

Involving the patient's family

Each step of the nursing process must be coordinated with the patient and his family if it is to succeed. For example, nurse and nutritionist may devise the ideal diet for a patient with elevated blood sugar levels. But if his wife does not understand how to change her methods of meal planning and preparation, the prescribed diet will be useless.

Some patients do what the nurse suggests while in the hospital but return to normal habits when back at home. The nurse must therefore investigate carefully to find out exactly how the patient feels about his therapy and what can be done to ensure his cooperation. Almost all patients are capable of becoming effectively involved in their own care. Exceptions are babies, senile adults, the unconscious, or the acutely psychotic.

Skills required in the nursing process

Intellectual skills

The intellectual skills needed in the nursing process are **critical thinking, problem solving,** and **decision making.** (These skills have also been called lateral, vertical, and discriminative thinking.)[7] These skills have much in common but are nevertheless distinct.

It is vitally important to cultivate these skills and to maintain them through practice. The experienced professional as well as the nursing student must constantly maintain her ability to think critically, solve problems, and make decisions.

[7]Marlene G. Mayers. 1972. *A systematic approach to the nursing care plan,* p. 6. New York: Appleton-Century-Crofts.

The nursing process
is based on the four
principles of the
scientific method.

Critical thinking. Once the nurse has assembled a body of facts, she uses critical, or lateral, thinking to sift through the information and start generating ideas about what it means. The best critical thinker is the person who is able to consider several alternatives when trying to extract meaning from a group of facts.

Critical thinking is important largely because without it the quality of care the patient is receiving may deteriorate. If the nurse approaches her patient's problems prematurely, without taking time to think out the situation clearly, she may find herself moving half-blindly through motions that are not appropriate.

Problem solving. After extracting a series of possible meanings from a collection of facts, the nurse is ready for problem solving, or vertical thinking. This is the thought process used to define problems based on interpretations made in the critical thinking phase. Both levels of thinking are essential when a nurse is faced with an unstructured situation.

Many educators feel that the problem-solving technique gives organization and direction to the various elements of nursing practice. Problem solving also allows for better assessment and planning because it focuses the nurse's thinking on the individual rather than the tasks involved in his care. It also helps in the planning and use of written **nursing care plans.**

As mentioned earlier, the nursing process is based on the four principles of the scientific method. The thought process of problem solving follows the same order in its steps:

1. Recognize and define the problem
2. Collect data from observation and experimentation
3. Formulate and implement a solution
4. Evaluate the solution

A situation may be complex and the plan chosen to approach it may be extensive, but the process of problem solving in itself is not complicated. It does not change and can be applied to any situation.

Problem-solving ability is directly related to how much a nurse has learned about the problems of patients and their solutions. It is impossible to use knowledge one does not possess. Both students and seasoned nurses should seize every opportunity for increasing their knowledge and skills.

Decision making. The third major type of thought process—decision making, or discriminative thinking—is used for deciding a particular course of action. The phases of the process have been divided into deliberation, judgment, and choice.[8]

---

[8]Jeannette Schaefer. 1974. The interrelatedness of decision making and the nursing process. *American Journal of Nursing* 74:1853.

During the deliberation phase, the nurse searches for conditions that call for action. Which is the most important situation for which a decision is demanded? What alternative actions can be explored? What are the probable consequences of a particular alternative?

During the judgment phase, she analyzes each alternative and its consequences. She then decides which is the most effective and efficient. Although decisions become more effective as the skills of deliberation and judgment increase, there are limits to rationality because there are limits to our knowledge. The choice phase of decision making occurs when one alternative and its consequences are selected as the course of action.

The phases of decision making are an interrelated cycle of activities. They demand both a constant search for situations that require action and a decision as to which are the most important. The factors that go into the choice of clinical alternatives may be numerous and may appear in varying combinations. Although there is no one "right" choice for all situations, there are definitely better or worse choices for each situation. To a given patient, the difference between better and worse may mean the difference between life and death.

With training, these parts of the intellectual process (critical thinking, problem solving, and decision making) will begin to operate at almost the same time. The result will be better decisions and methods for patient care.

Interpersonal skills

Developing interpersonal skills is as important as developing intellectual skills. It is these skills which distinguish the knowledgeable technician from the complete professional.

Self-knowledge and self-image. In order to be capable of reaching others, we must first be in touch with ourselves. Self-knowledge is therefore first on the list of interpersonal skills. The better a nurse understands herself and her own needs, the more insight she will bring to the problems of patients.

The term **self-image** refers to the way we see ourselves or believe ourselves to be. Some people are able to see into the mirror clearly, but many are not. Those who are unable to perceive their own defects are often incapable of giving to others except in a very limited way.

At the other extreme are those people who are constantly finding fault with themselves. They are equally unable to give love and attention. The mature person is aware of both his shortcomings and his abilities. The more a person knows himself, the better friend he can be to himself, and the more capable he will be of developing good relationships.

Communication. No matter how self-aware a nurse is and how deep her ability to empathize with others, her resources will be useless unless she

Self-knowledge is first on the list of interpersonal skills.

is capable of communicating. In the nursing sense, **communication** does not mean merely talking to the patient and answering his requests. There is a difference between everyday social conversation and the therapeutic communication of a professional.

Certainly, nurses will find themselves exchanging casual remarks with a patient just as they would with any other human being. Yet, basically, a nurse is concerned with establishing a rapport that makes her more aware of the patient's needs. Her attitude must encourage him to express his fears and anxieties, to voice his reaction to his illness, or to express his feelings about his dependency on others. Through the use of therapeutic communication, the nurse helps the patient to make his own decisions and to come to his own conclusions.

Patients often feel that the nurse's time is limited. They therefore hesitate to push a conversation beyond an exchange of pleasantries. For this reason, the nurse must utilize a variety of techniques to encourage therapeutic communication. (These techniques will be discussed more fully in chapter 10.)

All communication is not verbal. A patient learns much about the nurse's attitude toward him from her expression and mannerisms.

The ability to listen is basic to communication. The nurse must be able to pick up on faint signals the patient may broadcast; she must be able to draw him out.

The ability to listen is based on an attitude of acceptance. This attitude tells the patient that whoever he is or whatever his problems, the nurse is ready to hear him. She accepts his congenial and uncongenial qualities, his constructive and destructive attitudes, his positive and negative feelings. Her attitude helps free him of undesirable defenses and enables him to deal realistically with his problems.

Acceptance comes out of a knowledge of human personality, patterns of behavior, factors influencing change and growth in personality, and the patient's potential for self-help.[9] A patient senses acceptance from a nurse who spends time with him and tries to find out how he really feels about his illness.

A nonjudgmental attitude does not mean that the nurse must reject her own value system. It does mean that she refrains from judging the patient's values. If a patient is hospitalized as a result of an overdose of drugs, for example, it is not the nurse's role to air her opinions on drug abuse.

The nurse's objective in evaluating behavior is not to judge but to understand. This is not necessarily an easy task. Often a nurse who believes herself to be an accepting person will be surprised to encounter situations in which she is not. Eventually she will learn to recognize that the response

[9]Mary Grace Connolly. 1960. What acceptance means to patients. *American Journal of Nursing* 60:1754.

of an individual within a specific situation is often the best he is capable of making at that moment. When she understands this, she will concentrate on collecting data that will help her learn about him.

Other interpersonal skills

A fourth set of interpersonal skills that the nurse is asked to develop is the ability to convey interest, compassion, knowledge, and information.

In the case of a patient who is facing a tremendous change in his life as a result of illness and who is progressing slowly, the best thing a nurse can do is demonstrate interest and compassion. She does so by being kind, gentle, gracious, humane, and thoughtful. Each nurse will develop her own particular style of conveying these qualities.

In addition to being able to convey an emphathetic attitude toward the patient, the nurse must know how to transmit knowledge and information about his condition. This is usually of great concern and often of embarrassment to him. Nurses, like other people, may tend to respond in clichés when hearing another person's problems. They will comment, "Don't worry, you'll be all right," or, "You're lucky it wasn't worse." Such remarks offer little consolation to the patient and are actually more soothing to the nurse. Instead of comforting the patient, they make him feel the nurse is washing her hands of him.

Technical skills

In order to make each patient as comfortable as possible, a nurse must be familiar with a wide range of technical skills. For example, in the case of a patient with chronic obstructive pulmonary disease, the nursing plan might include simple measures such as providing two pillows and avoiding tight bed linens across the chest. In addition, the nurse will limit conversation and help him get to the bathroom. The plan would also include skilled procedures such as maintaining the IV flow rate; describing and recording sputum amount, color, and consistency; and recording fatigue, pulse, and respiratory response.

Without adequate professional expertise, the nurse will be a helpless bystander to the progression of disease. This will be the case no matter how well she has mastered the skills of communication and emotional support.

SUMMARY

In this chapter we have been concerned with the scientific basis of professional nursing, the nursing process. It is on this well-defined concept that the entire practice of nursing is built.

The nursing process provides a rational, scientific, and time-tested basis for administering care. It is a combination of intellectual activities and physical actions. It provides a systematic means of analyzing the patient's problems, determining how to solve them, and then implementing and evaluating the plan. Essentially, it follows the same method used by scientists. The difference is that the nurse is looking for answers to immediate problems and not for new knowledge.

In applying this process, the nurse will avoid the extremes. These are represented by the "cookbook" technician who has expertise but lacks humane qualities, and the compassionate, sympathetic nurse who cannot handle a health emergency. The nursing process demands the combination of intellectual and interpersonal skills to provide the best patient care. These skills can be learned, developed, and continually improved upon throughout the nurse's professional career.

Four steps have been identified in the process: assessment, planning, implementation, and evaluation. In reality, these do not occur in clear-cut succession, but rather they overlap. Especially for the nursing student, it is important to exhaust the possibilities of each step before continuing to the next. In this way, the temptation of jumping to obvious conclusions will be avoided. At all points in the process, careful record keeping will make for maximum dependability and accuracy.

Obviously, the nurse is expected to know the techniques of her profession and to do as much as possible to make the patient safe and comfortable. However, her ability to perform also depends on the development of intellectual skills. Of these skills, the most vital are critical thinking, problem solving, and decision making. Once these skills are learned they will serve as a point of reference throughout a lifetime.

At the same time, the nurse should be developing interpersonal skills. These can be divided into four groups: self-understanding and insight into attitudes and behavior; communicating; listening; and the conveying of interest, compassion, knowledge, and information. The nurse must learn how to empathize with the patient and how to let him know that she cares. She must also discover how to draw him out in a way that is most beneficial to his medical progress.

Although the nursing process is an established fact and the techniques are well known, each nurse will interpret the process in her own way. She will provide care in her own style, always following the basic precepts of the profession.

STUDY QUESTIONS

1. What are the steps involved in the scientific method of investigation?
2. What is problem solving? Define the types of reasoning used in this process.
3. What is the nursing process? Define and give examples of each step in the process.

4. Name and define two of the intellectual skills used by the nurse in applying the nursing process. Name and define two interpersonal skills.
5. In the light of what you know and what you believe about the nursing process, how would you respond to the following comments?
   a. "True nursing comes from within—from a desire to help people in need. It is only when training is combined with this desire that patients benefit."
   b. "Nursing care plans are fine for students, but they're too time-consuming for a busy staff nurse. Who's taking care of the patient while the nurse is sitting at the desk, writing out the care plan?"
   c. "I don't know why Mr. Jones is so uncooperative. I've tried everything, but he just won't listen when I tell him he should be getting more rest."

SELECTED BIBLIOGRAPHY

Carlson, Sylvia. 1972. A practical approach to the nursing process. *American Journal of Nursing* 72:1589–91.

Daubenmire, M. Jean, and King, Imogene M. 1973. Nursing process models: A systems approach. *Nursing Outlook* 21:512–17.

McCain, R. Faye. 1965. Nursing by assessment—not intuition. *American Journal of Nursing* 65:82–84.

Mayers, Marlene G. 1972. A search for assessment criteria. *Nursing Outlook* 10:257–64.

Yura, Helen, and Walsh, Mary B. 1974. *The nursing process: Assessing, planning, implementing, evaluating,* 2d ed. New York: Appleton-Century-Crofts.

5 Assessment

What is assessment?

When two people meet, they usually size up each other's personality traits, strengths, weaknesses, and particular characteristics. They do this in order to help guide themselves in dealing appropriately with one another. This sizing up occurs in the health care situation between nurse and patient, and it is vital in enabling the nurse to help the patient adapt to his problems and changing environment. It is a process called **assessment.**

Assessment differs from most social sizing-up. It is not a haphazard and informal collection of isolated facts and intuitive evaluations of another person based on a few exchanged words and glances. Rather, it is, in its most effective form, a systematic, purposeful, and complex gathering of data about the patient's present and projected needs and problems.

Usually the nurse initiates the assessment as soon as possible after she meets the patient. The nurse will continue to gather data, assess, and evaluate as long as she is in contact with the patient in order to develop a diagnosis that will serve as the basis for the patient's health care plan. Occasionally, collecting data and administering care are carried out simultaneously. This is particularly true in emergency situations when the patient is in acute need.

Patient assessment can serve as a useful and constructive tool if it takes into consideration the whole patient, not just his medical condition and immediate needs. This means that data must be obtained not only about his physiological condition, but also about his life-style, expectations of health care, view of his own health and/or illness, and what he expects of the health care practitioners. It means that data must be sought about the patient's social, emotional, and physical status.

By considering each patient as a distinct and unique individual, the nurse can help to individualize the care he will receive. This individualization of care is a very important goal in today's health care setting, where institutionalization and specialization have tended to depersonalize care. The nurse always has been and continues to be in a strong and vital position to promote a personalized type of health care. Assessment of the patient provides a sound basis for this kind of care. It also gives the nurse the opportunity to show the patient that someone cares, that someone is taking a personal interest in his wants and needs.

Assessment as an ongoing process

People are a complex combination of qualities, and they act and react to changing conditions around them. Because of this, collecting data for a useful patient assessment is necessarily much more than a passive gathering of facts. Rather, it is a complex intellectual process that must go on continuously. It must take into consideration the day-to-day needs of the patient and his response to care as well as the long-range view of the total health care plan. It must also consider the patient's capacity for change, the adequacy of his environment, his relationships with others, and the services he needs.

Effective assessment of the patient's needs requires much skill, sound judgment, sensitivity, and creativity. Things may not always be as they seem on the surface, and data are not always readily available or reliable. Even when they become available, they must be evaluated and put into a perspective that will aid the development of a helpful nursing care plan.

To evaluate patient data intelligently, the nurse must have a broad knowledge of people in general. She must understand basic human needs, human anatomy and physiology, and human behavior. She must be familiar with the major causes of morbidity and mortality, human growth and development, and basic pathophysiology and psychopathology. Knowledge of various cultures with their beliefs and social patterns, the major religions of the world and the obligations and rituals of their followers, family and social organization, and the economic patterns for that segment of society in which the nurse practices are also needed.[1]

With time, creativity, and these skills, the nurse should be better able to take isolated symptoms and facts and put them into a meaningful perspective and relationship in the nursing process.

Assessment vs. intuition

In recent years, the assessment process has become a more accepted tool for evaluating patients' needs. For many nurses, intuition has always been a major tool for assessing patients. At best, intuition means a haphazard collection of observable data; at worst, it provides an incomplete, subjective, and often misleading way of viewing the patient's needs.

The growing acceptance of systematic assessment as a nursing tool has not, however, led to the establishment of a standard or prescribed way

---

[1] Helen Yura and Mary B. Walsh. 1973. *The nursing process: Assessing, planning, implementing, evaluating,* 2d ed., p. 72. New York: Appleton-Century-Crofts.

of collecting data. The nursing literature is filled with suggested formats, categories, and questions prepared and recommended by nurses, nurse educators, and administrators. There is much variance in the length, scope, and priorities given to certain patient characteristics. Some formats are generalized and designed to apply to all nursing situations in a broad sense; others are geared to specific nursing situations such as acute or outpatient care. Most, however, share some basic approaches and characteristics about sources of data, techniques for obtaining data, and what data are important. This chapter will deal with those basics that are common to all effective nursing assessments.

Sources of data

Information about the patient's past and present health and social status in all the dimensions discussed above will probably come from a number of sources. The patient is usually the primary source of information. Other sources, such as family members, friends, other members of the health care team, significant members of the community, and available records and reports, can help enlarge, clarify, and substantiate the information obtained from the patient. The methods most often used for obtaining data are interviews, observation, and inspection. Of course, the specific nature of the situation will determine the *ways* in which the nurse obtains the information and *which* information will be sought from *whom*.

The patient will usually be the first source of information about himself. Very often the patient will offer a clear and concise picture of his needs and problems, his history, how he feels about his illness and hospitalization, and what he expects in terms of recovery and nursing care. However, even with the most cooperative of patients, the nurse must remember that the patient is a very subjective source of information about himself and that, whenever possible, information should be corroborated by a second source.

The patient's view of himself, his real or imagined needs and problems, his reasons for seeking health care services, and his anxieties about his condition will certainly color his response to questions about his condition. The patient who is a habitual complainer may exaggerate the frequency and severity of certain symptoms. The stoic patient, on the other hand, may provide few clues about the physical and emotional discomfort his condition is causing. Attempts to gather information about the patient's history will often depend on the patient's memory, which can be sketchy or unreliable due to anxiety or discomfort.

Other circumstances may inhibit the patient's desire or ability to supply information: feelings of embarrassment, fear of criticism, legal implications, or the possibility of jeopardizing his employment. For instance, a pilot may fear revealing aspects of his history that may impair

The patient is usually the primary source of information.

[Photo courtesy Gertrude M. Lee, R.N.]

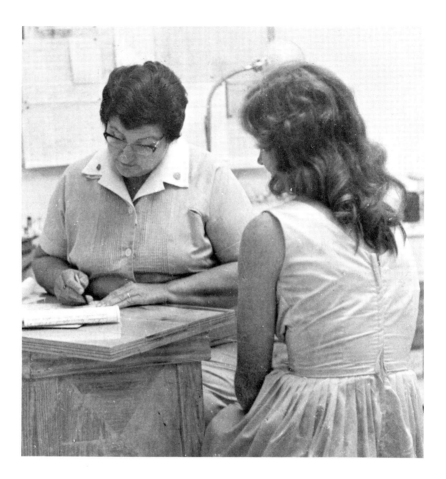

his ability to retain his status, or a teen-age patient may be unwilling to discuss a drug or sexual experience for fear of legal or parental reprisal.[2]

Because of age or condition, some patients will not be able to provide any verbal information about themselves. Data about an infant, a senile individual, patients who are incoherent, unconscious, or otherwise unable to speak will have to be obtained by the nurse through direct observation and reliance on others who are significant to the patient.

Family and significant others are sources of information, not only for those unable to offer data about themselves but for all patients. Family and friends can provide information about the patient's home environment and relationships with family members, stresses and strains the patient may have undergone prior to illness, and the family background of illness and health. They may also be aware of other aspects of the patient's physical,

---

[2]William C. Fowkes, Jr., and Virginia K. Hunn. 1973. *Clinical assessment for the nurse practitioner,* pp. 10–11. St. Louis: Mosby.

emotional, or social status that the patient may have avoided or forgotten to discuss. Here, too, the nurse must consider the motives of these informants and their relationships to the patient. Anxiety or other distorting factors may affect the data provided by even the most well-meaning individual.

Members of the health team, including other nurses, physicians, and auxiliary personnel such as physical or speech therapists, psychologists, and others, may provide valuable and insightful information. They should be consulted for information about the patient's medical history, his physical and emotional reactions to treatments they may have administered, social and emotional reactions they have observed, and contingencies for care. Information gathered by other members of the health care team for their specific purposes must also be assessed for relevance to the nursing care plan. Care must be taken to put the specialized information into its proper perspective.

Records and reports may provide factual and observed data that have been collected by other health care professionals during previous medical visits. Using such data will help the nurse avoid overburdening the patient with questions about vital statistics and factual background. It will also provide the nurse with information that can be used to refresh the patient's

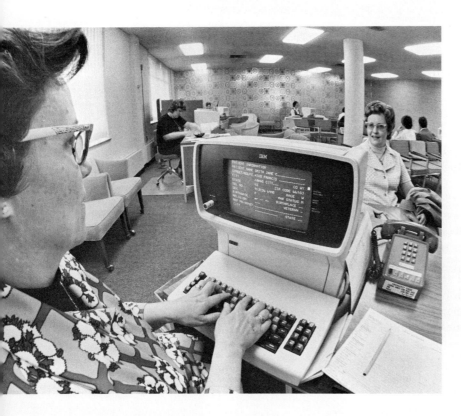

Sophisticated computers are playing an increasingly important role in record keeping.
[Photo by James E. Lubbock, courtesy International Business Machines Corporation]

memory about past events or to verify and confirm data that the nurse may obtain from the patient and other people.

Records of all types are currently being used and developed to supplement traditional medical and nursing records. Sophisticated computers and data banks permit rapid retrieval of information about a patient or a population group in a given area that might otherwise take hours or days to collect.

One example of the extensive use being made of computerized health records is a program for the 9,000 members of the Papago Indian tribe.[3] An automated and centralized data base and remote-control terminals that obtain information give the health team access to complete patient, family, and community health information whenever it is required. The community health nurse can obtain a medical summary by entering a patient's identification number on a teletypewriter at one of the remote terminals at the reservation health center. The computer provides a typed summary that includes information about the patient's recent clinical and field contacts, diagnosis made, medications prescribed, chronic problems, and current immunization status. Since the nurse is able to visit the community only once or twice each month, this information is especially important because it alerts her to any medical attention received between her visits.[4]

This example illustrates the value of records in patient assessment. Of course, such information is only as accurate as the people entering it, but with increasing utilization of comprehensive patient records may come a growing awareness and understanding of the potential of computer technology and a growing appreciation for the importance of accuracy.

Pertinent facts and conceptual knowledge not otherwise obtained from any of the above sources may be available from members of the community in which the patient lives or from a religious leader with whom the patient may have had contact. Newspapers (particularly in the case of illness resulting from a publicized accident) and eyewitnesses may also be helpful. Finally, there may exist other documents the patient may have written relevant to his condition.

In addition to information obtained from the patient and other concerned individuals, the nurse can use her knowledge of physiology, psychodynamics, pathology, etc., to make inferences concerning the patient's condition and probable responses to treatment. In this regard, current textbooks and journals are useful references that should be utilized extensively.

In cases where the nurse has difficulty obtaining adequate information from all the above sources, the possibilities for other sources of data are as extensive as the imagination and perseverance of the person pursuing them.

---

[3] Virginia B. Brown, William B. Mason, and Michael Kaczmarski. 1971. A computerized health information service. *Nursing Outlook* 19:158–60.
[4] Ibid., p. 159.

Means of collecting data: The interview

How the nurse goes about gathering all this information from a patient and others will depend very much on the situation, the established procedures of the health care unit, and other factors. Sometimes the patient is simply given a printed form to fill out, with routine questions about some of the above-mentioned factors. The patient is asked to fill in the blanks, or the nurse may do it for him. While such an approach may be efficient and easy, it is far from ideal. It provides little opportunity for patient-nurse interaction and little adaptability to the patient's specific characteristics.

Ideally, the **nursing history** should be developed during interviews with the patient and others. The interview allows the nurse to establish a verbal and nonverbal relationship with the patient and to convey an attitude of interest and caring. At the same time, she can convey information to the patient, help identify and clarify needs and goals, and answer questions which may be troubling him.

If the patient's condition is critical, with life-threatening problems, the nurse will first participate in relieving the crisis and then focus on the patient's participation. Should the patient be otherwise unable to express his needs because of age or mental capacity, a person who knows the patient well should be the subject of the primary interview. However, all efforts should be made to involve the patient as much as possible and as soon as possible.

Knowledge of interviewing techniques and the ability to interview are necessary for every nurse. Just as the role of the nurse has evolved to embrace the concept of the patient as a total person, the nursing history interview has evolved as a way of learning about the total person in order to individualize his care.

Who the nurse is seeking information from will determine to a large degree *how* the interview will be structured. Nonetheless, the patient is always the focus, and helping the patient is always the goal. But whether the interview is conducted with the patient, significant family members, or friends, the nurse is a stranger to them and will have to assist respondents in verbalizing feelings and identifying needs and goals. With other members of the health care team—colleagues of the nurse—the communication is between professionals and is necessarily different. The nurse's task here is to obtain information that is the most relevant to the nursing care plan for the patient.

Where the interview for the nursing history should take place will again depend on the situation, but it is essential that the patient have privacy. Whether in a hospital room, a physician's office, the client's home, an inner-city clinic, factory, school, camp, or community mental health center, the patient should feel comfortable and open about talking freely and uninhibitedly.

The nurse's attitude will also determine the patient's (or other respondent's) willingness to talk freely about needs and problems. Encouragement, patience, understanding, an unhurried and relaxed manner, and interest in and concentration on the patient and his feelings will have a positive effect. Annoyance, disgust, disinterest, or a hurried attitude on the part of the nurse will often tend to make a patient "clam up." The nonverbal messages that nurse and interviewee transmit to one another are often as important and revealing as the verbal messages. Smiles, frowns, grimaces, nervousness, or calmness lend essential meaning to words.

The interview should be a two-way process in which the nurse gains information about as well as gives information to the patient. In giving information, however, the nurse must be discriminating and professional, yet friendly. It would be inappropriate to use technical terms which the interviewee does not understand—terms that can be misinterpreted or that are frightening. It is unnecessary to give unasked for or extraneous information, just to demonstrate evidence of nursing knowledge, without being fully aware of the impact on the listener. While trying to be helpful and anticipate the needs and questions of others, it is easy to fall into the trap of the teacher who starts expounding on some aspect of her specialty. As the teacher rambles on, one student whispers to a second, "What question is she answering?" to which the second replies, "I haven't asked it yet."[5] Where medical information is concerned, the nurse may also provide information that the respondent may not be ready to accept or absorb. On the other hand, the nurse should seek out questions, doubts, and confusions, and focus on clearing up any distortions or misunderstandings of facts and attitudes before they aggravate a situation.

All the information collected through interviews and research will be of little help unless it is carefully sorted out and unless the question is asked, What does it all mean? To answer this, the nurse must *start* by integrating the data. Data will change, as will the patient's reactions to treatment and to the conditions around him. Thus, data must be continuously explored and recorded, even after the care plan has been initiated.

Data must also be continuously evaluated for accuracy and validity. Who has provided the data, what data they have provided, and what their motives or reactions may have been in serving as a source of information are all factors that influence the significance of the data to the overall nursing care plan.

The nursing history

Once the nurse has established *where* to get information about the patient, using some or all of the sources discussed in the previous pages, the next step is to determine *what* information is needed.

---

[5]Loretta Sue Bermosk and Mary Jane Mordan. 1964. *Interviewing in nursing,* pp. 10-11. New York: Macmillan.

The time used in
obtaining a nursing
history is well
spent. . . .

Whether the patient presents complaints that are fairly easy to identify, such as a twisted ankle, or those not so clearly pinpointed, such as general malaise, the nurse must gather information that will be helpful in planning both the physical and nonphysical care of the patient. It is not enough to know that the X-rays reveal no broken bones, that a temperature reading registers 101 degrees, or that the patient has felt extremely tired for 2 days. A complete and clear picture of the patient may turn up other factors that will verify, clarify, and yield information necessary for the development of an effective nursing care plan.

The process of collecting such information is called taking a nursing history. Many guidelines and formats for taking a nursing history have been developed to aid the nurse. Any one of them may be satisfactory. In order to be most effective for patient and nurse, it should be systematic, comprehensive, efficient, and adaptable.

When to take the history. A specific time should be designated to take the history, usually at the first occasion that patient and nurse come into contact with one another. It can be the sole activity of the moment, or it can be carried out in conjunction with other nursing activities. However, the amount of time spent should be adequate to obtain as much information as possible in an unhurried manner. There should also be time allowed for the nurse to give information to the patient. The time used in obtaining a nursing history is well spent for it may be a significant factor in saving time or avoiding problems later when the patient has already begun to receive treatment.

Consider, for example, the case of Mr. S., a middle-aged diabetic who was admitted for removal of gallstones. During his first few days in the hospital, he was unwilling to conform to any of the basic hospital routines. At mealtimes, he did not want to eat; at bedtime, he insisted on wandering around the halls. Any attempt by the nurses to deal with him was met with increasing hostility and lack of cooperation. It was only after 4 days that the nursing staff found out why. For 35 years, Mr. S. had worked as a night watchman. He was simply unable to adjust his schedule overnight to that of the hospital.[6]

A format that is systematic and efficient will be useful for obtaining the greatest amount of data in the least amount of time. If it is organized in a logical, systematic way, it will not be confusing to either patient or nurse. It will focus on one area, such as physical symptoms, and once those have been thoroughly recorded, it will focus on another area, such as personal habits. In this way, the nurse will not have to belabor points with the patient, and repetition of essential data can be kept to a minimum.

While a general framework that examines certain factors common to all persons is useful as a guide, the nurse should be able to adapt and

[6]Yura and Walsh, pp. 84–85.

adjust this general framework to include specifics that will accommodate the unique characteristics of the patient and his situation.

Initially, the nurse can start with a prescribed and standard list of questions applicable to all people and groups with health problems. The setting and particular situation will determine which areas assume primary importance and will thus modify the amount and kind of data collected. These will differ for the hospital nurse, clinic nurse, public health nurse, community nurse, school nurse, nursing home nurse, the nurse in the rural or urban setting, in an acute care or chronic care setting. Different factors will have different priorities for infants, adolescents, or older patients, for men or women, for those with special problems such as blindness, deafness, or mental retardation.

The nurse working in a community mental health center, for example, may focus more on the patient's abilities in the psychosocial, mental, and sensory-motor areas than on the condition of the skin.[7]

Basic content areas. Since the nursing history is intended for use in planning immediate and long-range nursing care, there are some basic content areas that are relevant regardless of variations in patient characteristics and the health care setting. These basic elements include:

1. Patient perceptions and expectations
2. Basic needs
3. Unspecified information that the patient may want to offer
4. The nurse's impressions and suggestions[8]

Specifically, the factors to be considered will generally break down into the following areas: age, sex, education, growth and development, socioeconomic, cultural, and religious background, biological and physical status, emotional status, coping patterns, interactional patterns, life-style, and employment. Additional important factors are the client's view of health and illness as it relates to himself and his family; his expectations of health care; his awareness of the roles of the health care practitioners (particularly that of the nurse); the social, emotional, physical, and ecological environment in which he lives; and the human and material resources available to him.[9]

These factors are all intricately bound to the person's health needs and may be assessed simultaneously. For purposes of discussion, however, they will be dealt with individually here.

Information about *age, sex, growth and development, socioeconomic and cultural background* is important in order to identify the patient's position

A nursing history format that is systematic and efficient will be useful for obtaining the greatest amount of data in the least amount of time.

[7]Pamela Holsclaw Mitchell. 1973. *Concepts basic to nursing,* p. 77. New York: McGraw-Hill.
[8]L. Mae McPhetridge. 1968. Nursing history: One means to personalize care. *American Journal of Nursing* 68:68–69.
[9]Yura and Walsh, pp. 80–81.

relative to others. Since models for wellness may differ for different age groups, for men and women, and for persons from varied backgrounds, knowing what is "normal" or expected for physical and mental functions in a particular grouping gives the nurse a standard against which to gauge the patient's status.

Racial and religious factors will help the nurse identify and accommodate the patient's habits and needs as they are influenced by rites, rituals, and culturally determined attitudes. Some practices and beliefs may affect the patient's reaction to health care, such as specific codes about immunization, blood transfusion, dietary laws, and beliefs about the causes of disease.

Since certain diseases are hereditarily linked to racial or religious background (sickle-cell anemia is linked to blacks, Tay-Sachs disease to Jews of Middle European origin, Cooley's anemia to individuals of Mediterranean origin), it is necessary to identify the patient's background. Similarly, the health condition or causes of death of family members will influence the patient's potential health problems and should be recorded.

The patient's perceptions and expectations will also be influenced by his feelings regarding *previous nursing care experiences.* The patient's answers should provide clues to the development of a specific plan of care based on his desires as well as his impressions of ineffective nursing behavior. They also may offer some ideas as to his perception of the nurse's role so that the nurse may foresee potential conflict.

An understanding of *goal expectations* related to the patient's prognosis and rehabilitation is crucial to the formulation of the care plan. The expressed expectations of the patient are clues to how he understands and accepts his condition, whether his goals are unrealistic in light of the diagnosis or expected response to therapy, whether he understands the plan of treatment, and whether his health priorities are consistent with those of the staff.

Mr. P., for example, who has been scheduled for an amputation of his right leg in 2 days, states that he came to the hospital to clear up the infection in his foot. The nurse, wondering if he has been told of the surgery, phones the physician to share this information with him and to determine what the patient has been told. The nurse learns that the patient has indeed been told of the amputation, that it has been discussed fully with him, and that he has agreed to the procedure. The nurse does not know whether he did not understand what was said, but agreed to the operation anyway. Or, is the patient denying the reality of this traumatic experience? Perhaps he is testing the nurse's knowledge of his case. In any case, the nurse is alerted to a nursing care problem.[10]

Effects of the illness on the patient's usual way of life and on his family will vary greatly, but information about these effects will aid in the development

---

[10]Dolores E. Little and Doris L. Carnevali. 1969. *Nursing care planning,* pp. 164–67. Philadelphia: Lippincott.

of a care plan. For one patient, illness may mean economic disaster; for another, dependence on others to an extent he finds very distasteful; for still another, the most significant effect of the illness is sexual impotence for several months.[11]

The patient's posthospitalization plans and expectations will help determine nursing needs. Statements by patients will help the nurse determine whether the patient's understanding of his illness is realistic. One woman, for example, who had a hysterectomy for a benign condition and presumably would be considered cured upon discharge, said that she expected to go to bed indefinitely after leaving the hospital and would be unable to do anything for herself. To help this patient plan realistically, the nurse must know not only what the patient thinks, but why. If this patient's response is based on fear of cancer, one kind of nursing action is indicated. If her answer reflects an exaggerated dependency need, an entirely different nursing measure is required.[12]

Attitudes about and relationship with family and friends can be determined by asking questions about the patient's family members and friends, what their attitudes are toward his illness, and whether he anticipates their visits. Sometimes the patient may want to have a say in the number and frequency of visitor contacts and which visitors he particularly wants to see or avoid. By becoming aware of the effect that the presence or absence of visitors may have on the patient *before* any problem arises, nurses can take appropriate action.

Sometimes the problem is one of too few visitors, particularly for the patient in a specialized institution distant from his home. The patient might become extremely lonely and depressed if deprived of friendly contact, and if the nurse anticipates this situation, appropriate intervention can be planned.

Basic needs of the patient are explored in order to determine whether nursing intervention will be necessary in order to insure safety, comfort, proper hygiene, nutrition, and rest. Illness, health care, and, particularly, hospitalization jeopardize the continuity of daily living habits and patterns. Yet, with a little modification of basic hospital routine, it is often possible to make adjustments that take the patient's habits into consideration.

Personal *sleep habits,* for example, are bound to be interrupted in the hospital. While rest and sleep form an important part of the healing process, the long-standing, half-joking comment about hospitals is that nobody goes there to rest. There are disruptions tied in with therapy; the environment is new; roommates may be disconcerting; unfamiliar noises, people, and beds all disrupt a person's regular sleeping habits. The nurse can help to individualize patient care by providing the patient with opportunities to maintain as many of his usual sleep habits as possible, including

[11] McPhetridge, p. 70.
[12] Ibid.

A knowledge of the patient's activities, hobbies, and interests may open doors for a better interpersonal relationship between patient and nurse.

an evening glass of milk, a reading period prior to bedtime, or whatever he prefers. This is a particularly important consideration when working with children.

Food and eating habits of patients are also highly individualized, influenced as they are by cultural and geographical factors, custom, physical status, age, likes and dislikes, occupation, and socioeconomic status. For many patients there are dietary restrictions that make the adjustment problem even more difficult. Whether or not the patient's diet is restricted, meals in the hospital often become the focus of a great deal of attention and are a frequent source of dissatisfaction or satisfaction. As an obviously important area of concern to the patient, it must then become an area of concern to the nurse. Information about eating patterns should focus on three areas of inquiry: patterns of meals, food and fluid likes and dislikes, and food allergies.[13] (Maintaining the patient's nutritional status will be discussed in more detail in chapter 19.) Knowledge about the patient's *personal hygiene habits,* such as patterns and rituals related to bathing and grooming, can be used to accommodate the patient's preferences with a minimum of disturbance to the hospital routine. Such flexibility will go a long way in helping the patient feel comfortable.

Because one important index of a patient's progress during illness is clinical data about elimination, it is important for the nurse to know what the patient's normal elimination habits are, such as how often and when he has bowel movements and whether he normally relies on laxatives.

Other special habits or characteristics of the patient should be recorded to aid the nurse in providing effective care. Perhaps a patient finds certain positions in bed more comfortable than others; perhaps because of vision or hearing problems on one side, the patient's telephone and belongings should be placed on the other side. A knowledge of the patient's activities, hobbies, and interests may open doors for a better interpersonal relationship between patient and nurse.

The patient's *physical condition* and needs can be assessed by an in-depth physical examination, which will be discussed in a later section of this chapter. However, through observation and inquiry, much information can be gathered by the nurse about the patient's general and obvious physical condition.

Use of a basic format

For the nursing student or beginning practitioner, it is helpful to have a basic standard format around which to work in compiling the nursing history. Such a format should only serve as a guide, however, for it is easy

---

[13]Little and Carnevali, p. 75.

to fall into the trap of becoming too rigid about a guideline and therefore overlooking relevant factors about a particular patient. Using a standardized form also tends to depersonalize the process of taking a nursing history, whose very purpose is to personalize the care the patient is to receive. Checklists and questionnaires that have been devised to save time and increase convenience are often inadequate because they elicit information only about the items included on the form. One faces the danger of fitting the patient into a generalized or stereotyped picture.

Nonetheless, keeping in mind the dangers and temptations of using a standard form, it is worthwhile studying one to gain a good idea of its scope and content. Figure 5-1 is an excellent example of a comprehensive and personalized form that is flexible enough to cover many different types of situations.

Nursing vs. medical history

The principles discussed above should provide the nurse with a basis for history taking. How do these principles compare with those involved in taking a medical history, another component of patient assessment that is usually undertaken by the physician?

Basically, the techniques of taking a medical history are quite similar to those involved in a nursing history. The physician makes use of information gained from interviews, open-ended questions, and observation, with consideration given to assisting the patient in conveying his concerns. The major difference between the medical and nursing history lies in the focus. From the nursing viewpoint, the meaning of health, illness, and hospitalization to the patient and the patient's family is the basis for planning much of the care; from the medical viewpoint, the pathology of the patient is the major basis for planning care.

During an interview with the patient, the nurse may obtain much of the same information as does the physician, but the primary concern of the nurse is how impairment of the patient's arm movement affects his functional abilities, physically and emotionally. For the patient with motor difficulties there are many implications for daily living. The nurse will attempt to find out about the patient's adaptive mechanisms—how the illness affects the patient's self-image and how the hospitalization affects his adaptive processes. This information is then used as the basis for a nursing care plan that will help the patient and his family cope with his new life situation.

The nursing history is as important a part of planning patient care as is the medical history. But the collection of data in and of itself will be of little value unless this information is evaluated and applied intelligently to subsequent patient care procedures. (The techniques of planning and implementation will be discussed in the next chapter.)

FIG. 5-1 (*next page*) *An example of a comprehensive and personalized nursing history form.*

[From L. Mae McPhetridge, Nursing history: One means to personalize care. *American Journal of Nursing* 68 (1968):71–74. © 1968 by the American Journal of Nursing Company. Reproduced by permission of the American Journal of Nursing Company.]

Nursing History

Date __February 18, 1975__   Medical Diagnosis: __Toxoplasmosis, Detached__
Name __Meg Rogers__   __Retina, rt. eye__
Hospital Number __123-34-0155__   _____
Address (*city or county*) __Sunnyside__   _____
Age _32_____ Sex: M _____ F _X_____   Information obtained from Patient _X_____
Occupation __Teacher's Aide__   Other _X_____
_____   Relationship __husband__
Religion __Methodist__   History needs to be rechecked at later date
Race/National Origin __American Negro__   Check postsurgical

I. Patient Perceptions and Expectations Related to Illness/Hospitalization

1. Why did you come to the hospital? (or go to the doctor?) __Spots in front of right eye and__ __diminished vision.__

2. What do you think caused you to get sick? __Toxoplasmosis, which preceded detached retina__ __(patient thinks it was caused by eating raw or rare meat or having a cat).__

3. Has being sick made any difference in your usual way of life? If so, how? __The medication I have__ __been taking has made me tired. I am now more careful about the way I use my eyes__ __and try to read for shorter periods of time.__

4. What do you expect is going to happen to you in the hospital? __I will be operated upon for re-__ __attachment of retina, and I will remain in hospital for 4 days' recuperation.__

5. What is it like for you being in the hospital? __It's neither good nor bad. I want to get this__ __operation over with quickly and have the problem taken care of so that I can go__ __back to a normal life. The doctors and nurses are professional and answer questions,__ __but brusquely. The surroundings are comfortable.__

6. How long do you expect to be in the hospital? __3-4 days__

7. With whom do you live? __Husband and 2 children (ages 3 and 7)__

8. Who is the most important person(s) to you? __Husband and children__

9. What effect has your coming to the hospital had on your family? (or closest person?) __The normal__ __family routine has been upset in many ways. Friends, relatives, and babysitters are__ __all pitching in to help out during hospitalization by cooking meals, getting chil-__ __dren off to school, helping husband with house chores. However, house seems to be__ __in a "holding pattern" until my return.__

10. Are any of your family (or close persons) able to visit you in the hospital? __Yes, husband and__ __friends will visit. Children will not. Husband can only come on weekend because of__ __working hours.__

11. What do you enjoy doing for recreation? (to pass the time?) __Reading, writing, sewing, sports,__ __card-playing.__

12. How do you expect to get along after you leave the hospital? __I think it will be difficult be-__ __cause of the demands on my time and services (housework, cooking, taking care of__ __children, dependency on car to get around and to chauffeur kids). I realize it will__ __be difficult to do all these things as before, and I guess I will have to get some__ __help, but I don't know where.__

4) What, if anything, do you use on your skin? Moisturizer on face morning and evening; body lotion on body after bath.

5) How often do you prefer to bathe? Daily

                 Morning X   Afternoon _____   Evening _____

                                                   No Preference _____

6) Do you prefer a   Tub bath X   Shower _____

      This question is not pertinent _____

2. Safety
   a. Locomotion
      1) Do you have any difficulty in walking about? Yes X   No _____
         If yes, describe Have trouble judging distances, especially on stairs. Have to hold on to railings because of problems with depth perception.
      2) Did you have any difficulty in walking before you came to the hospital?
                                                                    Yes X   No _____
         If yes, describe Since onset of toxoplasmosis in right eye, have had problems on stairs.
         How did you manage? Walk carefully, using railing; avoid carrying packages and children on stairs wherever possible.
      3) Has anyone said anything to you about staying in bed (or getting out of bed) since you came to the hospital? Yes X   No _____
         If yes, what? Some friends who have had surgery for detached retina have told me that I would have to lie still in bed for about a week with sandbags around my head to prevent it from moving.
         What do you think about staying in bed? (or getting out of bed?) I think I would go crazy if I had to lie in bed like that, and I hope that I can get out of bed right away. My doctor said nothing about staying in bed after surgery and I hope I don't have to.
      4) Do you expect to have any difficulty getting about after you leave the hospital?
                                  Yes X   No _____   Don't know _____
         If yes, how do you expect to manage? By not trying to do as many things, by relying on friends and neighbors to help.
   b. Vision
      1) Do you have any difficulty in seeing? Yes X   No _____
         If yes, describe No peripheral vision in right eye, poor vision in left. Can't see anything at distance without glasses; have trouble seeing anything on right without turning head to side. Driving is difficult because of vision pr'
      2) Do you wear glasses? Yes X   No _____
         If #1 is yes, in what way does your limited sight handicap you? Not being well; reading is difficult; close work is difficult.
         How do you manage? Have gotten used to limitations, t'
   c. Hearing
      1) Do you have any difficulty in hearing? Yes X   No
         If yes, describe Poorer hearing in right ear
      2) If yes, do you wear a hearing aid? Yes X   No _____

II. Specific Basic Needs

1. Comfort, Rest, Sleep
   a. Pain/Discomfort
      1) Have you had any pain or discomfort since admission?   Yes __X__   No _____
         If yes, describe __Severe headaches and nausea__
      2) Did you have any pain or discomfort before coming to the hospital?
                                                          Yes __X__   No _____
         If yes, describe __Severe headaches, occasional nausea, dizziness, sharp shooting__
         __pains through right eye region; more than usual fatigue.__

         How long? __3 months__
         What did you do to relieve the pain/discomfort? __Take aspirin or other similar pain-__
         __killer, take a nap, lie down.__
         Was the pain/discomfort relieved by treatment?
                   Completely _____   Partially __X__   Not at all _____
      3) If you have pain/discomfort while in the hospital what would you like the nurse to do to relieve it?
         __Give me pain-killer, cold compresses on forehead and eyes, turn down overhead__
         __lights, turn off phone.__
   b. Rest/Sleep
      1) Are you having any trouble getting enough rest or sleep since you came to the hospital?
                                                          Yes __X__   No _____
         If yes, describe __The noise in the halls and from other patients is disturbing and__
         __keeps me up, wakes me up in middle of night and early in morning. The medical__
         __and nursing procedures (temperature and pulse-taking) wake me.__

      2) Do you usually have trouble going to sleep?   Yes _____   No __X__
         Do you usually have trouble staying asleep?   Yes __X__   No _____
         If yes, describe __Ever since the beginning of cortisone treatment for the toxo-__
         __plasmosis, I have had occasional nightmares and have awakened in the middle of__
         __a sleep. Then it is very hard for me to get back to sleep.__

         What have you done in the past to help you get enough rest or sleep? __Cup of hot tea before__
         __going to bed, listening to the radio or reading a book; in really bad cases,__
         __taking a warm bath.__
         Was it effective?
            Always _____   Usually __X__   Sometimes _____   Never _____
      3) What would you like the nurse to do to help you get the rest and sleep you need while in the
         hospital? __Turn lights off and close door to room at night. Bring cup of hot tea.__
         __Avoid taking temperature early in morning. Leave window in room open for air.__
   c. Personal Hygiene
      1) Do you need help with your bath while in the hospital? __No, unless eyes will be patched__
         __after operation, in which case I will need to be taken to the bathroom.__
      2) Do you need help with brushing your teeth? __No, unless head movements will be re-__
         __strained after surgery. In that case, I will need help with brushing my teeth,__
         __or at least toothbrush, paste, and rinsing water brought to my bed.__
      __s__ your skin usually Dry __X__   Oily _____   Normal _____

4) What, if anything, do you use on your skin? Moisturizer on face morning and evening; body lotion on body after bath.

5) How often do you prefer to bathe? Daily

               Morning X   Afternoon _____   Evening _____

                                                          No Preference _____

6) Do you prefer a   Tub bath X   Shower _____

     This question is not pertinent _____

2. Safety

  a. Locomotion

    1) Do you have any difficulty in walking about? Yes X   No _____

       If yes, describe Have trouble judging distances, especially on stairs. Have to hold on to railings because of problems with depth perception.

    2) Did you have any difficulty in walking before you came to the hospital?

                                                        Yes X   No _____

       If yes, describe Since onset of toxoplasmosis in right eye, have had problems on stairs.

       How did you manage? Walk carefully, using railing; avoid carrying packages and children on stairs wherever possible.

    3) Has anyone said anything to you about staying in bed (or getting out of bed) since you came to the hospital? Yes X   No _____

       If yes, what? Some friends who have had surgery for detached retina have told me that I would have to lie still in bed for about a week with sandbags around my head to prevent it from moving.

       What do you think about staying in bed? (or getting out of bed?) I think I would go crazy if I had to lie in bed like that, and I hope that I can get out of bed right away. My doctor said nothing about staying in bed after surgery and I hope I don't have to.

    4) Do you expect to have any difficulty getting about after you leave the hospital?

                             Yes X   No _____   Don't know _____

       If yes, how do you expect to manage? By not trying to do as many things, by relying on friends and neighbors to help.

  b. Vision

    1) Do you have any difficulty in seeing? Yes X   No _____

       If yes, describe No peripheral vision in right eye, poor vision in left. Can't see anything at distance without glasses; have trouble seeing anything on right without turning head to side. Driving is difficult because of vision problems.

    2) Do you wear glasses? Yes X   No _____

       If #1 is yes, in what way does your limited sight handicap you? Not being able to drive too well; reading is difficult; close work is difficult.

       How do you manage? Have gotten used to limitations, to a certain extent.

  c. Hearing

    1) Do you have any difficulty in hearing? Yes X   No _____

       If yes, describe Poorer hearing in right ear

    2) If yes, do you wear a hearing aid? Yes X   No _____

II. Specific Basic Needs

1. Comfort, Rest, Sleep

   a. Pain/Discomfort

     1) Have you had any pain or discomfort since admission? Yes _____X_____   No _____

      If yes, describe _Severe headaches and nausea_____

     2) Did you have any pain or discomfort before coming to the hospital?

                                          Yes __X_____   No _____

      If yes, describe _Severe headaches, occasional nausea, dizziness, sharp shooting____
pains through right eye region; more than usual fatigue._____

      How long? _3 months_____

      What did you do to relieve the pain/discomfort? _Take aspirin or other similar pain-____
killer, take a nap, lie down._____

      Was the pain/discomfort relieved by treatment?

               Completely _____   Partially __X_____   Not at all _____

     3) If you have pain/discomfort while in the hospital what would you like the nurse to do to relieve it?
Give me pain-killer, cold compresses on forehead and eyes, turn down overhead
lights, turn off phone.

   b. Rest/Sleep

     1) Are you having any trouble getting enough rest or sleep since you came to the hospital?

                                          Yes __X_____   No _____

      If yes, describe _The noise in the halls and from other patients is disturbing and____
keeps me up, wakes me up in middle of night and early in morning. The medical
and nursing procedures (temperature and pulse-taking) wake me._____

     2) Do you usually have trouble going to sleep? Yes _____   No __X_____
Do you usually have trouble staying asleep? Yes __X_____   No _____

      If yes, describe _Ever since the beginning of cortisone treatment for the toxo-____
plasmosis, I have had occasional nightmares and have awakened in the middle of
a sleep. Then it is very hard for me to get back to sleep._____

      What have you done in the past to help you get enough rest or sleep? _Cup of hot tea before
going to bed, listening to the radio or reading a book; in really bad cases,
taking a warm bath.

      Was it effective?

           Always _____   Usually __X_____   Sometimes _____   Never _____

     3) What would you like the nurse to do to help you get the rest and sleep you need while in the
hospital? _Turn lights off and close door to room at night. Bring cup of hot tea.
Avoid taking temperature early in morning. Leave window in room open for air.

   c. Personal Hygiene

     1) Do you need help with your bath while in the hospital? _No, unless eyes will be patched____
after operation, in which case I will need to be taken to the bathroom.

     2) Do you need help with brushing your teeth? _No, unless head movements will be re-____
strained after surgery. In that case, I will need help with brushing my teeth,
or at least toothbrush, paste, and rinsing water brought to my bed._____

     3) Is your skin usually Dry __X_____   Oily _____   Normal _____

3) If #1 is yes, in what way does your limited hearing handicap you? Sometimes can't hear conversations too well. Have to ask people to repeat things often.

How do you manage? By sitting closer to people talking, by asking people to repeat themselves, by listening more carefully.

3. Fluids

1) Has the amount of fluid you usually drink been changed since you got sick?

Increased X   Decreased _____   Unchanged _____

2) What fluids do you like to drink?

Water X   Fruit juice X   Tea X

Milk X (skim)   Coffee _____   Soft drinks _____

Other Wine, ice cream sodas

3) What fluids do you dislike? Coffee, soft drinks, especially orange and grape sodas.

4. Nutrition

a. Teeth/Mouth

1) What is the condition of your teeth?

Good _____   Cavities X   Other _____

2) Do you wear dentures? No

Upper _____   Lower _____   Partial _____

3) Is eating limited by the condition of your teeth?   Yes _____   No X

If yes, describe _____

4) Do you have any soreness in your mouth?   Yes X   No _____

If yes, does it interfere with your eating?   Yes _____   No X

b. Do you consider yourself to be

Overweight X   How much 30–40 lbs.

Underweight _____   How much _____

About right _____

c. Appetite/Food Preference

1) Has being sick made any difference in your eating?   Yes X   No _____

If yes, describe Sometimes more hungry than usual; other times much less. Always very thirsty.

2) What foods do you eat mostly? Meat, vegetables, fruit, salads, cakes, ice cream.

3) Are there any foods you do not eat?   Yes X   No _____

If yes, which foods do you not eat and why? Eggs, because I don't like them. Chocolate, because it makes me sneeze.

d. Diet

1) Are you on a special diet?   Yes X   No _____

If yes, what kind? Low salt

2) Were you ever on a special diet before you came to the hospital?

Yes X   No _____

If yes, what kind? Low salt

Did you have any problems with your diet?   Yes X   No _____

If yes, describe Love to pour salt on food and can't stand the taste of food without salt. Have been using salt substitute.

3) Have you had any problems with your food since you came to the hospital?

Yes ___X___   No _____

If yes, describe ___No salt substitute is available and food tastes too bland.___

If yes, what do you think would correct the problem? ___Getting some salt substitute or___ ___adding other spices to food.___

4) Do you expect to be discharged on a special diet?

Yes _____   No ___X___   Don't know _____

If yes, how do you expect to manage? _____

5. Elimination

a. Bowels

1) Has being sick changed the way your bowels function in any way?

Yes ___X___   No _____

If yes, describe ___Urinate less often than I used to. Frequently constipated. Before,___ ___bowels moved every day regularly.___

2) Do you usually have   Constipation ___X___   Diarrhea _____   Neither _____

3) How often do you usually have a bowel movement? ___Now, once every 3-4 days___

4) What time of day do you normally have a bowel movement? ___no usual time___

5) Do you take a laxative   Regularly _____   or an enema?   Regularly _____

Frequently ___X___   Frequently _____

Occasionally _____   Occasionally _____

Never _____   Never ___X___

If yes, what kind? ___Senokot or something similar___

6) Do you do anything else to help you have a bowel movement?

Yes _____   No ___X___

If yes, describe _____

7) Do you expect to have any problem with your bowels after you leave the hospital?

Yes ___X___   No _____

If yes, how do you expect to manage? ___Will continue to take lots of laxatives.___

b. Bladder

1) Have you had any difficulty in passing your urine (water) since you came to the hospital?

Yes _____   No ___X___

If yes, describe _____

2) Did you have any difficulty with your urine before you came to the hospital?

Yes _____   No ___X___   Don't remember _____

If yes, describe _____

How did you manage? _____

3) If #1 is yes, what do you think would help you pass your urine (water) while in the hospital? _____

_____

4) Do you expect to have a problem with your urine after you leave the hospital?

Yes _____   No ___X___

If yes, how do you expect to manage? _____

6. Oxygen

1) Has being sick caused any change in your breathing? Yes ___X___   No _____

If yes, describe ___More frequent shortnesses of breath.___

2) Did you have any difficulty with your breathing before you came to the hospital?

Yes _____   No __X_____

If yes, describe _____

If yes, how did you manage? _____

3) If #1 is yes, what do you think would make it easier for you to breathe while you are in the hospital?
__Don't know_____

4) Do you expect to have any difficulty with your breathing after you leave the hospital?

Yes _____   No __X_____   Don't know _____

If yes, how do you expect to manage? _____

7. Sexuality (Ask according to marital status and appropriateness to the patient.)

1) (If Married) Has being sick made any difference in your being a
husband _____   wife _____   Yes __X_____
father _____   mother _____   No _____
If yes, describe __Less able to do things with and for husband and children. Feel inadequate for the situation.__

(If single and appropriate) Has being sick made any difference in your relationship with other people, particularly the opposite sex?   Yes _____   No _____
If yes, describe _____

2) (If appropriate) Has being sick caused any change in your sexual functioning (sex life)?

Yes __X_____   No _____

If yes, describe __Diminished sexual functioning because of more frequent fatigue. Increased fear of pregnancy and passing illness on to a child has put restraints on sex life.__

3) Do you expect your sexual functioning (sex life) to be changed in any way after you leave the hospital?   Yes _____   No _____   Don't know __X_____
If yes, describe _____

4) Do you expect your ability to function as a husband, wife, father, mother, or in a socal relationship to be changed in any way after you leave the hospital?

Yes _____   No _____   Don't know __X_____

If yes, describe _____

III. Other

1. Do you have any known allergies?   Yes __X_____   No _____
If yes, what kind? __Chocolate, pepper, sun (direct summer sun)__
How have you managed? __Try not to eat chocolate or pepper. Try to stay out of sun on beaches, etc.__

To what extent does the allergy handicap you? __In summer, can't go to beach as often as I would like.__

2. How far did you go in school? __Two years college__
Can you read and write? (Ask only if indicated)   Yes _____   No _____

3. Is there anything else you wish to tell me that would help us with your nursing care? __Have fears about losing vision and being less and less able to see; that it will affect hearing; that it will affect other parts of body. Am afraid of the side effects of medication.__

IV. Nurse's Impressions and Suggestions

1. In your judgment which word(s) best describe this patient?

Alert __X__	Disoriented _____	Passive _____
Angry _____	Distrustful _____	Questioning _____
Answers questions readily __X__	Embarrassed __X__	Quick to comprehend __X__
Answers questions reluctantly ____	Euphoric _____	Secure _____
Anxious __X__	Fearful __X__	Seeks support __X__
Confident _____	Homesick _____	Slow to comprehend _____
Confused _____	Hyperactive __X__	Talkative __X__
Cooperative __X__	Hypoactive _____	Trustful _____
Critical _____	Lethargic _____	Unable to comprehend _____
Demanding _____	Nonquestioning __X__	Withdrawn _____
Depressed __X__	Nontalkative _____	

2. Summary of findings that are significant for nursing care. __Patient is very afraid of the out-__
come and long-term results of operation; she needs information about what is most
likely to happen and how the condition is likely to affect her. Patient changed subject and avoided eye contact when nurse attempted to give her information about condition, particularly in those areas that frighten her. Otherwise, she is bright,
verbal, and understands what is said to her. Stutters occasionally when talking about
things that trouble her.

Nursing examination

Up to this point in the nursing assessment, much of the data about the patient will have come from verbal communication with the patient and others, reading of records, and observation of the patient's general appearance and reactions.

By now, the nurse will have developed a feeling for the patient's physical and emotional state. The next step in the assessment process is to examine the patient for physical signs that may help to better define the patient's condition and therefore help the nurse in planning the patient's care. Where and how does the nurse start the patient examination?

Systematic head-to-toe assessment

Rather than making scattered observations about the patient, the nurse should have an organized plan for carrying out a thorough examination. There will be less chance of overlooking signs that may not, at first appearance, be related to the patient's complaints, but may, in the final analysis, be significant.

A thorough examination is best accomplished in a systematic way, beginning at a logical starting point and progressing to a logical ending point. In humans, the logical progression would seem to be a head-to-toe order.

Each region should be exposed and examined separately, with all structures within the area being considered at one time. When examining the patient's neck, for example, the nurse should check the trachea, thyroid gland, pulses, and lymph nodes, rather than tracing all the pulses or lymph nodes in the body at one time. The latter approach would necessitate several changes in position and draping and would be less efficient. While examining each region, the nurse should consider the underlying anatomical structure and possible abnormalities that may be present.[14]

Since the body is normally symmetrical on left and right sides, the nurse should compare findings on one side with those on the other.

Moving from head to toe, the nurse should focus on the following factors during the examination: *The head, face, and neck* can easily be the most revealing areas, especially for the newborn.[15] They may provide equally important information in adult patients.

Scalp. Feel the scalp for any unusual scars, abrasions, bulges, swellings, or malformations. Check for skin tone of scalp. Is it dry and scaly? Are there signs of dandruff? Is it oily? Look for signs of ticks, ringworm, and other sources of inflammation or infection.

Hair. Check the hair for color, texture, distribution, and thickness or sparseness. Is the hair excessively dry or oily? Is the color of the hair consistent or are there signs of albinism or pigment variations? Is the hair dyed? In what condition is it kept? Is hair evenly distributed over the entire scalp or are there bald spots?

Head. Note the size and shape of the head. Is the head unusually large or small? Is it abnormally shaped? In infants, the nurse should record the circumference of the head at each visit, since the rate of growth at that age is significant. Check the proportions of different parts of the head with one another. Prominent foreheads or frontal bulges, for example, may be signs of rickets or syphilis. Note the way the patient holds his head and the amount of head control. If the head is always held at an angle, there may be hearing or vision difficulties or muscle problems. Movement of the head is also important. Test for the patient's ability to turn the head up and down and from side to side. Watch for jerking, tremors, and failure or difficulty in moving in some direction.

If the patient has indicated problems due to frequent headaches, have him locate and trace the usual progression of the headaches.

[14] Fowkes and Hunn, p. 29.
[15] Mary M. Alexander and Marie Scott Brown. 1974. Physical examination, part 6: The head, face, and neck. *Nursing '74* (January): 47.

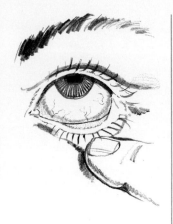

Face. Check whether the face is symmetrical, whether there are any signs of muscle weakness or paralysis. Watch the facial expressions when the patient laughs, furrows his brow, grimaces, and talks. Check color of skin for evidence of jaundice, pallor, cyanosis, or other abnormal infections, irritations, or unusual scars.

Eyes. Examination of the eye includes an evaluation of its function as well as its appearance. Visual acuity can be tested with a letter chart placed 20 feet from the patient. (Visual acuity is expressed as a fraction: the reading 20/40 vision indicates that the person is 20 feet from the chart and can read the lettering that a normal eye can perceive at 40 feet.) The examiner tests vision by covering each eye one at a time.

If the patient wears corrective lenses, the testing should be done with and without the lenses. Testing for refractive errors in vision, such as myopia, hyperopia, or astigmatism, is done with a pinhole test to determine the degree of diminished visual acuity.

The movements of the eyelids and eyeballs should be observed for muscle weakness or imbalance. Testing can be done by having the patient hold his head fixed and straight while following the movements of the examiner's fingers. Question the patient about blurring of vision or spots in front of his eyes.

The appearance of the eyes should be assessed for symmetry, shape, size, position, and general features. Look for inflammation, infection, discharge, or unusual appearance. Excessive tearing (lacrimation) may indicate infection or inflammation. Lack of tearing may indicate nerve injury or vitamin A deficiency.

The pupils should be checked for size. Pupils that are unequal in size or unusually dilated or constricted may indicate other conditions. The whites of the eyes should be checked for color, since such abnormalities as a yellowish tint may indicate jaundice or hepatitis. The eyeball should be checked for abrasions, hemorrhages, and swelling. For a more extensive eye examination, an ophthalmoscope is used.

Eyebrows and eyelashes should be checked for amount, distribution, condition, and position. Conditions such as hypothyroidism may result in loss of hair from the lateral portion of the eyebrows. The absence of eyelashes may be caused by congenital conditions or inflammatory disease.

Ears. Check the ears for appearance and hearing acuity. Appearance should include the position, shape, size, and symmetry of the ears. If the presence of wax (cerumen) obstructs the view of the ear canal, it may be removed simply with moist cotton, or the ear may have to be drained and irrigated. For a complete ear examination, an otoscope or ear speculum, which fits into the ear canal, is used. It can help the nurse detect abnormalities of the ear drum, such as perforations, bulging, or scars, or abnormalities in the canal, such as foreign bodies, discharge, swellings, or unusual color.

The patient's hearing acuity can be checked by seeing if he can follow conversation in normal tones and also in whispers. An individual with normal hearing can hear a whispered word from approximately 15 feet, a spoken word from 20 feet. The ear not being tested is covered during the procedure. If the patient wears a hearing aid, check on the degree of his hearing loss.

To test hearing balance—whether one ear hears sound louder than the other—a tuning fork may be used. Strike it on the heel of the hand and place it on the midline of the skull above the patient's forehead. The patient with normal hearing balance hears sound equally in both ears. The tuning fork can also be used to test for nerve deafness by placing it on the mastoids, right behind the ear. The examiner should record how much time elapses before the patient can no longer hear the tuning fork's sound.

Nose. The nose should be examined for appearance, shape, size, and symmetry of left and right sides. The nurse should also check the condition of the nasal passages, mucous membrane, and sinuses as well as for the presence of discharge, obstruction, colds, allergies, and trauma. The instrument most often used for nasal examination is an otoscope or a flashlight. The maxillary and frontal sinuses should be felt for tenderness since these may be affected by allergies or infection.

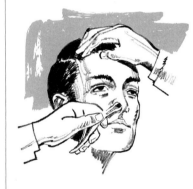

Mouth and throat. The patient's lips should be inspected for color, moisture content, lesions, fissures, or crusts. Examine the oral cavity itself by using a tongue depressor and flashlight. Observe the mucous membranes, gums, and teeth, taking care to note the presence of bleeding, soreness, cavities, or dentures. Problems such as swelling or bleeding gums may be caused by poor dental health or may be the first signs of a more serious hematologic problem. The tongue should be inspected for color, moisture content, markings, symmetry, coating, and mobility. Ulcers of the tongue may be indicative of syphilis, tuberculosis, or carcinoma.

Examine the palate for abnormalities. The palate, uvula, and tonsils can be checked by having the patient say "ah" and gently applying the tongue depressor to the middle of the tongue.

The amount of saliva in the mouth should be checked, since reduced or excessive saliva may indicate early manifestations of complicated illness.

The presence of hoarseness may indicate a mild inflammatory condition involving the vocal cords or a more severe situation, thus warranting a more extensive laryngeal examination.

Neck. The neck should be checked for presence of pain, stiffness, or limitation of movement, injury, thyroid enlargement, or lumps. Stiffness or tenderness of the neck may be related to benign local muscular problems or to more serious pathological conditions such as meningitis. The patient should be asked to swallow while the nurse looks for evidence of an enlarged thyroid gland (goiter)—a relatively common occurrence in areas having iron-deficient diets.

The strength of the major cervical muscles is tested by having the patient turn his chin against the examiner's hand and shrugging. The nurse should feel the neck for any enlargements in the nodes, a condition that may indicate an upper respiratory infection or more serious infectious neoplastic disorders. Other lymph nodes in the axilla should also be checked at this time for enlargement.

Chest and lung area. To examine the cardiopulmonary area, the patient should be questioned about the presence of chest pain, shortness of breath, palpitations, cyanosis, cough, night sweats, edema, murmur, and difficulty in breathing (dyspnea). The chest area should be examined for shape, symmetry, abnormal bulges, condition of skin, slope of the ribs, characteristics of the intercostal spaces, and position of the bones. This part of the examination can be carried out while the patient is in a sitting position.

Evaluate the characteristics of the respiratory movements, observing the rate and rhythm of respiration. Since the chest normally moves when air is inhaled and exhaled, the nurse should observe the chest movements while the patient takes deep breaths. The diaphragm should be checked for position and movement by having the patient take a deep breath and hold it while chest movement is observed.

Examination of the cardiovascular system at chest level primarily involves listening for abnormal sounds of the heartbeat. Listening at the chest is an important part of the chest examination. There are not only heartbeat sounds but breath sounds and voice sounds that "vibrate" within the chest cavity. An experienced ear will be able to distinguish sounds and detect minor irregularities that indicate problems. A stethoscope, frequently used for chest and back examinations, can pick up and amplify these sounds greatly.

Breasts. With the patient in a sitting position, check the nipples for discharge, crusting, or unusual pigmentation. The breasts should be observed for symmetry of size, skin color, and vascular patterns, and the presence of swelling, bulging, or masses noted. Then ask the patient to lie on her back and examine her in that position for masses or swellings. If a mass is found, the consistency, elasticity, location, size, tenderness, mobility, and attachments to adjoining tissues should be checked.

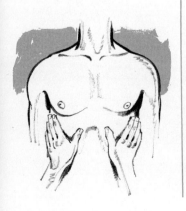

Abdomen. Since the abdominal symptoms may be caused by conditions outside of the abdomen, accurate assessment of any abdominal problem must include examination of the chest, heart, genitalia, and rectum.[16]

[16]Fowkes and Hunn, p. 76.

Generally, the examination is performed with the patient in a supine position with knees slightly flexed to enhance relaxation.

The nurse should evaluate the condition of the abdominal skin, noting the presence of scars and superficial dilated vessels. Normally, the abdomen will be symmetrical, and any signs of asymmetry suggest underlying organ enlargement. The nurse should feel for signs of enlargement, swelling, tenderness, abnormal pulsations, and peristaltic activity. This can be done by using both hands, with a "passive" hand placed against the abdominal wall and an "active" hand applying pressure to the passive, or "sensing," hand. This examination should take place with the patient breathing in and out normally.

Also included in this examination is location and palpation of the liver, kidney, and spleen. The inguinal lymph nodes should also be located and checked for inguinal or femoral hernias.

Genitals. The male genitals should be examined at the time the inguinal and femoral areas are examined, with the patient either lying down or standing. Examine for signs of discharge, tenderness, swelling, or inflammation. The scrotal sac should be examined for unusual masses.

The female genital organs should be examined while the patient is in the lithotomy position (knees bent, legs apart). Examine the external organs for infection, color, and type and amount of discharge. The internal organs should be examined manually for signs of cysts, obstructions, swelling, or tenderness. For the internal manual examination, the nurse should first lubricate the index and middle fingers of the hand to be inserted into the vagina, and then place the other hand on the abdominal wall, gently moving around to examine the reproductive organs. Size and location of uterus, ovaries, and tubes should be checked, and the position and consistency of the cervix evaluated. Usually, a smear of the vaginal canal will be taken for a Papanicolaou test.

Rectum. Examine the patient rectally for signs of thickened skin, inflammations, lesions, or rashes in the anal area. The sphincter muscle should be assessed for muscle tone and the anal canal for masses, tender areas, or swellings. Occasionally, complaints from the patient about bowel abnormalities will indicate the need for a more extensive examination by the physician.

Extremities and back. The extremities and the back are considered together because of their relationship to joint mobility.[17] In the extremities, the nurse is concerned with bone, joint, and muscle evaluation as well as arterial and venous circulation and lymph nodes.

The posture, gait, and movements of the patient should be noted.

[17] Ibid., p. 88.

Inspect the upper and lower extremities for size, shape, symmetry of musculature, temperature, and color of skin. The extremities should be examined for generalized swelling, localized bulges and swelling, the presence of varicose veins, and the appearance of the circulatory vessels in general.

The joints should be examined for swelling, tenderness, erythema, and temperature. Joints that are inflamed may be warm to the touch.

Range of motion should be checked by having the patient move arms and legs at the different joints in several directions. If the patient complains of hip or knee problems (common sites of injury), they should both be examined for interrelated problems.

The spine should be checked for contour, limitations on mobility, the occurrence of pain, and deformity and tenderness.

Neurological system. Much of the neurological examination is done during the routine check of other organs and systems. Initially, the nurse should evaluate the patient's mental status from data derived during the interview. The nursing history will provide information about the patient's feelings, behavior, and thoughts. The medical assessment will indicate the presence of mental illness in the family and the presence of organic brain disease. In addition, the patient's reactions will provide the nurse with information about his conscious thought processes.

Endocrine system. The patient should be questioned and examined about temperature intolerance, his history of growth and development, excessive thirst or hunger, hirsutism, and changes in secondary sex characteristics.

Observational skills

In conducting a thorough and accurate physical examination of the patient, the nurse will have to rely on the use of several tools. Some of these tools are the nurse's own senses—sight, touch, hearing, and smell. An enormous quantity of information can be gathered just by using these senses. However, these senses and the nurse's observational skills must be developed, since, just like with any fine tools, dexterity comes with practice. Without knowing exactly what to look, listen, touch, and smell for, it is easy to "look without seeing" and to "listen without hearing."

The observational skills of the nurse will be used simultaneously during the examination while the nurse is talking and reassuring the patient or performing such tasks as applying the sphygmomanometer. But for purposes of discussion, the observational skills will be considered separately below.[18]

[18]Yura and Walsh, Appendix B.

Observations made by seeing

By looking at the patient as a whole, the nurse is able to observe his general appearance and visible mood expression; age appropriateness; nutritional state (obese, lean); and visible emotions (anxious, eager, alert, tearful, depressed).

1. Visible physical factors
   a. Head and neck area: macrocephalic, microcephalic, normocephalic, tumors, swelling, infections, paralysis, scars.
   b. Hair: amount, distribution, color, length, and condition.
   c. Eyes: shape, size, symmetry, size of pupils, color, swelling of lids, muscular reactions like blinking or twitching, use of eyeglasses or contact lenses.
   d. Nose: shape, size, symmetry, position of septum, shape of nostrils, type of discharge (bloody, thick, thin).
   e. Ears: size, shape, deformities, drainage, swellings, presence and amount of wax.
   f. Lips, mouth, and teeth: position of tongue, coating on tongue, condition and color of teeth and gums; full dentition, primary or secondary, number of fillings, presence of dentures; color and condition of gums, swellings, inflammations, presence of food; presence of harelip or cleft palate and type of repair, if any; facial expressions and presence of paralysis.
   g. Skin: color, contour, integrity, hygiene, texture, secretions, distribution of pigment; presence of chafing, sunburn, peeling, rashes (type, size, and color); scars, swellings, tumors.
   h. Posture: position, presence of supports such as braces, cane, crutches; gait (rigid, shuffling, foot dragging); sitting position, standing position; unusual movements (convulsing, writhing, palsy, shaking chills, stiffness).
   i. Extremities: absence of any portion or all of an extremity (fingers, toes, part of arm); artificial limbs; size, shape, and symmetry of limbs; presence of unusual folds or shape (such as mongoloid palm); movement of limbs; wringing hands, tapping feet, tremors, twitching, clenching; color (occupational dyes, nicotine tan); physiological discoloration from gangrene; condition of finger- and toenails, presence of hangnails, cracks, chips, bandages, dirt, blood; amount of muscle development and control.
   j. Trunk area: shape and size; barrel chest, protruding ribs, absence of ribs; symmetry; tumors, burns, scars, abrasions, distortions; in female, size, shape, and condition of breasts, discharge or lesions on nipples; degree of breast development in males and children; shape of abdomen, scars, swellings; presence of incisions, punctures, hernias; gross abnormalities in back.

k. Pelvic and genital area: congenital anomalies, discharge, tumors, swellings, signs of menstruation, stool, urine and its color and consistency; color, size, and shape of genital organs.

Other factors about the patient that can be visibly observed concern outward physical appearance. What type of clothing is the patient wearing—work or casual apparel? Is it appropriate to the climate? In what condition is it, and has it been appropriately buttoned, fastened, and put on? What attachments and prostheses does the patient have, such as jewelry, eyeglasses, hearing aid, dentures, artificial limbs? Is the patient attached to any therapeutic supports such as catheters, intravenous tubes, dialysis monitor leads? The external environment of the patient will also provide visual clues about his possessions. It will give the nurse clues about unusual or noteworthy habits, about hobbies, about necessities for the patient. Observations of people with the patient will provide information about significant others.

Observations made by hearing (including auscultation)

General characteristics of the patient can be noted by listening to the way the patient talks, breathes, and moves. The patient's environment will provide auditory clues about the way the patient lives. Specifically, some of the auditory clues to listen for may be

1. Patient's physical factors
   a. Voice and speech: quality, tone, and degree of loudness. Is speech calm, excited, demanding, loud, soft, inaudible, stammering, strained, hoarse, tongue-tied, singing, grunting? Is the patient's voice screeching, gasping, muffled, complaining, or hysterical? Does the patient have a dialect, speak in jargon, a foreign language? Auditory clues about *what* the patient is saying provide information about the patient's needs, problems, hopes, fears, concerns, and attitudes.
   b. Breathing: abnormal sounds such as wheezing, whistling, blowing, diversions through tracheostomy, gasping, burping, hiccuping, panting, or rales; rate of breathing and whether it is shallow or deep.
   c. Heart sounds: listen for regular heart sounds and for abnormal or irregular beats, murmurs, or absence of sound.
   d. Abdomen: listen for presence of peristalsis, hyperactive or hypoactive peristalsis, and gurgling or flatus.
2. Patient's environment
   a. Immediate environment: listen for sounds of music, for sounds from radio, television, phonograph, for mechanical sounds of creaking, banging, squeaking doors, elevators, utensils.
   b. Neighborhood: clues about the patient's physical environment come

General characteristics of the patient can be noted by listening to the way the patient talks, breathes, and moves.

partially from neighborhood noises. Is traffic heavy or light? Are there noisy and bothersome sirens, horns, animals, external music, crying, screaming, or construction noises?

Observations made by touching (palpation and percussion)

Touch, which is used extensively during the physical examination of the patient—as opposed to hearing and seeing, which can be used extensively during the interview phase as well—will help provide many clues about the patient's condition. In fact, **palpation** and **percussion** are ways of feeling and touching the patient to test for normalities and abnormalities. Touching may mean gently resting the hand on the patient, or it may mean probing with the fingers, lightly hammering or vibrating the skin, or pushing against internal organs to test for tenderness or swellings. By touching, the nurse can evaluate general factors about the patient: texture, temperature, and secretions of the skin and sensitivity to touch. Specifically some of the factors that can be examined by touch are

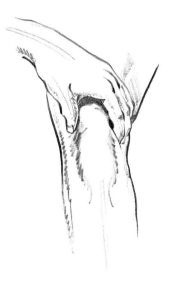

1. Patient's physical features
   a. Hair: texture—dry, coarse, soft
   b. Skin: texture and temperature; abnormalities such as lumps, warts, moles, tumors; pulsations, whether weak, strong, regular, intermittent; sensitivity to pressure
   c. Chest: shape and size of rib cage; presence of masses and determination of their pressure sensitivity; condition of breasts—lumps, engorgement, size; type of pulse; presence of enlarged nodes
   d. Abdomen: degree of hardness or softness; presence of tumors, distention, painful reaction to pressure; degree of uterine contractions or peristaltic action
   e. Skin secretions: degree of moistness and temperature; location on the body where secretions are taking place
   f. Muscle tension: degree of muscle relaxation; presence of throbbing, chills, twitching, spasm
2. Patient's immediate environment
   a. Bedding: condition of bedding, whether dry, moist, hard, or soft
   b. Prostheses: appropriateness and comfort of fit
   c. Temperature and humidity of immediate environment

Observations made by smelling

The nurse's sense of smell can supply information about usual or unusual odors that the patient may give off because of food, drugs, or products ingested or because of a particular infection or illness that produces an odor. Body secretions that should be checked for abnormalities of smell include general body perspiration and perspiration specific to the feet, axilla, and genitals. Mouth odors may indicate tobacco, alcohol, mustiness, sweetness, or use of chemicals such as commercial mouthwashes or those less easily recognizable. Odors of body discharges such as feces, urine, and vomitus should be noted, as well as those emanating from wounds, infections, or dead tissue.

Vital signs and special tools

Often the nurse augments basic observational skills with special tools and equipment such as a **thermometer, stethoscope,** and **sphygmomanometer.** These are used for checking the patient's **vital signs**—bodily functions that are basic indicators of a person's health condition. These vital signs are the **pulse rate, respiration, temperature, blood pressure,** and sometimes the **apical beat.** It is essential that the nurse measure and record vital signs during a nursing examination. Vital signs should be taken periodically to evaluate any change in the patient's condition.

While the techniques for measuring vital signs will gradually become routine, it is helpful to understand the significance of the vital signs, the tools and procedures used in their measurement, and common technical errors that occur in the measurement and interpretation of the vital signs.

Since a person's vital signs are influenced by many factors—both internal and external—the nurse should give consideration to these factors when taking vital sign readings. For example, a person "at rest" will generally have much lower readings than a person performing or having recently completed some form of activity. The more strenuous the activity, the more an increase is likely in readings.

Some medications, such as digitalis, will alter the values of the blood pressure, apical beat, and other signs. The nurse should know the effects that prescribed medication and treatments have on vital signs.

Outside influences, including temperature and humidity of the room, will influence the patient's body temperature and cardiac rate. Noise, distraction, and anxiety- or fear-provoking incidents will often raise the blood pressure.

In order to interpret the readings of the vital signs accurately and effectively, these factors must be considered and related to the levels that are considered "normal" for the person being examined. "Normal" for the patient is a relative reading, since the patient's normal readings in a satisfactory state of health may be higher or lower than readings considered typical for the patient's age, sex, body type, and condition.

Before the nurse takes the patient's vital signs, she should make him comfortable and, if possible, relaxed. Often the nurse can use this period to converse with the patient in order to obtain information for the nursing history and to convey reassurance and concern for the patient.

Temperature. Since a person's temperature is often a barometer of his state of health, even small variations from one recording to the next can indicate serious physical changes.

Temperature can be measured centrally and superficially. Superficial temperatures are indicated by feeling the skin, usually the forehead, or a particular problematic spot on the body. A localized area may be particularly hot or cold, or particularly dry or moist.

Central temperature is measured orally, rectally, or in the axillary region. The rectal thermometer, which is least subject to extraneous influences, is the most accurate.

Temperatures are graded on a thermometer in Fahrenheit or centigrade measure. Before the temperature is taken, the position of the liquid in the column should be shaken down to below the usual body temperature. In Fahrenheit measurement, it is usually 98.6°; in centigrade, 37°. To convert Fahrenheit to centigrade, subtract 32 from the Fahrenheit reading and then multiply by $\frac{5}{9}$. The formula is simple: $C = \frac{5}{9} (F - 32)$.

The principle behind the thermometer is that heat causes liquids such as mercury, which is often used, to expand, and since the mercury is confined to a narrow column in the thermometer, it expands by moving upward.

There are several factors that will affect a patient's temperature and that may alter the reading by several degrees without indicating a fever. External factors, such as room temperature, humidity, and clothing, may affect a person's temperature. This is also true—for oral readings—of recently ingested food that is hot or cold (thus, temperatures are usually taken prior to mealtimes). Because of cyclic variations, body temperature is usually lowest in the early morning and highest in the evening. Thus, if a single daily reading is taken, it should be taken at the same time every day, usually in the late afternoon or early evening when it is at its highest point.

Another factor affecting temperature reading is the method used. Rectal temperatures average 0.7°F higher than oral temperatures, and axillary temperatures average 1°F below the oral temperature. Thus, it is important to indicate on the patient's record which type of measurement was taken.

Women's temperatures during the latter half of their menstrual cycle are usually one-half a degree higher. Infants' temperatures are generally higher than those of adults.

Readings will also be affected by the amount of time the thermometer is left in place. Generally 2 minutes is considered minimum for oral readings; 3 minutes for rectal. However, studies show that some patients require at least 5 minutes for an accurate reading. Such problems of inaccuracy are considerably diminished with the use of electronic thermometers, which register the patient's temperature in a few seconds, and with infrared fever thermometers, which give an instant reading without even touching the patient. Eventually, more and more nurses will have access to these types of thermometers, but for the moment, because of their cost and, in some cases, experimental status, their accessibility is somewhat limited.

Respiration. How often and how a patient breathes should be observed, preferably while the patient is unaware that he is under observation, because a person can exercise a certain amount of voluntary control over respiration rate and rhythm. By careful listening, certain normal and abnormal patterns can be detected. While occasional sighing respiration (a periodic deep breath) is normal, irregular patterns with dyspnea or hyperpnea may indicate such problems as congestive heart failure. Normal respiratory sounds are soft rustling noises that are most typically heard with a stethoscope over the back of the chest. They may be inaudible unless the patient breathes deeply through his open mouth. Abnormal sounds, such as wheezes, groans, whistles, or bubbles, are usually the result of accumulated secretions in air spaces and passages.

Since examination of the respiratory process by auscultation can yield a great deal of information about a patient and can help to establish a baseline from which to determine improvement or deterioration, it is a procedure that nurses should perform even on patients without known or obvious respiratory problems.

More and more frequent use is being made of the stethoscope for respiratory auscultation since it is useful for detecting respiratory congestion and irregularities, and it magnifies sounds that can be heard less clearly by the unaided ear.

The stethoscope consists of two earpieces connected to flexible tubing that is approximately $\frac{1}{4}$ inch in diameter and 10 to 15 inches long. The tubing is connected to the head, which is the portion applied to the patient. The head consists of a diaphragm or bell, and some stethoscopes have a combination head with both variations. The diaphragm is a flat, circular disc that tends to screen out low-frequency noises, making it easy to hear high-frequency sounds such as pulmonary breath sounds or heart murmurs. The bell corresponds, for all practical purposes, to the old-fashioned trumpet-type hearing aid,[19] and is used for low-pitched sounds such as gallop rhythms or rumbling murmurs.

Generally, nurses use the closed diaphragm type or the combination piece. Both can pick up most heart and lung sounds, provided that the earpiece fits snugly and correctly. Ill-fitting earpieces can make the best stethoscope unsatisfactory since they will allow outside noises to interfere.

To use the stethoscope for chest auscultation, the nurse should place the warmed head of the stethoscope directly on the skin over the area to be examined.

[19]David Littmann. 1972. Stethoscopes and auscultation. *American Journal of Nursing* 72:1239.

Care must be taken to differentiate between sounds caused by friction between the instrument and the skin or body hair and those sounds actually related to respiration.

The stethoscope is also used for auscultation of heart sounds, including the apical pulse, and, in most cases, for taking blood pressure readings.

Pulse. The pulse may be taken at several sites (for example, the temple, neck, thigh, or foot), but the most common site is the wrist, where it is called the radial pulse. It is taken by placing the pads of the second, third, and fourth fingers on the area of the patient's wrist just below the thumb. If the rhythm feels regular, the number of beats in a 30-second period should be recorded. For irregular rhythms, a reading of a minute is preferable. Some factors that cause the pulse rate to increase are anger, fear, and fever; the rate is decreased by pain, faintness, and reduced cardiac output. Normal pulse rates in adults at rest are 60 to 100 impulses per minute, while in children the rate is generally more rapid.

The pulse rhythm should be noted for irregularities and later followed up by taking an apical pulse rate by placing a stethoscope over the apex of the patient's heart and counting the heart rate by auscultation.

Variations in the volume, contour, and quality of the pulse are of clinical importance for their potential cardiovascular implications.

The stethoscope is used for auscultation of heart sounds, including apical pulse.

[Photo by Sandor Acs]

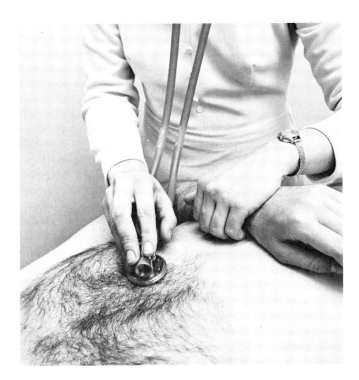

Blood pressure. Blood pressure is actually an indirect measurement of the variation in the pulsatile pressure within the arterial system.[20] Blood pressure is measured with an instrument called the sphygmomanometer. The sphygmomanometer is actually a rubber bladder that can be wrapped around an extremity (usually the upper arm) and into which air can be pumped manually. This bladder is connected by means of rubber tubing to a pressure recording device that usually measures pressure in the cuff in millimeters of mercury (mm Hg). The bulb is attached to the bladder by rubber tubing and is equipped with a valve that allows air to be directed into or out of the cuff. This allows the operator to vary pressure gradually in the cuff upward or downward. After the cuff has been snugly wrapped around the patient's extremity, the bladder is gradually filled until a pressure in excess of expected **arterial pressure** (usually 200 mm Hg) is registered. The air is then gradually released from the bladder through the escape valve.

This change in pressure on the artery affects the normally smooth and noiseless blood flow and causes it to become turbulent and noisy **(Korotkoff's sounds).** The beginning of flow after the pressure has been applied, and the point at which the Korotkoff's sounds are first noted, represents the **systolic pressure.** The end of the turbulent flow is recorded at the disappearance of the sounds and represents **diastolic pressure.**

Normal blood pressure varies in different individuals, with the usual range being from 140/99 mm as the upper normal limit and 90/50 or 90/60 mm as the lower safe limit. As aging occurs and the compliance and elasticity of the larger vessels decrease, systolic pressure generally increases.

Sounds are heard by placing the head of a diaphragm-type stethoscope over the nearest superficial artery just distal to the cuff, unless one of the newer models of electronic sphygmomanometer is being used to measure pressure. These instruments have a microphone built into the cuff, thus eliminating the need for a stethoscope.

They also help to eliminate, or at least diminish, some of the errors that commonly occur in blood pressure recording—reading mistakes due to the examiner's hearing acuity, misinterpretation of sounds, and problems with visual and auditory correlation.

Most cuffs are available in different sizes for use with adults or children and for different extremities. An appropriate size should be used since errors in determination may occur if the cuff is too small or too large.

Apical beat. The apical beat, evaluated through use of a stethoscope, measures rhythm, rate, and quality of the heartbeat. The nurse places the stethoscope on the patient's skin over the **cardiac apex.**

[20]Fowkes and Hunn, p. 34.

The normal rate is 60 to 100 beats per minute, though it is usually more rapid in children. The rhythm is usually a double tone that sounds like the syllables "lup-dup."

Collecting and testing specimens

Additional information about the patient may be obtained through samples of body fluids such as urine, blood, sputum, vomitus, and wound drainage. Some of these specimens, such as urine or sputum, can be collected directly by the nurse, to be analyzed by laboratory personnel or by using chemical kits or tapes. The value of specimens for diagnostic clues depends not only on accurate analysis in the laboratory but also on the use of proper collecting techniques. Appreciation of the importance of collecting techniques is enhanced by the nurse's understanding of the significance of certain specimens.

Urine. Urine, which can be collected in a clean or sterile container while the patient is voiding, can yield information about blood sugars, hormones, protein levels, disease-causing bacteria, and many others. Changes in a patient's condition are often rapidly detected by urinalysis. There are several standard tests that may be conducted on a urine specimen:

1. *The pH level.* The **pH level** of the urine indicates the balance between **acidity** and **alkalinity.** A reading under 7.0 indicates acidity; a reading over 7.0 indicates alkalinity. The normal range of pH readings for urine is 4.5–8.0, with an average reading of approximately 6.0. Various pH indicators may be used, including **litmus paper.** The indicator is dipped in the urine, and the resulting color is compared with a chart.
2. *Specific gravity.* The **specific gravity** is an indicator of the kidney's ability to concentrate and dilute urine. To test the specific gravity, the patient's fluid intake should be restricted for approximately 12 hours, after which three urine specimens are collected at hourly intervals. If the kidneys are functioning normally, the specific gravity of the urine should increase with each specimen.
3. *Sugar.* The level of sugar **(glucose)** in the urine is an important indicator of the presence of **diabetes mellitus.** As in the case of pH level, commercial indicators are available that may be dipped into the urine and the resulting color compared with a chart.
4. *Acetone.* Like the level of glucose, the **acetone** level of urine is another indicator of the presence of diabetes mellitus. Since individuals with uncontrolled diabetes mellitus are unable to metabolize sugar, the fatty acid and ketone bodies in the blood are also elevated and spill over into the urine. The procedure for testing the acetone level is the same as that for sugar and pH, with commercial indicators and accompanying charts readily available.

Stool. Stool, which can be collected while the patient is defecating or transferred from a bedpan to a specimen container, can yield information about disease-causing bacteria or parasites that invade the bowel. Where there are gastrointestinal problems, feces are often the source of many clues to diagnosis.

Blood. Blood can be tested in several forms—whole, serum, or plasma. The value of blood analysis is important for typing, so that, in the event of transfusions, the patient receives compatible blood. Additionally, the blood carries signs of bacteria and other disease-causing organisms that generally can be isolated in the blood earlier than in fecal or urine specimens.

During the actual collection of the specimen, which may be through a finger prick or from a vein in the antecubital portion of the arm, the area must be thoroughly washed with soap and water, dried with a sterile towel, and cleaned with surgical spirit or iodine. The blood specimen should be exposed to air as little as possible, in order to leave the test specimens as uncontaminated as possible. There are special collection vessels designated for the purpose that will, if properly used, help ensure this.

In order for the above specimens, and any others such as vomitus, sputum, or secretions from wound drainage, to be viable for laboratory examinations, they should be sent for analysis as soon as possible after they have been collected. The risk of decomposition increases with time, and such decomposition tends to diminish the accuracy and value of the lab findings. The actual time of collection of a sample should always be noted on the label to facilitate interpretation of the result.[21] Sometimes dietary control is required prior to collection, or fasting specimens are required. As well as the normal variations due to age and sex, there is a **diurnal variation** in the concentration of some specimens. The serum iron level in blood, for example, will be higher in the morning than in the afternoon.[22]

Yet another observational tool which the nurse can use to assess the patient is the recording of intake and output, both of solids and liquids. The patient who is ill usually takes in decreased amounts of food and water, and may be vomiting or experiencing diarrhea and/or excessive moisture loss through sweating or increased urination. Such disturbances to the usual intake and output of fluids can cause serious shifts in fluid and electrolyte balance and should be watched carefully. If these shifts are allowed to continue uncontrolled, there is danger of heart failure or other serious effects. (The maintenance of fluid and electrolyte balance will be discussed

[21]John Hatcher. 1972. It begins at the bedside. *Nursing Mirror* 134:35.
[22]Ibid.

Time Interval		11-7	7-3	3-11	11-7	7-3	3-11	11-7	7-3	3-11	11-7	7-3	3-11
INTAKE	Oral		200 cc	500 cc	100 cc	700 cc	500 cc	100 cc	800 cc	500 cc			
	Other	800 cc	850 cc	150 cc									
	Total	800 cc	1050 cc	650 cc	100 cc	700 cc	500 cc	100 cc	800 cc	500 cc			
OUTPUT	Urine	150 cc	1200 cc	1000 cc	200 cc	1100 cc	800 cc	200 cc	500 cc	400 cc			
	Suction	50 cc											
	Other												
	Total	200 cc	1200 cc	1000 cc	200 cc	1100 cc	800 cc	200 cc	500 cc	400 cc			

in chapter 22.) Excessive retention of fluid, on the other hand, will cause such conditions as puffiness of the face, edema of the extremities, or pulmonary edema.

A typical intake and output sheet is illustrated in this chapter. If the patient is able, he should be taught how to keep the record himself.

FIG. 5-2 *Sample intake-output record.*

What is a nursing diagnosis?

Armed with information about the patient's unique characteristics, the nurse must now put all this knowledge together and use it productively in developing the nursing care plan. Florence Nightingale in her *Notes on Nursing* expressed the real significance of nursing observations when she wrote:

In dwelling upon the vital importance of sound observation, it must not be lost sight of what observation is for. It is not for the sake of piling up miscellaneous information or curious facts, but for the sake of saving life and increasing health and comfort.[23]

The process of evaluating observable data about a patient and finding a pattern in the data that will determine the nursing care plan is called **nursing diagnosis.** For many years, diagnosis was regarded exclusively as an activity of the physician. Now it has achieved a broader meaning and is seen as an appropriate activity for the nurse as well.

[23]Nancy Myers. 1973. Nursing diagnosis. *Nursing Times* 69:1129.

A nurse has some responsibilities dependent on and others that are codependent with other members of the health care team. Determining nursing care based on the patient's needs is a function of the nurse alone. It is important, therefore, that the nurse develop diagnostic skills and an understanding of the purpose of the nursing diagnosis in order to successfully devise a nursing care plan appropriate to the patient's actual needs.

The diagnostic process is not unique to any one profession. Nurses, physicians, social workers, and teachers are all responsible for gathering facts and using them as the basis for defining the client or patient's situation and needs. Recently, several states have given specific legal recognition to the diagnostic responsibility of nurses. In the state of Washington, the law serves the purpose of legitimizing what nurses have been doing for a long time, but now, "Playing with words is gone; if a nurse says that it's measles, then it's measles. The nurse no longer has to say it's a nursing judgment or evaluation," said a Washington state public health officer in relation to the law.[24]

While both the recognition and acceptance of a nurse as a diagnostician are gradually becoming more widespread, there is still misunderstanding about the definition of a nursing diagnosis and how it differs from a **medical diagnosis.**

Actually, there are similarities. Both types of diagnoses begin with a gathering of facts. The facts may be a blood pressure reading of 120/80, the presence of a blood clot, the tendency to stutter, or the fact that a father of four has lost his job. In all diagnostic processes, at some point during or after the fact-gathering, the practitioner will look for and recognize a pattern, and then state a conclusion.

Differences in diagnoses arise from each practitioner's view of his responsibilities and from the knowledge necessary for the practice of each profession.[25] The nursing diagnosis may be the same as the medical diagnosis, for example, in emergency situations, when the nurse's therapeutic actions will be the same as the physician's.[26] An initial diagnosis for cardiac arrest may be both a medical and nursing diagnosis calling for immediate respiratory and cardiac resuscitation. Following emergency treatment, the two diagnoses will change, however, so that the medical one will become "ventricular fibrillation" or "myocardial infarction," and the nursing diagnosis may become "ineffective cardiac output" or "fear of pain."

The process of nursing diagnosis, like the medical diagnosis, begins as soon as the patient comes under care. But the nursing diagnosis changes as the nurse learns, for example, that a patient's fear and anxiety about

---

[24]Where R.N.s can diagnose and prescribe. *RN* 36 (August 1973): 31.

[25]Mary Durand and Rosemary Prince. 1966. Nursing diagnosis: Process and decision. *Nursing Forum* 5:51.

[26]Ibid., pp. 56–57.

a surgical procedure have become fear and anxiety about the possibility of cancer.

While the medical diagnosis is usually stated in terms of disease or physiological condition, the nursing diagnosis may take several different forms, depending on the circumstances. The diagnosis may be descriptive, such as "communicates exclusively through gestures," or it may be etiological, such as "lessened intestinal peristalsis" or "inadequate understanding of hospital environment because of problems in understanding English."[27] As more and more information is obtained about the patient, the diagnosis tends to become more etiological, indicative of the causes of the patient's condition. This type of diagnosis tends to identify more pertinent nursing care.

Some nursing diagnoses may be similar for patients with totally different medical diagnoses because of the nature of nursing diagnosis in general. In two patients with vastly different medical diagnoses, similar psychological and social problems of adjustment may exist, and similar nursing actions may be appropriate.

Identifying needs and problems

Once the facts have been collected, it is necessary to pull them together and examine what they reveal. Identification of the patient's basic **needs** and **problems** is the forerunner of identifying the patient's nursing requirements. The nurse may use a variety of theoretic guides about basic human needs to help identify them. While categories of needs are general in nature, the nurse should assess individual and particular aspects of each. Basic human need refers to those needs that all people must satisfy to enhance their images of themselves as persons. One model of human needs commonly encountered in nursing has been proposed by Maslow.[28]

In Maslow's "hierarchy of needs," five basic categories of needs are identified and discussed.[29] They are

1. Physiological: the need for food, oxygen, physical activity, rest, elimination, water, and sexual satisfaction. All are present at birth, except the need for sexual satisfaction, which differs because it is active only intermittently and can be satisfied by substitute measures.
2. Safety and security: the need for sameness, sureness, familiarity, and trustworthiness in people, things, places, and events.
3. Love or belonging: the need for affection, warmth, kindness, and consideration in human relationships.

[27] Ibid., p. 56.
[28] Abraham H. Maslow. 1970. *Motivation and personality*, 2d ed., pp. 35–46. New York: Harper & Row.
[29] Yura and Walsh, pp. 73–76.

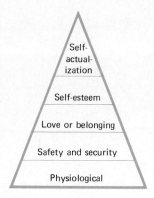

FIG. 5-3 *Maslow's hierarchy of needs.*

4. Self-esteem: the need for respect, status, prestige, and a good reputation. A sense of accomplishment carries with it feelings of adequacy, competency, and mastery.
5. Self-actualization: the need and ability to control oneself, one's destiny, and one's needs, rather than to be controlled by them.

In times of stress or illness, problems may arise in meeting all or some of these needs. Illness does not mean that these needs do not have to be satisfied; in fact, it may be even more important for the individual that they are fulfilled, and the demands for fulfilling them may be even greater than usual.

While the physiological needs must be met before others in life-threatening situations, under normal life-sustaining situations all needs should be considered. To focus on only one or several of the needs, to the exclusion of others, may be destructive, because what affects any one aspect of any individual inevitably affects all other aspects. Thus, the nurse, in developing the nursing plan, must avoid developing a limited perspective about the patient's problems.

It is true, however, that all needs do not carry the same weight at the same time. During illness, some needs may take on a greater importance for the patient than others. A starving person will concentrate on physical needs, rather than intellectual, social, and economic pursuits, until his hunger drive is satisfied. So, too, the ill person may be totally absorbed by depression and low self-esteem. Attention to physical needs for improved health status can be achieved only when the nursing care plan tries to help the person develop a more positive self-image.

Need vs. problem

"Need" and "problem" are terms that are often used interchangeably. In the diagnostic process, it is important to differentiate between those things that a patient needs and those things that are causing a patient problems. A need may be defined as that which the individual must have in order to survive or function within the limits that society considers normal.[30] These include the essentials of Maslow's first category (physiological) and the needs of his other categories, which allow a person to function effectively on an emotional plane.

Simply stated, a problem is a barrier to a goal, an obstruction of some kind that prevents a need from being met. The patient's responses to his problems—his symptoms—may be emotional or physical, verbal or nonverbal. In nursing situations, a problem is a condition that the nurse can

[30]Thora Kron. 1971. *The management of patient care: Putting leadership skills to work,* p. 11. Philadelphia: Saunders.

help alleviate by meeting the underlying need or helping the patient meet his own need.

The patient's problems may be obvious and discernible (overt) or not directly recognizable (covert). Sometimes a patient will make many minor requests—for a glass of water, a readjustment of his bedding. These requests may tend to obscure his real problems—feelings of insecurity, a desire for attention, etc. The nurse must develop the ability to analyze the patient's behavior in order to determine the cause of his actions.

Sometimes the patient and the nurse do not see the same problems or identify the same conditions in the same ways. Patients may consider a condition or situation a problem, but the nurse might dismiss or overlook it as irrelevant or trivial.

However, the nurse, as a helping and supportive person, can be effective only by trying to understand the patient within his own frame of reference. That which is real and meaningful to the patient must be of concern to the nurse, and nursing care must be structured around that which is of concern to the patient.

The patient should never be made to feel that the nurse or other health care personnel are disapproving or in any way judging his feelings and expressed needs. Such attitudes are inhibiting to the patient and counter-productive to supportive care. What counts in the development of a nursing plan for the patient are the needs that the patient perceives *as well as* the needs that the nurse perceives. Whether the need is recognized by both patient and nurse, or by just one or the other, the nursing care plan must take into consideration these different perceptions.

Identifying the patient's own resources

Many patients have sufficient internal and external supports and resources to meet some of their own needs. In assessing the patient, the nurse should identify the patient's strengths and assets as well as his limitations and liabilities to meet his own needs or solve his own problems. Once they have been identified, the nurse should help the patient to mobilize these resources in his own behalf, by organizing and utilizing them in the most effective manner possible.

The patient's resources should be assessed in the following spheres: (1) physical, (2) emotional, (3) intellectual, (4) spiritual, (5) social, and (6) economic.

Whatever his medical diagnosis, it is important to consider the patient within his environment in order to identify areas where nursing influence or intervention may prevent problems or improve the situation. *Physical functioning* of the patient should be considered in terms of his basic health status, as well as what he can and cannot do for himself. If he has limited mobility, and therefore is unable to perform some of the essential activities of daily living to which he was formerly accustomed, adjustments will have

That which is real and meaningful to the patient must be of concern to the nurse. . . .

to be made in the nursing care plan. The patient who will be unable to prepare his meals, for example, may be referred to a social welfare agency that provides meals for the homebound. Tasks of personal care, such as bathing and dressing, may be hindered if the patient is incapacitated. Responses to such situations may involve bringing in support personnel or teaching the patient to make his own adjustments.

The *emotional* status of the patient will greatly affect his ability to deal with his needs and problems. The nurse should assess the patient's emotional status by viewing such feelings as the patient's general mood; whether the patient's feelings of dependence or independence are likely to be constructive or destructive to his treatment; what his motivation and morale are and how variable they may be from day to day. The nurse will pattern behavior and care around the patient's emotional status and ability to deal with his own illness. Some indicators of impairment in the patient's mental health, which could dramatically affect his ability to meet his needs, are forgetfulness and inability to follow a train of thought. Also important are inappropriate behavior, inability to orient himself, paranoia, apathy, depression, low frustration tolerance, and demonstrations of faulty judgment.

The *intellectual* capacity of the patient will determine to a large degree the patient's ability to meet his needs. Can the patient actually understand the medical and nursing recommendations? Can he understand directions about medication? About personal self-care? Does he have the intellectual capacity to make choices and judgments that are appropriate to his needs and problems? (The nurse should not confuse intellectual ability with amount of formal education or even with literacy since these characteristics are not necessarily synonymous.)

Spiritual, social, and economic resources are determining influences in the patient's capacity to adapt successfully. The nurse should assess spiritual needs and resources on an individual basis, rather than dealing with the patient strictly on a denominational or ritualistic level. Otherwise she may make the wrong assumptions because of her generalizations.

The social environment of the hospital, or the community or home in which the patient lives, may exert positive or negative forces on his coping abilities. An evaluation of any of these factors that may have contributed to or aggravated the illness will be important to the nurse in establishing nursing priorities.

The patient's economic resources may be so strained by illness that the patient's perception of his condition, his rehabilitation, and his treatment may be largely altered. The patient's prognosis may affect his earning capacity, may disqualify him for a job he formerly held, or may make employment prospects unclear. It is of concern to the nurse that the means and opportunity be provided to enable the patient to reach a fulfilling level of economic independence. If this is not possible, provisions should at least be made to make necessities available to the patient.

Stating the diagnosis

Once the pattern of a patient's problem has been recognized, the actual statement of the diagnosis must be made. The actual diagnosis is a statement of conclusion. It should be precise, concise, and highly personalized to apply to the individual patient.

A diagnosis that meets all these requirements and that would be of help in developing the nursing care plan would, for example, state: "Limited ability to communicate by vocal sounds or writing; anxiety because of limited ability to communicate." This diagnosis was derived from information about a patient who had a temporary tracheotomy, who had difficulty covering the opening of the tracheotomy tube with his finger in order to speak, who used gestures extensively in communicating, and who made little effort to communicate with the nurse or other health care personnel.

An unsatisfactory diagnostic statement about the same patient might, on the other hand, simply state "Poor reaction to tracheotomy."

Using common terminology

In stating diagnoses that can be helpful and useful to all nursing care personnel, and not just to the particular nurse who is diagnosing the patient, terms that are readily understandable and identifiable must be used. "Limited ability to communicate by vocal sounds or writing" is specific enough to indicate the nature of the patient's problem to anyone reading the diagnosis. However, all too often, vague terminology is used that can be interpreted in many different ways by different people.

Although an acceptable standard list of terminology for nursing diagnosis has not yet come into use, many nurses are promoting the idea of developing such a classification. In medicine, such a standardized classification system does exist in the *International Classification of Diseases,* and its existence and use have greatly facilitated communication between physicians and other health care practitioners. When, for instance, the word "appendectomy" is used, there is no question as to what it means.

As a first step in developing a nursing classification system, a group recently met for the First National Conference on the Classification of Nursing Diagnoses to begin laying the groundwork for such a system.

The prerequisites for developing such a classification would be to identify all those factors that nurses locate or diagnose in patients—that is, the patient problems or concerns most frequently identified by nurses and most amenable to nursing intervention. These would then have to be given standard names so that nurses could quickly identify a concept or activity by a common name.

Although a standard system of classification is still a nursing tool of the future, present methods of nursing can still become much more efficient and workable by using precise, concise terms in defining diagnoses.

SUMMARY

Assessing the patient is perhaps the most vital and critical step in the nursing process. Investigating the facts and interpreting those facts is what nursing assessment, simply stated, is all about. The process is anything but simple, however, for it demands a wealth of knowledge and common sense from the nurse, as well as an ability to weigh and evaluate many factors.

Assessment is not only invaluable as a method of finding out more about the patient, his needs, his problems, and his fears, but is also a way of establishing interaction between patient and nurse. During the assessment process, the patient should be encouraged to voice his feelings, to ask questions, and to express attitudes. The nurse, in turn, should take advantage of the opportunity to convey interest, concern, and respect for the patient.

The intelligent and creative use of the assessment process is one of the most effective ways by which the nurse can personalize care for the patient. The aim of personalized and individualized care, which is central to the whole focus of the nursing process, can be effected during the diverse phases of the assessment process. The process of obtaining information from patient, family, and others involves interviews, examinations, and observation. All these methods offer the nurse opportunities to obtain a multidimensional picture of the patient as a social, emotional, and physical being with a unique life-style and personality. The nursing history, because it does not focus solely on the patient's symptoms and the physical manifestations of his conditions, deals with the patient as a total person.

Here lies the very core of the assessment process, for its purpose is to see the patient as a complex combination of needs, concerns, and problems related to the medical diagnosis but sometimes treatable in quite a different manner. The nursing diagnosis, which is derived from an evaluation of all the data obtained about the patient, then serves as the basis for a nursing care plan aimed at helping the patient deal with the social, emotional, and physical implications of his medical diagnosis.

STUDY QUESTIONS

1. Briefly define the role of assessment in the nursing process.
2. What are the major sources of data used in the assessment process?
3. What is a nursing history? What are the four basic content areas covered by a nursing history?
4. Briefly list the steps used in a systematic physical examination.
5. Name and define the vital signs. How are they measured?
6. What is a nursing diagnosis? How does it differ from a medical diagnosis?
7. Refer to the nursing history on pp. 82–88. Based on the information given there, formulate an appropriate nursing diagnosis for this patient.

SELECTED BIBLIOGRAPHY

Durand, Mary, and Prince, Rosemary. 1966. Nursing diagnosis: Process and decision. *Nursing Forum* 5:50–64.

Chambers, Wilda. 1962. Nursing diagnosis. *American Journal of Nursing* 62.

Fowkes, William C., Jr., and Hunn, Virginia K. 1973. *Clinical assessment for the nurse practitioner.* St. Louis: Mosby.

Harrison, Cherie. 1966. Deliberative nursing process versus automatic nurse action. *Nursing Clinics of North America* 1:387–97.

Little, Dolores E., and Carnevali, Doris L. 1969. The nursing history. In *Nursing care planning,* pp. 66–97. Philadelphia: Lippincott.

McCain, R. Faye. 1965. Nursing by assessment—not intuition. *American Journal of Nursing* 65.

McPhetridge, L. Mae. 1968. Nursing history: One means to personalize care. *American Journal of Nursing* 68:68–75.

Maslow, Abraham H. 1970. A theory of human motivation. In *Motivation and personality,* 2d ed., pp. 35–58. New York: Harper & Row.

Medical Programs Incorporated. 1970. Patient assessment: Taking a patient's history (programmed instruction). *American Journal of Nursing* 74:293–324.

Yura, Helen, and Walsh, Mary B. 1973. *The nursing process: Assessing, planning, implementing, evaluating,* 2d ed. New York: Appleton-Century-Crofts.

6 Planning, implementation, and evaluation

Upon completing this chapter, the reader should be able to:

1. Define the three phases required for patient care, following patient assessment: planning, implementation, evaluation, and possibly modification.

2. Discuss the need for the joint efforts of the patient, the nurse, the patient's family, and the health care team in the phases of planning, implementation, evaluation, and modification (if needed) for successful patient care.

3. Describe the process of assessment, planning, implementation, evaluation, and modification as continuous and ongoing until the patient is discharged from the nurse's care.

Relevant information about the patient has been gathered. An assessment of the patient's problems (or lack of them) has been made, and his needs have been identified. Now, it would seem, the nurse can at last get down to the job of meeting those needs.

But how will they be met and who will meet them? Which needs will be met first? When and where will they be met? What evidence will be used to determine whether the patient is making progress?

Planning

Obviously, there is a big step between *knowing* the patient's needs and *meeting* them. That step is the **planning** step, an integral and important phase of the nursing process. The written **nursing care plan,** which is developed during this stage of the nursing process, is a guide or blueprint for the care of the patient. It is based on the nurse's assessment of the patient's problems and is aimed at resolving or reducing those problems.

If every patient with a given problem were to be treated in exactly the same way, the nurse would simply have to be familiar with a "standard formula" for the treatment of that problem. However, as every nurse comes to realize, each patient is different and unique. The nursing process is used to provide care that is appropriate for each individual. Thus, "standard nursing plans" are (hopefully) seldom used.

Consider, for example, two patients facing hysterectomies. They may undergo similar medical and surgical procedures. But if one is a 20-year-old, recently married woman without children and the other is a 59-year-old, postmenopausal woman, their nursing needs are bound to be vastly different. The hysterectomy will have a different meaning and effect for each. It therefore follows that if their care is to be therapeutic, it must also differ.

114

In addition to providing for individualized care, planning also helps the nurse to:

1. Set goals or objectives for patient care
2. Assign priority to the problems diagnosed
3. Determine who can best deal with the patient's problems
4. Designate specific actions and the immediate, intermediate, and long-term goals for these actions[1]

Setting goals for patient care

Planning nursing care does not simply mean designing a time schedule of isolated activities. A scheme whereby temperature and pulse are taken at 7 A.M., breakfast served at 8 A.M., bath given at 9 A.M., and treatment begun at 10 A.M. would guarantee that necessary nursing procedures are performed. But the long-range purpose of all these activities would be unclear. In order to make treatment more meaningful for both patient and nurse, it is important that the goal of all these procedures be clearly defined. The nursing care goal is the sum total of what all nursing actions are directed at accomplishing. It is the reason that these actions are performed. It is also, and perhaps more importantly, the aim toward which the patient himself will be striving.

In the case of a healthy person, the goal or objective is to remain healthy. For a stroke patient, a goal may be to minimize muscle atrophy or increase mobility. Even terminally ill patients may aim toward goals of increased independence, regularity of function, or enjoyment of a favorite activity.

Working with the patient. Nursing care may be either *for* the patient or *with* the patient. Planning what is best for the patient, based on knowledge of his condition, scientific considerations, and a desire to help is a task that some nurses try to undertake alone. While it is well-intentioned, it is not always the best or most effective way to help the patient. Because the road to attaining planned goals is often long and difficult, it is essential that the patient and nurse plan the goals jointly. When both are motivated by the same goals, both will be willing to invest the time, effort, and energy necessary to attain them. Energy used in this way is far more productive than energy expended in frustration or anxiety because of misunderstood goals.

Including the patient in planning for his care serves several purposes. It allows the patient to learn beforehand what types of care are to take place, thus preventing him from being taken unawares. It also helps the

[1] Helen Yura and Mary B. Walsh. 1973. *The nursing process: Assessing, planning, implementing, evaluating,* 2d ed., p. 93. New York: Appleton-Century-Crofts.

patient better understand the whys and wherefores of planned nursing action. He will know the reasons for instituting and continuing certain therapeutic measures. The patient who is involved in planning his own low-sodium diet is more likely to follow it than the person who is merely presented with a written list of recommended foods and portions. The patient who is involved in planning has a better opportunity to make individual and family arrangements in accordance with the nursing care plan. It also gives him a chance to inform and teach the nursing staff about special measures he must observe and methods of care that have been used in the past. Finally, he can let the staff know what his reactions are to a proposed plan of action.[2]

In order for patient and nurse to work together toward goals, they must be realistic. Perhaps serviceable ambulation is the ultimate goal for a patient with a stroke. But the thought of the long struggle involved may depress him in his present state of helplessness. He may be able to work purposefully toward a goal that is more realistic: for example, to lift the heel of the affected extremity one inch off the mattress, the first step in relearning ambulation. (See below for a discussion of short-term and long-range goals.)

Working with other members of the health care team. The cooperation not only of the patient but also of other members of the health care team is necessary in establishing workable goals. While some objectives might be met primarily through the efforts of the physician or other health team members, they rarely exclude all involvement by the nursing team. Similarly, some objectives that are primarily of a nursing nature may require supporting activities by other health team members. For instance, keeping the patient's skin intact is mostly a nursing objective. This goal cannot be accomplished, however, without the assistance and cooperation of the physician, the nutritionist, and other specialists.[3]

Short-term and long-range objectives

Some goals defined by the patient and nurse will be reached fairly rapidly. Others will require a long time and many intermediate steps. To avoid frustration and give the goals a further focus, they should be defined in terms of the time span needed for their accomplishment.

Long-range goals give perspective to the nursing care plan, while short-term goals give direction to individual patient contacts. When these goals are meaningfully stated, each nursing action will be planned and

[2]Laurel Archer Copp. 1972. Improved patient care through evaluation, part 3: Your plan of nursing care. *Bedside Nurse* 5:28.

[3]Berniece M. Wagner. 1969. Care plans: Right, reasonable, and reachable. *American Journal of Nursing* 69:983.

purposeful. The results can be easily evaluated and the orders changed if necessary.

A long-range goal, such as "takes competent care of her baby," will involve many short-term objectives. These may include "is relaxed when feeding baby," "knows how to give baby a bath," and "keeps baby's skin free of diaper rash." The short-term objectives might be determined weekly or even daily, depending on the circumstances. As each short-term goal is accomplished, it contributes toward the realization of the long-range objectives.

Wording objectives or goals

Talking about defining goals is easier than doing it.[4] Wording objectives clearly and concisely, so that everyone involved will understand the goals that the patient and nurse have set, provides clear direction for nursing action. It also provides a means of determining whether the objectives were attained. Stated objectives should therefore be concrete, specific, and unambiguous. They should clearly communicate their intent to health team members, the patient, and his family.[5]

Because the focus of the goals is the patient, objectives should be worded in terms of observable patient behavior rather than nursing action. The goal is something the patient is moving toward; nursing actions only help it happen. For instance, "provide arm mobility exercises" for a mastectomy patient is not a goal. It is a nursing action designed to achieve the goal, "patient raises shoulder to a 45-degree angle," or, "patient brushes hair."

Another pitfall in wording nursing objectives is to state too few objectives and to state them too generally. Many objectives are so general as to be meaningless. "Achieves optimal recovery" is certainly desirable but it is not measurable or specific. A more meaningful goal would be, "Can sit up for five minutes without change in pulse rate." Being specific also makes it easier for other health team members to use their time more efficiently because they will know exactly what the desired goals are.

Establishing priorities

Nurses cannot know or expect to meet all of a patient's needs at the same time. Nor do all needs require prompt attention. For example, the more life-threatening a situation is, the faster it requires attention and resolution. Some objectives are unattainable until progress has been made toward prior goals. Some objectives require help from other health team

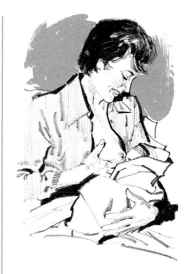

A long-range goal, such as "takes competent care of her baby," will involve many short-term objectives.

---

[4]Ibid., p. 989.
[5]Dorothy M. Smith. 1971. Writing objectives as a nursing practice skill. *American Journal of Nursing* 71:319.

members. Other needs and problems only come to the surface later in treatment and obviously can only be dealt with when they appear.

The nurse must decide the order in which problems are to be dealt with. By assigning low, medium, and high priorities to problems and goals, the nurse is less likely to waste time and energy.

How does the nurse assign priorities? An important element in assigning priorities is the nurse's understanding of the patient's needs. As was discussed in chapter 5, human needs may be broken down into five basic categories. They are listed below in the order in which they must be satisfied:

1. Physiological
2. Safety and security
3. Love or belonging
4. Self-esteem
5. Self-actualization[6]

Using this hierarchy of human needs, one can consider a patient with acute pulmonary edema who has trouble breathing and is anxious. The first priority would be for the patient to be able to breathe (a physiological need). Only after this need has been met would it be possible to reduce his anxiety (a safety need). If the patient is afraid that he will be unable to return to work, his need for safety will take precedence over his need for self-esteem. The short-term objective should reflect this priority even though increased self-confidence might be the long-range goal.

Just as the patient and nurse work together in formulating goals, they also work together to establish priorities. The patient is often able to express what is really most important for him. In some cases, the nurse may be concerned about a problem that the patient has not yet recognized. Eventually, however, nurse and patient will have to agree on which problem will be given prime consideration.

As high-priority problems are resolved fully or in part, the order in which remaining problems are to be resolved may have to be reevaluated. In the course of treatment, new problems may arise that have to be integrated into the nursing plan.

Identifying possible alternatives

To travel from point A to point B, one can go by foot, bicycle, car, train, bus, etc. Any number of alternatives are possible, though some are

---

[6]Abraham H. Maslow. 1970. *Motivation and personality*, 2d ed., pp. 35–43. New York: Harper & Row.

obviously more suitable than others at any given time. So, too, it is with nursing actions.

Identifying as many alternatives as possible, based on data collected about the patient, serves very definite purposes. Should the action selected prove ineffective, other options immediately become available because they have already been identified. A list of alternative actions also prevents rote or reflex nursing care whereby a patient's problem is always treated with the same nursing action.

Alternatives are based on the knowledge, experience, and resources available to the health care team. *Knowledge* of the patient's expectations and of cultural, social, and psychological influences on his responses will help to determine which actions are appropriate. If a patient is very self-sufficient, does the nursing action provide for as much patient participation and self-help as he is capable of giving?

Previous *experience* helps to answer other questions, such as: How predictable are the desired outcomes of a particular action? Will it be possible to identify results that are the direct outcomes of a specific action? Are there many variables in the situation that cannot be controlled? Is the action compatible with actions required to give other kinds of nursing care? (That is, will preventive measures, such as turning the patient and having him exercise in bed, negate other measures instituted to conserve the patient's strength?)[7]

Finally, the methods proposed will be affected by the *resources* available to the team and to the patient. These resources may be technical, financial, or human, but their availability must be realistically measured. For example, a mechanical aid for lifting a patient out of bed (Hoyer lift) may be very desirable, but is one available? Is a change of room assignment financially possible? Is there enough staff for someone to stop in to see the patient every 15 minutes?

Not only does the nurse consider personal and outside resources but those of the patient and family as well. The patient may have considerable health information. The family may know a great deal about the disease condition of the patient. A child may have developed considerable muscle coordination.[8]

Selecting the best alternative

Once all reasonable possibilities have been proposed, the nurse should select the approach that seems to have the best chance of succeeding. The alternative selected should be the most realistic for the particular time and place in which the nurse and patient find themselves. It is usually helpful

[7]Grace K. Eckelberry. 1971. *Administration of comprehensive nursing care: The nature of professional practice*, p. 82. New York: Appleton-Century-Crofts.
[8]Ibid., p. 83.

There is rarely an occasion when any one action is the absolutely right answer.

to consider the causes of the problem at hand when choosing the best alternative. For example, the problem "inadequate milk intake" may have come about because the patient does not like the taste of milk. But it also may be due to his being unable to afford its price. The action that appears to have the best chance for success will depend on the underlying causes of the problem.

There is rarely an occasion when any one action is the absolutely right answer. A nurse can only select the one that *seems* best. An element of trial and error will always remain. In dealing with human beings, there are all kinds of unknowns operating in any given situation. The ability to select the best of several alternatives comes gradually as more and more knowledge and experience are acquired. This ability is enhanced by having accurate data with which to work and by systematically considering the available options.

Prescribing nursing activity (writing nursing orders)

How to help the patient move from where he is to where he is going (his goal) must be clearly understood. Everyone involved in his care must know not only the goal but also how the patient can best get there. This understanding is the purpose of written nursing orders. (This topic will be discussed more fully in chapter 7.)

To be truly useful, nursing orders must have several characteristics:

1. *They must be clear and specific.* It is not enough to prescribe "frequent exercise." To one person that may mean three or four times a day; to another, once an hour.
2. *They should be written in words that have the same meaning for everyone.* If there is any doubt on this point, terms should be defined.
3. *They should be realizable and adaptable to the particular life situation, beliefs, and expectations of the patient.*

Formulating and writing the nursing orders and making sure they are carried out are generally the responsibilities of the professional nurse. But the professional nurse alone does not usually provide *all* the care a patient receives. Nonprofessional health team members round out and supplement information about the patient. They should be encouraged to contribute ideas for possible nursing approaches. They are also an excellent source of information that the professional nurse can use in determining whether or not the plan is effective.

The patient should have a voice in the type of nursing activity he prefers or dislikes. Perhaps he finds relief in a morning backrub or prefers to take a nap just prior to visiting hours. Such requests should be worked into the nursing orders whenever possible.

Implementation

Using the nursing care plan as the blueprint and having the immediate, intermediate, and long-range goals clearly in focus, recommended actions are put into practice. This carrying out of planned actions is the **implementation** phase of the nursing process.

There are many nursing actions that may take place during the implementation phase. These include inserting, withdrawing, turning, cleansing, rubbing, massaging, irrigating, manipulating, teaching, exercising, offering, awakening, cuddling, holding, drying, applying, communicating, and administering. Also involved may be influencing, altering, relieving, supporting, cooling, warming, providing, accompanying, sitting with, listening, walking, moving, touching, soothing, pulling, pushing, straightening, and flexing—to mention just a few.[9] These actions are used to resolve, dissolve, and diminish the patient's problems.[10]

Implementation is obviously more than a blind carrying out of orders in the nursing care plan. Providing a patient with help in reaching goals challenges the imagination, creativity, and observational powers of the nurse. Often the nurse must look beyond the straightforward requirements of the nursing orders and decide what, when, how much, or in what manner the implementation action is to be carried out.

For example, specific nursing action planned to relieve pain should follow a careful assessment of physiological manifestations of the pain. Its location, quality, and character must be considered. Also important is an understanding of what the pain being experienced means to the patient. Factors such as sociocultural background, age, sex, religion, and body part involved may also influence the patient's reaction to pain and his resulting behavior. Psychological factors, too, influence the patient's feeling of pain, particularly if the patient hopes to gain attention by complaining or has had past experience with pain.[11] Thus, nursing action to relieve pain may not always take the form of medication. It may involve changing the patient's position or simply paying him an added bit of attention.

To make decisions and judgments about how to implement care does not necessarily involve spending a lot of time with each patient. The time spent with each patient may vary significantly, but each interaction should be goal-directed and purposeful. A few minutes spent observing, listening, and talking with the patient while he is being bathed can help far more than a prolonged bath and massage with no other communication or interaction.

Personalizing implementation action with conversation, encouragement, and attentiveness should not be limited only to fully aware patients.

9 Yura and Walsh, p. 117.
10 Ibid.
11 Ibid., pp. 116–17.

Providing a patient with help in reaching goals challenges the imagination, creativity, and observational powers of the nurse.

It is also important for those who cannot respond in the usual or expected manner. Talking to an infant, an unconscious patient, or a patient with cognitive disturbances will help to maintain **sensory integrity.** Many patients who are gravely ill do, in fact, have reduced awareness and reasoning ability because their illness absorbs so much of their attention and energy. The nurse can use the implementation period to stimulate them verbally.

Nursing action with Mrs. M., who suffered from nephrotic syndrome, shows how a problem situation can be alleviated.[12] Mrs. M. would not look at or talk to anyone entering her room. Part of the nursing intervention was designed to increase Mrs. M.'s verbalization. This was intended not only to help her interact more with her environment but also to reduce the anxiety that contributed to her cognitive disturbances. The nurse used a persistent, structured, and optimistic approach, conveying the belief that Mrs. M. could and would speak or act. The nurse spoke slowly and deliberately, often repeating questions, while giving the patient plenty of time to respond. The questions required more than a one-word answer, and the nurse pursued any response the patient made. Initially, the nurse questioned Mrs. M. about her activities and condition. Then the nurse got Mrs. M. some books that were of interest to her. Eventually, Mrs. M. and the nurse began discussing the books, chatting about other things, and focusing less on Mrs. M.'s discomforts and anxieties.

Working with other members of the health care team

Implementation may be carried out directly and independently by the nurse. Often, however, the patient's needs are such that other members of the health care team must also become involved in the therapy. Physicians, social workers, dieticians, and teachers—all with a focus and orientation somewhat different from the nurse's—will deal with aspects of the patient's problem not within nursing's realm.

Usually, the implementation actions of other members of the health care team overlap with nursing actions. Both the nurse and the social worker, for example, are prepared to give supportive care. Both are concerned with the inter- and intrapersonal needs of the patient and his family. Both use their ability to work with the patient.

Effective cooperation among members of the health care team during the implementation phase depends upon the following factors:

1. *All members of the team must know and understand the goals of treatment.* To ensure this, the goals must be written clearly and precisely into the nursing care plan. In this way, all members of the team will be able

[12]Noreen Meinhart and Mary Jo Aspinall. 1969. Nursing intervention in hypovigilance. *American Journal of Nursing* 69:996.

to structure their own plans and actions around the intended treatment goals.

2. *The activities of all members of the team must be coordinated.* In order to do so, the concept of **vertical planning** should be implemented.[13] Vertical planning aims at timing actions to coordinate with the patient's biological rhythms and to complement other actions. For example, treatment should not be scheduled to begin just as the patient is about to eat or just as a visitor enters the room of a lonely patient.

3. *Information must be freely and frequently shared among members of the health care team.* Only in this way will everyone understand the goals of treatment and work together to ensure continuity and consistency of care. For a patient who needs to learn how to adjust to diabetes mellitus, for example, a nurse may begin a series of learning experiences intended to increase his independence. If the nurse fails to communicate her implementation of these actions to the other members of the team, there may be a lack of support on their part, or even a breakdown in the treatment. If the teaching plan is not clearly laid out, the patient may be forced to listen to different members of the team give the same lesson several times over, perhaps with variations. This may very well lead to irritation, confusion, or both. It is also possible that one nurse may assume responsibility for carrying out all the diabetic routines herself, negating the original plans for increased patient independence.[14]

4. *All efforts should be made to ensure that the patient and his family understand the plan of action that is being carried out.* For example, the nurse should call in social workers and other professionals only after considering the way the patient and family view these resources. Do they associate the social worker with financial inadequacy? Perhaps they feel the use of social services implies the existence of poor family relations.

Evaluation

The real test of a good nursing plan comes in the **evaluation** stage. On paper and in the initial planning phase, the plan may have looked tailor-made for the patient. In the implementation of the plans, everything may have seemed to go smoothly.

But there are several questions that must be asked: Is the patient moving toward his goals—and at the expected rate? If he is, is it because of the nursing action or in spite of it? Does the nursing action appear to be ineffective, or not as effective as anticipated, in helping the patient?

No one would purposely continue bailing out a water-filled canoe with

[13] Yura and Walsh, p. 116.
[14] Dolores E. Little and Doris L. Carnevali. 1969. *Nursing care planning*, p. 6. Philadelphia: Lippincott.

a bucket that had a big hole in it. It would be just as senseless to continue a nursing action that was not working as well as planned. The worst that a damaged bucket could do to the bailing-out process is make more and longer work for those emptying the canoe of water. But an ineffective, inefficient, or improper nursing action can be far more damaging. It can frustrate both patient and nurse. It can delay the implementation of a more effective nursing action and the achievement of the patient's goals. It can jeopardize a good cooperative working relationship between patient and nurse. An ineffective nursing action can also jeopardize or work against a therapeutic action being used by another member of the health care team. And worse yet, it can jeopardize or delay the patient's psychological or emotional recovery.

The evaluation phase of the nursing process is used to avoid such consequences. The purpose of evaluation is to determine whether the patient has reached the goals previously established jointly by nurse and patient. It will also pinpoint errors in the assessment, planning, and implementation stages. The giving of medication may have helped the patient achieve the desired goal of sleeping through the night without waking in pain. But if the patient still complains about restless and uncomfortable nights, a new goal should be established. This would be to eliminate nighttime restlessness, perhaps by relieving the patient's anxiety about his illness.

The outcome of the evaluation is essentially a report card on how the patient is doing. It may reveal several things:

1. The patient has responded as expected.
2. Short-term goals have been reached, but intermediate and long-range goals have not been achieved.
3. None of the stated goals have been achieved.
4. New problems have arisen.

The answer to how well the patient is doing may not be clear from just inspecting or asking the patient. By using appropriate criteria for making the evaluation, the process becomes more logical for nurse and patient, and the answers will be more accurate.

Criteria for evaluation

It is essential that all expected outcomes be evaluated in terms of the goals originally established. Just as these goals should always be formulated in terms of the patient, judgment about how these goals are being met should originate with the patient. Appropriate criteria for evaluation involve how the patient feels, how he thinks he is doing, and what behavior he demonstrates.

Appropriate criteria will be determined by the specific patient or group

The purpose of evaluation is to determine whether the patient has reached the goals previously established jointly by nurse and patient.

of patients in a particular setting. For neurological patients, criteria for evaluation may include control of infection, skin irritations, muscle integrity, and bladder and bowel functions. Other criteria, related to the goals of conservation of energy, may include maintenance of respiratory function, weight, fluid and electolyte balance, and sleep patterns.[15]

Criteria for a patient evaluation in a prenatal clinic, on the other hand, may focus on maintenance or control of other factors. These include a protein-rich diet, water retention, and the mother's ability to care for the newborn. Many basic formats for criteria and evaluation have been developed that are appropriate for specific nursing care situations.

All workable formats have certain characteristics in common. The criteria they use are observable, quantifiable, and useful.[16] "Observable" means that the criteria are stated in terms that enable the nurse to determine unequivocally whether or not they have been met. "Quantifiable" means that the degree of goal achievement can be measured. "Useful" means that the presence or absence of the criteria can lead to some type of corrective action. (See Fig. 6-1, which is an example of a general, systematic format for evaluation.)

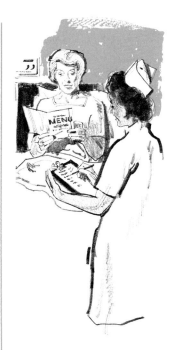

Working with the patient

The patient's responses to treatment are the most important factor in the evaluation process. His responses may or may not be clear, however, depending on his ability to verbalize, reason, and focus on the evaluation. The nurse is thus challenged to pick up clues from the patient. These may come from what the patient says or does not say or how the patient acts or does not act. Also important are what he can or cannot do and what clinical symptoms present themselves.

Verbal clues. When the patient is able to communicate verbally, he can give direct answers to such questions as: "Is your pain relieved?" "Do you breathe easily?" "How would you plan a low-sodium diet, and what foods would you include?" The answers to these questions help the nurse determine whether the following goals have been met: relief from pain, ease in breathing, ability to understand and plan appropriate diet.

The patient may also verbalize his degree of satisfaction with the nursing care being given him. He may feel he is not receiving enough attention. Perhaps too many different health care personnel are asking him the same questions and repeating the same directions. Verbalization of his annoyance, frustration, and anxiety can help the nurse determine the appropriateness or inappropriateness of health care personnel assignments. She can then adjust responsibilities and time schedules accordingly.

When the patient is able to communicate verbally, he can give direct answers to such questions as: "How would you plan a low-sodium diet, and what foods would you include?"

[15] Joyce Waterman Taylor. 1974. Measuring the outcomes of nursing care. *Nursing Clinics of North America* 9:345.
[16] Ibid.

FIG. 6-1 *A sample evaluation form.*

[From Dorothy Smith, A clinical nursing tool. *American Journal of Nursing* 68 (1968):2385. © 1968 by the American Journal of Nursing Company. Reproduced by permission of the American Journal of Nursing Company.]

1. Vital statistics:
   a. Name
   b. Hospital number
   c. Number of Shands Teaching Hosp. admissions
   d. Age
   e. Sex
   f. Race
   g. Marital status
   h. City of residence
   i. Medical diagnosis

2. Appearance on first sight.

3. Patient's understanding of illness and events leading up to the illness.

4. Some indications of the patient's expectations.

5. Brief social and cultural history including work, education, significant persons in patient's life.

6. Significant data in terms of:
   a. Rest and sleep patterns
   b. Elimination patterns
   c. Breathing
   d. Eating
   e. Skin integrity
   f. Activity and recreation preferences
   g. Interpersonal and communicative patterns
   h. Temperament
   i. Dependency and independency patterns
   j. Senses

7. What is important to this patient? What will tend to help him feel secure, comfortable, protected, safe, cared for?

8. What are the nursing goals for this patient?

9. What are the factors which inhibit the achievement of these goals?

10. What are the factors which enhance the achievement of these goals?

11. What methods (nursing orders) will be most likely to achieve the goals?

12. Evaluation of goals and methods in terms of each item through the use of progress notes.

13. Modification of goals and methods in light of the patient's progress.

14. Discharge summary.

Getting the patient to verbalize his feelings is not always easy. Some patients may be reluctant to admit dissatisfaction. Others, who are chronic complainers, may find it difficult to pinpoint verbally specific positive aspects of their situation. The methods and implications of effective nurse-patient communication will be discussed in more detail in chapter 10.

Nonverbal clues. Nonverbal clues are especially important in cases where the patient has sensory deprivation and cognitive problems. They are obviously the only means by which the reactions of infants, comatose patients, and others unable to communicate verbally can be judged. But they are also an important source of information even in the case of a patient who is able to talk. Recognition of these clues involves looking, listening, and otherwise observing patient behavior. Of prime importance are clinical measurements and patient reactions to external stimuli.

Clinical measurements offer fairly obvious clues about the patient's condition and are easily measurable against a baseline. For example, comparisons of original and present readings in temperature, pulse rate, blood pressure, urinalysis, blood sugar, and cholesterol may indicate change and degree of change. Other clinical measurements may include number of days in the hospital, duration of fever, postoperative treatment, and types and doses of narcotics, analgesics, and sedatives.

Reactions to external stimuli are often a mirror of the patient's mental and physical condition. Is the patient lethargic, unresponsive, irritable, or negative? Is the patient cheerful, responsive, enthusiastic, or smiling?

Some other measures for nonverbal clues that have been used in validation experiments[17] include degree of physical independence, mobility, skin condition, and patient reaction to nursing care he has been given. Patient activities are another source of measurement. These include time spent in bed, in a chair, walking, interacting with others, and in occupied leisure.

In order to be useful in validation, the criteria chosen must be sensitive to changes in the patient's condition. They must also take into account differences among individual patients. Once the characteristics of a particular individual are familiar to the nurse making the evaluation, changes in condition and behavior can be estimated and even predicted. However, such evaluative judgments run the risk of being influenced by the nurse's biases and opinions. Thus, it is much more accurate and helpful to the evaluation process for the nurse to absorb these verbal and nonverbal clues carefully and then see if a pattern emerges from them.

The cause-and-effect relationship is far more difficult to evaluate when psychosocial behavior is involved, as the following example indicates.[18] As a supportive measure, the night nurse decided to look in frequently on a patient who often signaled for trivial requests or "by mistake." If she found him awake, the nurse would ask him to take a walk down the hall with her. After the third night, the patient's light was no longer flashing and he slept soundly through the night. This change may indeed have been caused by the nurse's action. But it might simply have been the result of the patient's finally having become accustomed to the hospital's routine.

> Nonverbal clues are especially important in cases where the patient has sensory deprivation and cognitive problems.

[17] Eckelberry, p. 86.
[18] Ibid., p. 85.

Even when cause and effect are difficult to establish definitely, continued evaluation and reevaluation can help to determine whether or not the patient is, in fact, progressing. This evaluation can also establish whether or not specific nursing actions seem to have been influential in changing the patient's condition.

Barriers to goal fulfillment

Sometimes the patient does not make the anticipated progress toward his goals. This may be due to factors specific to the patient himself, to the nurse, or to other members of the health care team. The patient's family may also be involved. The patient may develop allergic reactions to a prescribed treatment. He may be unable to cope with adjustment to illness because of the combined effects of financial worries, loss of job, and adverse reaction to therapeutic agents.

The nurse's actions may contribute to the failure to achieve desired goals. Such actions include overlooking data, assigning priorities inappropriately, or failing to consider the medical plan when formulating the nursing care plan. Failure may also be due to the nurse's not involving the patient in planning his own care.[19]

Also, other health team members may be responsible for the failure of the patient to achieve planned goals. There may be a lack of continuity in planning or implementation due to lack of communication. There may have been too much concentration on the purely technical aspects of a therapy to the exclusion of interpersonal aspects.

With so many variables at work, it is little wonder that many originally defined goals and planned actions are later found to be inappropriate, ineffective, or ill-defined. The evaluation phase of the nursing process serves to indicate where such weaknesses are. Most importantly, it enables the nurse and other members of the health care team to pinpoint how the plan should be modified.

Modification

When the evaluation phase indicates that there is something wrong with the original plan, modification is necessary. Nursing care plans may need modification for a variety of specific reasons. There are, however, two general reasons that underlie the need for plan revision. These are changes in the patient's status or response and/or changes in the nurse's knowledge or perception of the patient and his problems.[20]

[19]Yura and Walsh, p. 132.
[20]Little and Carnevali, p. 161.

Changes in the patient's status

The patient may have entered the hospital hemorrhaging profusely. The primary goal of all actions would be to arrest the bleeding and stabilize the patient. Once the life-threatening situation is under control, new goals and needs may arise, such as pain control and maintenance of stable vital signs. As a patient's condition stabilizes, even temporarily, the original life-saving therapeutic measures may no longer be necessary. The change in the patient's condition may either be very dramatic or almost imperceptible.

Unless the care plan is appropriately modified to take into account the patient's new condition, the nursing staff will be unable to work effectively with the patient. The patient cited above may need his vital signs monitored hourly during the first few days following admission. If this hourly procedure is continued beyond the time it is necessary, it may needlessly tax the patient both physically and psychologically.

Changes in the nurse's knowledge and perceptions

The need for modification may result from the accumulation of more data about the patient or new insights into his condition. More data are often collected about the patient as the nurse and other staff members spend more time with him. They will become familiar with his expectations, perceptions, and responses to a wider variety of situations. This additional information should supplement, validate, or invalidate the original judgments made about the patient and his needs. It should, of course, influence the type of nursing intervention that will be used.[21]

Modification of nursing care plans may take different forms, depending on the patient's condition. Modification may be necessary, for instance, in the stated goals or in the time schedule for accomplishment of the goals. The patient may have adjusted to his illness much more rapidly than anticipated, or much more slowly than hoped for.[22]

Consider the following two patients and their needs for revised nursing care plans. Mr. R. was originally assessed as an incontinent, confused, and dejected hemiplegic. He was incapable of following even simple directions. Yet, only 6 months later he had progressed to the point where he was cheerful, walking, meeting friends, and playing checkers. His progress exceeded everyone's original expectations. He might have progressed even faster, had his original goals not been limited for a long period to such short-term basics as "is able to wash himself" and "can feed himself."

On the other hand, Mrs. H., a patient with similar problems of hemi-

---

[21]Ibid.
[22]Doris Schwartz. 1965. Toward more precise evaluation. *Nursing Outlook* 13:44.

plegia and confusion, seemed not to have progressed much beyond her original state after the same 6-month period. For her, a total reevaluation was necessary to determine more precisely the reasons for her lack of progress.

It may be necessary to reevaluate only part of the nursing care plan. Or, as in the case of Mrs. H., the whole plan may need reworking. All areas of the plan should be open to change, including the statement of the problem, the patient's and staff's goals, the nursing orders, and the assessment, implementation, or evaluation stage. The modification step involves reentering the assessment-planning-implementation-evaluation cycle at the appropriate point and continuing from there.

The original assessment may have provided insufficient information to define all the problems explicitly. For instance, the first contact with a preoperative patient may have shown that the patient was highly anxious or frightened. At this point, the problem may have been stated as "appears anxious." However, after learning the specific object of his discomfort—fear of death or of dependency—the problem can be stated more definitely as a basis for selecting nursing intervention.

When the problem is stated too generally, as above, specifics need to be supplied. When the problem is stated too narrowly, on the other hand, the extent of the problem and the range of actions leading to a solution may be overlooked. Thus, definitions of problems that are too narrow also need modification.

Goals, too, may have to be redefined because they are unrealistic, or because they run contrary to the patient's own objectives, values, or norms. Often goals are either too broad and ambiguous or too narrow in their perspective, making designation of nursing action equally difficult.

The nursing orders are usually subject to the most revision. Changing patient responses to nursing action, changing priorities in the patient's needs, and the need to narrow or enlarge the scope of nursing actions will all result in modification of the nurse's planned interventions.

As the patient responds to modifications in the nursing care plan, evaluation must continue to take place. The patient may be responding and moving toward his goals, or the plan may need yet further modification because of insufficient response. This ongoing process of assessing the patient, planning, implemention, and evaluation continues until the patient is discharged from the nurse's care.

SUMMARY

After making an assessment of the patient and his needs, the nurse enters into the final phases of the nursing process—planning, implementation, evaluation, and, if necessary, modification.

Planning the goals and method of treatment should be a joint effort on the part of the nurse and the patient. It will also often involve other members of the health care team, as well as the patient's family. Effective cooperation and communication among all these people will go far to ensure that the plans made will be appropriate and successful.

Because good nursing care is patient-oriented, goals of treatment should always be stated in terms of patient achievement, rather than nursing action. Not all goals are reachable at the same time, so priorities must be assigned, based on the patient's needs. These priorities, which designate goals as short-term, intermediate, or long-term, should also be determined jointly by nurse and patient.

Since there is never any single perfect solution to a problem, all possible alternatives for achieving the planned goals must be explored. These alternatives should take into account the knowledge, resources, and experience of the patient, his family, the nurse, and the health care team.

Implementation of the plan that is arrived at in this way may be carried out directly by the nurse. More often, it will require a cooperative effort with other staff. It will always require the cooperation of the patient. The nurse must always be sure that all those involved in caring for the patient, and the patient and his family, know and understand the methods and goals of treatment.

The evaluation phase of the nursing process enables the nurse to determine whether or not the desired goals are being achieved. An important factor in evaluation is the response of the patient himself. This response may be verbal or nonverbal. Nonverbal responses take the form of test data, behavior and attitudes, and comparisons made when the patient was admitted.

The evaluation phase may have several outcomes. It may reveal that the patient's needs have been met, that only some have been met, or that the plan of action has not succeeded in meeting any of his needs. It may also reveal that new problems have arisen. Unresolved problems may be due to changes in the patient's condition and reactions, or they may result from new observations by the nurse and other members of the health care team.

If evaluation reveals that there are problems that are not being resolved, modification of the original plan will be necessary. Modification may involve the redefinition of patient problems, the formulation of new goals, or the selection of alternative means of treatment. Modification essentially involves reentering the assessment-planning-implementation-evaluation cycle. Each time the patient and nurse work together through the nursing process, the patient comes closer to receiving effective, personalized care.

STUDY QUESTIONS

1.　What is a nursing care plan? What is its function in patient care?
2.　Referring to the nursing history on pp. 82–88, and the nursing diagnosis you made as a result (see p. 112), devise a nursing care plan for this patient.

3. What are long-range goals in patient care? Give examples. Define and give examples of short-range goals.

4. What patient behaviors, both verbal and nonverbal, would indicate to you that the following goals have been met?
   a. Patient will increase range of motion of right shoulder each day.
   b. Patient will increase protein intake to 70 grams per day.
   c. Pain in patient's left hip will be decreased during ambulation.

5. How can the nurse involve the patient, his family, and other health team members in the planning phase of patient care? in the implementation phase? in the evaluation phase? Give examples.

6. What factors should the nurse consider when evaluating the results of a nursing care plan?

SELECTED BIBLIOGRAPHY

Copp, Laurel Archer. 1972. Improved patient care through evaluation, part 3: Your plan of nursing care. *Bedside Nurse* 5:25–29.

Eckelberry, Grace K. 1971. *Administration of comprehensive nursing care: The nature of professional practice.* New York: Appleton-Century-Crofts.

Kramer, Marlene. 1972. Standard 4: Nursing care plans . . . power to the patient. *Journal of Nursing Administration* 2:29–34.

Mayers, Marlene Glover. 1972. The patient's response as a test of good planning. In *A systematic approach to the nursing care plan,* pp. 117–39. New York: Appleton-Century-Crofts.

Smith, Dorothy M. 1971. Writing objectives as a nursing practice skill. *American Journal of Nursing* 71:319–20.

Yura, Helen, and Walsh, Mary B. 1973. *The nursing process: Assessing, planning, implementing, evaluating,* 2d ed. New York: Appleton-Century-Crofts.

Zimmerman, Donna Stulgis, and Gohrke, Carol. 1970. The goal-directed nursing approach: It does work. *American Journal of Nursing* 70:306–10.

7 Record keeping and charting

Patient records have come a long way from those of a century ago. Then, details of a patient's development were communicated verbally between doctors. Instructions were only occasionally passed on to nurses, and care of the patient was often uncoordinated.

In the past hundred years the quality of nursing care has improved considerably. This is due in large part to the increasing emphasis on systematic assessment, team conferences, and communication among members of the health care team. Vital to this communication is the use of written patient records.

Why are written records necessary?

Written records have become so standard and important a part of patient care that sometimes they seem to be given more attention than the patient himself. The following story, although hopefully exaggerated, has become legendary. A patient is brought into the emergency room bleeding profusely. Before any emergency treatment is administered, he is expected to gasp out answers to questions about everything from his family history to his eating habits. Finally, the record is complete. Alas, it is too late to use any of this information—the patient has died.

Obviously, the purpose of maintaining thorough records has not been served in such a case. When properly used, however, written records can be invaluable for clinical, professional, and administrative purposes. And all of these serve the desired goal of better care for the patient.

The maintenance of patient records is sometimes viewed as an annoying "extra" part of nursing care. It is a task that some nurses feel takes them away from the job for which they have been prepared: taking care of the patient himself. However, taking care of the patient certainly involves planning the patient's care and analyzing and assessing his problems. Record keeping also involves communicating with other members of the health care team about the patient and about other behind-the-scenes

133

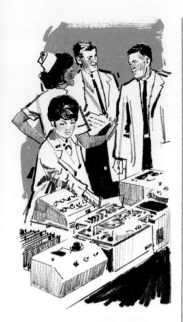

Complete and accurate
records allow every
member of the team to
know what the others
are doing to assist the
patient.

activities that the patient may not see. All of these are very much a part
of patient care and the nursing process. They are all more efficiently and
systematically carried out through the use of written records.

Communication

Communication among members of the health care team is the most
obvious and one of the most important goals served by the written record.
It is true that physicians, nurses, and others exchange information verbally
about a patient. Too often, these verbal exchanges take place during a crisis,
right after a crisis, or deal only with a specific problem. The aim, however,
of good nursing care is to treat the patient as a whole person and not as
a broken leg or a heart attack. To do so, communication among members
of the health care team should deal with all aspects of the patient's being.
The nurse should understand the technical details of a patient's surgery.
In turn, the surgeon and other attending physicians should understand the
patient's social and emotional background and nursing needs. A written
record of a patient's physical and psychological state following a colostomy,
for example, may provide revealing information about his rate of recovery.

The written record is also a means of saving time. It takes only a few
minutes per day to update records and read over those parts that are
maintained by others. This generally takes far less time than having to
repeat questions, examinations, or laboratory procedures that should have
been noted in the written record. It is certainly much less of a strain on
the patient.

Such communication among members of the team should make coordination of the patient care plan easier and more efficient. Complete and
accurate records allow every member of the team to know what the others
are doing to assist the patient. There is much less chance of questions,
procedures, or, worse yet, medications being repeated. There is a far
greater chance for an effective joint effort in treating the patient.

Research

Research material about any given patient is readily available when
written records are maintained and saved. The memory of a patient or
health care provider will never be as complete and precise as the record
of the event that is written at the time it took place. This is true whether
the record is of events that occurred yesterday or 10 years ago.

A flare-up of an ulcer or a parasitic condition, for instance, will be
much more readily identifiable if written records from the first appearance
of the condition are available. Similarly, a patient's condition and behavior
after an operation may be clarified or explained by referring back to written
information about his status before the operation.

Research into the causes of various illnesses and the development of new treatments can be carried out in part by the reading of patient records. The use of experimental drugs and procedures also demands the keeping of thorough and accurate records.

Statistical information

The written record generally provides statistical information about the patient's vital signs, results of laboratory tests, and other measures of his condition. Such basic information as the patient's age, sex, distinguishing features and characteristics, occupation, and home address may also serve a useful purpose in evaluating his condition. They can aid in developing comparisons with other patients in similar categories and in formulating such aspects of the patient care plan as the type and amount of medication he should receive.

The growing importance of computers in the health care field has also increased the value of the written record as a source for statistical data. For example, data for state, national, and international mortality figures are obtained from individual written records.

Legal records

The written record also plays a vital role in that it provides legal evidence concerning the patient's treatment and responses. Written records are the most admissible form of evidence in a court. Nurses' charting on patients is often used in medicolegal cases involving personal injury, insurance claims, workmen's compensation, criminal cases, and will probates. They are also vital in malpractice cases.[1]

There are casebooks full of legal decisions in malpractice suits where written records served to absolve or implicate the nurses involved in a patient's care. One lawsuit involved the death of a mentally ill girl. The record showed that the patient's temperature was 101.8° on March 13 and 104° on March 16. The record did not show any evidence of treatment or any other notes for March 14 and 15. This record was held to be evidence of the hospital's failure to provide ordinary and reasonable care for the patient.[2]

In an era when patient's rights are being more widely promoted, every provider of health care runs the risk of becoming involved in a legal proceeding at some point in his or her career. Failure to record thorough and accurate data about a patient's treatment and response may result in a weak defense or no defense of one's actions.

Research into the causes of various illnesses and the development of new treatments can be carried out in part by the reading of patient records.

[1] Helen Creighton. 1970. *Law every nurse should know,* 2d ed., p. 84. Philadelphia: Saunders.
[2] Ibid.

Audits

Finally, written records provide a means for auditing the care a patient is receiving and the competence of those providing it. **Audit committees** are being established to evaluate the performance of staff members. Patient records provide these committees with information about the completeness and relevance, judgment, and logic of a nurse's actions in patient-care situations.

Problem-oriented records

One of the problems in medical record keeping, however, is that many records do not meet any or all of the above needs. For a long time, nurses and physicians entered their records in separate parts of the patient's chart. Lab reports were placed elsewhere. Social workers and therapists entered their notes in yet another section of the chart. These records were based on a **source-oriented** approach. They separated the patient into medical problems, to which the doctor attended, nursing problems, etc. In the middle of this disjointed activity, the patient and his problems received attention that was often uncoordinated. To correct this situation, the problem-oriented record has been developed.

The **problem-oriented** approach to patient care is a system that emphasizes the whole patient and his problems. Popularized by Lawrence L. Weed,[3] it is an approach that integrates the care given by various providers into the patient's record. *The emphasis is not on who gives the care but on the problems for which the care is given.*

The problem-oriented system has been successfully used since its introduction in the 1950s in a broad spectrum of health care settings. These include inpatient and outpatient areas, preventive and rehabilitative medicine, pediatrics, psychiatry, etc. While each setting requires modification of the system to allow for special contingencies and needs, four basic components are always used. These are:

1. Baseline patient data
2. Needs or problems
3. Plans
4. Progress notes

The order in which the components are listed is significant. It indicates the chronological order in which they are recorded.

[3]Lawrence L. Weed. 1971. *Medical records, medical education, and patient care: The problem-oriented record as a basic tool.* Cleveland: Case Western Reserve.

Baseline patient data

The **baseline patient data** make up the first component of the problem-oriented record (POR). They consist of information about the patient at the time he presents himself to the health care setting. Included are physiological, social, and emotional data. For a general hospital patient, the elements would be his chief complaints, a description of his average day, of his present illness, and a past history and systems review. Also included would be a physical examination of standardized content and X-ray studies. The nursing history and observations about the patient's life-style and current status should also be part of the data base.

The following are the standard elements of baseline patient data:

1. *Historical*
   ID—Identification: demographic and administrative data (name, age, address, insurance information, etc.)
   PH—Past History: medical surgical, allergic problems, hospitalizations, previous exams and tests, dental records, eye records, etc.
   Rx—Past and current treatment, immunizations, coffee, cigarette, and drug usage
   FH—Family History: genetic and medical
   SH—Social History (patient profile): habits, hobbies, recreational activities, family situation, economic status, education, jobs, profile of typical day, religion, personal strengths and preferences, etc.
   ROS—Review of Systems: structured review of body systems relative to symptoms or possible problems

2. *Physiological*
   Body measurements (height, weight, etc.)
   Vital signs (heart rate, blood pressure, etc.)
   General physical examination (*not* including details on *problems*)
   Functional measurements—vital capacity, visual acuity, etc.

3. *Laboratory*—routine tests such as:
   Blood chemistry "battery"
   "Hemogram"
   Urinalysis
   Chest X-ray
   ECG
   PAP smear[4]

The data base is generated from many sources. These include interviews with the patient, relatives, and other key people; direct observation; reports

[4]Stephen Yarnall and Judith Atwood. 1974. Problem-oriented practice for nurses and physicians: General concepts. *Nursing Clinics of North America* 9:220.

from other doctors and nurses; and the traditional physical and psychological assessments.

The source of any information in the data base should always be identified. It has been seen, for example, in pediatric mental health clinics, that a father's description of his child may be quite different from the mother's. Both may be markedly different from the health care worker's description. Each description has its own importance.

Standardized forms for obtaining data base information have been developed by administrators, educators, and individuals. These ensure that patient data are obtained easily, completely, and in a standardized manner. These may be elaborate, multipage forms that require the interviewer to underline or circle appropriate information about the patient.[5] Others that are less regimented require open-ended information about the patient's personal and social history, family history, general health, habits, and other significant factors.

Use of a well-defined data base provides a number of advantages:

1. Information gaps may be more quickly identified and corrected. This permits earlier identification of the patient's problem and more rapid initiation of treatment.
2. Any member of the staff can review the information and add to it.
3. The format promotes the efficient use of staff skills.[6]

Needs or problems

In the course of compiling the data base, some of the patient's problems will be identified. The complete **problem list,** part two of the POR, is a carefully drawn up list of problems that require further observation, diagnosis, management, or education. The essence of the POR is the structuring of health care and written records around the patient's important problems.

The problem list is compiled by the admitting physician or the person assuming major responsibility for the patient's care. It is then attached to the front of the **chart,** where it remains as an index or table of contents to the rest of the chart. Each problem is designated by a number. All future references to that problem are identified by the number given to it in the original problem list.

Although the number assigned to each problem remains fixed, the problem list itself must be dynamic. Problems that are first designated as signs or symptoms may evolve into diagnoses as evidence accumulates.

[5]Richard E. Easton. 1974. *Problem-oriented medical record concepts,* pp. 69, 73. New York: Appleton-Century-Crofts.
[6]Henry J. Fay and Arthur Norman. 1974. Modifying the problem-oriented record for an inpatient program for children. *Hospital and Community Psychiatry* 25:27.

Over a period of time, new problems may be added. And some parts of the problem list may become outdated because problems may be resolved or become inactive. However, because problem lists are intended to be permanent records that can be referred to throughout the person's life, problems may be redefined or reclassified but never erased.

Not all abnormalities in the data base need to be included in the problem list. (Several relatively complicated approaches have been devised that involve listing past problems, inactive problems, temporary problems, etc.) One way of classifying a former problem that has been resolved is to give it a number and list it as inactive in the patient's complete problem list. Transient episodes (such as backache or severe heartburn) that may not turn out to be new problems should be listed as temporary problems. They are carried as such until resolved or transferred to the complete current problem list.

Figure 7-1 is a problem list that was formulated using the POR system. Each problem should have its own plan, numbered correspondingly. Any experienced observer reading the record can then see at a glance whether a problem is being dealt with by a complete and reasonable plan.

Plans

In preparing the initial plan, the patient profile and complete list of problems will serve as a basis for choosing appropriate action. The patient's life-style and entire problem list should be considered before planning measures to resolve any one given problem. For example, surgery may be beneficial for one person, while for another it may be disastrous to his physical and psychological state. Since there is no "standard" case of

PATIENT NAME _____ IDENTIFICATION # _____

No.	Problem	Date Entered	Status
1	Anemia a. Fatigue b. Shortness of breath on exertion	1/1/75	active
2	Joint pain, all extremities	1/1/75	active
3	Hematuria (last 2 days)	1/1/75	active
4	Worried about interrupting college term	1/1/75	active
5	Significant hypertension in several family members re- ported by patient	1/1/75	active

FIG. 7-1 *A typical problem list.* [Based on a case study in Mary Woody and Mary Mallison, The problem-oriented system for patient-centered care. *American Journal of Nursing* 73 (1973):1168-69.]

Nursing plans should
focus on identifying the
patient's nursing needs
and problems.

emphysema, angina, or pregnancy, the variables associated with each individual situation must be used in formulating the initial plan.

Specific plans developed for each problem fall into three separate categories:[7]

1. Plans for collection of further data in order to establish a diagnosis or aid in management
2. Plans for treatment with specific procedures or drugs
3. Plans for educating the patient about his illness and his part in managing it

Nursing plans should focus on identifying the patient's nursing needs and problems. They should define realistic goals specifically related to those problems and determine the nursing techniques that will have the most beneficial effect. The plans developed by physician and nurse should complement one another. In this way the nurse's decisions dealing with activity, diet, observation of vital signs, patient education, etc., will be coordinated with and supported by the medical plans.

Formulation of a nursing plan for a patient with Hodgkin's disease, for example, will take into consideration such problems as progressive weakness, confusion, and dealing with terminal illness. The plan might involve some of the following procedures, itemized in a format appropriate to the POR.

Progress notes

Once the patient's problems have been identified and a plan has been put into effect, the patient's response to the treatment program must be recorded. **Progress notes,** the fourth component of the POR, contain all the relevant data about the patient's responses. These include notes by everyone involved in the patient's care: nurses, physicians, therapists, and social workers. They also include special treatment sheets and records of vital signs and medications.

The SOAP format

To help those making the progress notes, and to ensure clarity and completeness, a systematic format for writing the progress notes is used in the POR. This is known as **SOAP,** which stands for **S**ubjective data, **O**bjective data, **A**ssessment, and **P**lan. The acronym was coined, it is said, by a British physician who explained, "In England, we're SOAPing the records—it helps to clean up the thinking, you see."[8]

[7]Weed, p. 43.
[8]Mary Woody and Mary Mallison. 1973. The problem-oriented system for patient-centered care. *American Journal of Nursing* 73:1172.

INITIAL PLAN

#1 Progressive Weakness:

Allow the patient to decide each day the amount of activity
he/she can tolerate. Allow rest periods after each nursing
procedure.

#2 Confusion:

Reorientation to time and place by everyone who enters
patient's room. Refer to wall calendar in patient's room while
giving care. Encourage family-patient dialogue that is
meaningful to patient's orientation.

FIG. 7-2 *Nursing plan for a patient with Hodgkin's disease.*

Subjective data is the term for information obtained by taking a history and asking the patient how he feels. This important information is recorded first in order to overcome the tendency of some physicians to concentrate on laboratory and X-ray data while overlooking the patient's own description of his symptoms. This also allows the health care team, in reading over the medical record, to see the patient and not just the X-ray. Separating the subjective and objective data also helps one identify, and therefore use more therapeutically, one's own emotional responses when angered, frustrated, or pleased in an encounter with a patient.[9]

Objective data include the physical signs, measurements, and results obtained from physical examinations, observation of the patient, EKGs, X-rays, and other diagnostic measures.

The difference between subjective and objective data is illustrated by the case of a patient who complains of a sore throat, inability to swallow, and dryness (subjective data). This patient speaks in a hoarse whisper, winces when eating or drinking, and coughs repeatedly (objective data).

The assessment portion is the analysis of the patient's problem. The nurse's assessment concentrates on an evaluation of the patient's ability to cope with his problem. The physician's assessment will emphasize the medical diagnosis. Again, both should complement one another.

The assessment portion of the progress notes has often been viewed as the most challenging and difficult to write. It demands creativity, a thorough understanding of the patient's problem, and insight into the reasons for the patient's responses. All these demands may seem intimidating to a new practitioner, particularly since the assessment becomes part of a permanent written record. But the value of the assessment step has many aspects:

1. It demands disciplined and logical thinking by the examiner.

[9]Ibid., p. 1173.

2. It enables others reading the chart to understand the diagnostic progression.
3. It allows each problem to be evaluated individually and clearly.

The plan is an extension or revision of the initial plan for each problem. The plan may include immediate and future nursing plans, what the patient was taught, and whether the patient understood the instructions.

Progress notes recorded by this method may deal in minute-by-minute responses if the patient is in intensive care, or in hourly or daily fluctuations for a hospitalized patient. Weekly or monthly changes will be recorded for an outpatient under treatment for chronic arthritis. Yearly changes are noted in preventive care checkups. Regardless of the time interval chosen, progress notes fall into three basic categories in the POR system formulated by Weed and others. These are:

1. Narrative notes
2. Flow sheets
3. Discharge notes

Narrative notes, which record the patient's progress on a regular basis, contain entries by all members of the health care team. In keeping with the POR format, narrative notes are keyed to problem numbers. A separate narrative note is entered for each current problem.

Sometimes certain data require ongoing observation and must be recorded repetitively in order to accurately follow the patient's progress. Because narrative notes would be lengthy and impractical in this case, the information is recorded on a chronological chart known as a **flow sheet**

FIG. 7-3 *Flow sheet used in a renal intensive care unit.*
[From Mary Woody and Mary Mallison, The problem-oriented system for patient-centered care. *American Journal of Nursing* 73 (1973):1174. © 1973 by the American Journal of Nursing Company. Reprinted by permission of the American Journal of Nursing Company.]

	B/P	P	R	CVP	TEMP	ORAL	INTAKE IV	BLOOD	GU IRRIGANT IN URINE	3-way FOLEY OUTPUT CASTRIC	RESIDUAL	NET OUTPUT OTHER	MED., RX.	OTHER
12 A	124/80	80	20	10.2	97⁶		155		100	130		30	Wt = 47.0 kg. Hct = 30	
1 A	122/70	80	16	9.0			95		100	145		45	Morphine 4 mg 1⁰ AM	M Shauln
2 A	124/90	80	18	9.			200		100	150		50		
3 A				9.5		Ice chips 15	150		100	130		30	Large clots now in urine	
4 A	126/80	82	16	9.5	97⁸		200		100	150		50	D5½NS hung	
5 A	122/88	74	16	10.			150		100	140		40		
6 A	110/70	76	14	12			200		100	150	30	50	BUN, Lytes, glucose, Ca, P, osmol, CBC & diff sent. Urine sent for C+S, osmol, K, Na	
7 A	112/78	74	16	12			100		100	50		50	Morphine 4 mg 7¹⁵ AM / bladder spasms	
TOTAL							1250		800	1045	30	345	Wt = 46.5 / Hct = 30.	M Shauln
8 A	120/80	76	16	12.5	97⁶	15	115		100	180		80	EKG done. Foley irrigated by A. O'Brien	
9 A														

STAMPED WITH PATIENT NAME
HOSP. NUMBER
DATE
(POST- KIDNEY TRANSPLANT Pt)
VITAL SIGNS

24 HOUR INTENSIVE CARE DATA SHEET

		BLOOD PRESSURE					
		NURSE'S NOTES - PATIENT INTERVIEW					
		CARDIAC CLINIC					
		GRADY MEMORIAL HOSPITAL					
		ATLANTA, GEORGIA					

Name
Number

Date	Medications	Subjective	Objective - (RA)				Assess & Plan
			at 30°	Immed'ly Standing	Standing To 5 Min		
8/23/72	Ismelin (25 mg. tab.) 87.5 mg. q.d. (3½ tab.) Lasix 40 mg q.d, KCl 2 tsp. q.d	Dizzy, weak Taking Ismelin 63.5 mg + Lasix 40 mg B.i.d.	200/90	160/84	152/84		1) ↓ Lasix to 40 mg qd per Dr. Fargo 2) Continue Ismelin 2½ tab. qd (62.5 mg) 3) R.T.C. 2 wk - BP
9/13/72	Ismelin 62.5 mg q.d Lasix 40 mg q.d. KCl 2 tsp. q.d.	Still c/o dizziness + weakness during day and on arising	180/90	160/82	150/80		1) ↓ Ismelin to 50 mg q.d. per Dr. Fargo 2) Reinstructed re: body's need for time to adjust to lower B.P. 3) R.T.C. 2 wk.
9/27/72	Ismelin 50 mg. q.d. Lasix 40 mg q.d. KCl 2 tsp. q.d.	"Taking meds as directed" Dizzy when walking about	194/120	164/110	190/120		1) Continue Ismelin 50 q.d. but add 2) ALDOMET 250 mg TID per Dr. Fargo 3) R.T.C. 1 wk - CBC

FIG. 7-4 *The episodic clinic flow sheet.*
[From Mary Woody and Mary Mallison, The problem-oriented system for patient-centered care. *American Journal of Nursing* 73 (1973):1174. © 1973 by the American Journal of Nursing Company. Reprinted by permission of the American Journal of Nursing Company.]

or **flow chart.** The flow sheet is particularly useful when several factors such as temperature, pulse rate, blood pressure, respiration, and reflexes are involved. A comparison of these factors may be important in measuring a patient's reaction to treatment. This comparison can be more easily made if the information is recorded in a tabular or graphic form.

Flow sheets are used most often in rapidly changing situations. They may also be used effectively to record infrequent office visits in which the comparison of such factors as weight change, blood pressure, and uremic protein is important.

Figures 7-3 and 7-4 are two examples of flow sheets. Figure 7-3 records hourly changes in a renal intensive care unit; Figure 7-4, biweekly readings in a cardiac clinic.

Discharge notes are the final phase of the progress notes. They focus on plans for management of the problem and give the information needed for future analysis of the problem. They should contain an overall assessment of the results of hospitalization or outpatient treatment. The discharge notes should also be keyed to the problem list and should offer information about the status of the problem—resolved, active, inactive, or whatever. For example, a diagnosed inflamed appendix that has been surgically removed without complication, with satisfactory healing of the incision, requires very little information in the discharge notes. Abdominal pain that was never completely understood or resolved should be described at length. In this way, should the problem recur, the new health care team will have as much help as possible in identifying and treating the problem.

Figure 7-5 is a summary prepared by a cardiovascular nurse-clinician in the case of 40-year-old patient who had a history of three myocardial infarctions. The patient, who was visited at home prior to being referred to another physician, had just heard about the loss of his job.

The problem-oriented system and the nursing process

The organization of the problem-oriented record system closely follows that of the nursing process itself. The step-by-step progress from data base

FIG. 7-5 *Home visit summary.*
[From Maureen B. Niland and Patricia M. Bentz, A problem-oriented approach to planning nursing care. *Nursing Clinics of North America* 9 (1974):244. Reprinted by permission.]

Patient: Mr. T.   Discharged: June 18, 1973

Date: June 26, 1973—11:00 AM   Diagnosis: Anterior Subendocardial MI
                                                        June 5, 1973

Job Loss
    S—"It's all over with the company." States will be able to get work at a
       service station run by a friend.
    O—Upset about news that opportunity to manage a station has been
       withdrawn.
    A—Does not seem to be worried about getting *A* job—upset that *THE* job
       he wanted is no longer available for him.
    P—Suggest Cardiac Work Evaluation Clinic to PMD.

Myocardial Infarction
    S—No C/O pain or SOB.
    O—Pulse regular @ 72—intermittent s4—no signs of failure.
    A—Cardiac status stable.
    P—Patient to continue with discharge orders until first office visit—
       appointment not yet made.

Inflammatory Process—Left Arm
    S—States area more tender and extensive than at discharge.
    O—Hot, hard, tender area of vein near left antecubital space.
    A—Inflammatory process 2° to ?
    P—Apply moist heat to area.
       Consult PMD when calling for first office visit.

Health Education
    S—"No questions."
    O—Daughter doing well with cooking; has resumed smoking; exceeding
       activity limitations in terms of auto ride to downtown for meeting re
       employment.
    A—Not a good time for counseling re above; patient preoccupied with
       news of unemployment.
    P—Follow-up phone call next week, follow-up visit at four weeks—
       assessment of problems with diet, activity, etc., at that time.

to problem identification, to care plan, to progress observation, helps the nurse to see the patient as a total person. It also helps her deal with his problems in a thorough and systematic manner.

The individual steps in preparing the problem-oriented record parallel the steps of the nursing process. The preparation of the data base, an information-seeking phase, is comparable to the assessment step in the nursing process. It requires a nursing history and diagnostic studies—both of which are central to the assessment process. The POR plan, involving diagnostic, treatment, and education factors, corresponds to the development of nursing orders and the nursing care plan. Finally, the progress notes or flow sheets of the POR are important to the process of evaluation.

Not only is the problem-oriented record compatible with the nursing process, but its use greatly increases the nurse's effectiveness. The physician's orders can be more readily understood and related to specific problems. Active and inactive problems are quickly identifiable. The nurse can assess and treat current problems without having to play Sherlock Holmes and search them out in the medical record. At the same time, the nurse can keep a lookout for the recurrence of resolved problems or the beginning of new ones.

Many nurses feel that it is useless to write detailed notes "because doctors and other health care workers never look at them." In the problem-oriented system, however, nurses' notes are an integral part of a coordinated record and are not written on separate pages in a separate part of the patient's chart. In this way, they are not overlooked.

Finally, the system gives the nurse an opportunity to involve the patient in his own care. This aspect of patient participation is particularly crucial to the nursing process. The patient may and, in fact, should introduce a great deal of information directly into the subjective data of the records. Much of this information, previously ignored by the health care team, will give an indication of the patient's real progress.

Not only is the problem-oriented record compatible with the nursing process, but its use greatly increases the nurse's effectiveness.

Traditional records

Traditional chart forms usually contain much of the same objective data as the problem-oriented system. Notations are made chronologically, however. Included are many of the patient's problems, his reactions to treatment, and progress reports on his condition. The patient's progress from day to day, or week to week, is of prime importance. The variables discussed are subject to the ability of the individual filing the report.

The Kardex system

The **Kardex** system provides general basic information and has become widely used for patient data. A sample Kardex form shown in Figure 7-6

FIG. 7-6 *Sample Kardex form.*
[From Maureen B. Niland and Patricia M. Bentz, A problem-oriented approach to planning nursing care. *Nursing Clinics of North America* 9 (1974):242. Reprinted by permission.]

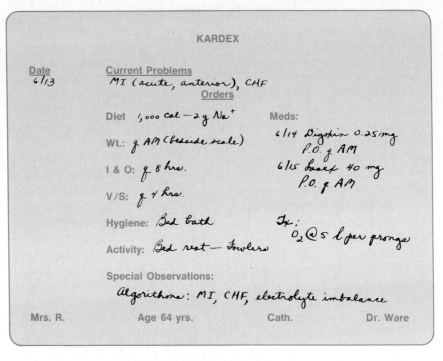

serves as a temporary concise summary and quick reference for pertinent information about the patient.

The Kardex, as opposed to the POR system, should have notations written in pencil. They can then be erased and kept up to date as the patient's condition changes. The cards are stored in a portable index file.

Writing nurses' notes

Writing nurses' notes is a skill that must be developed and practiced until it becomes second nature. Too many nurses' notes report that the patient is "better" day after day. Sometimes the patient leaves the hospital worse than or in the same condition as when he entered, despite the daily "better" reports. Other notes found in nursing records are equally uninformative: "had a good day," "complained of no pain," or "IV treatment continuing properly." Such comments are completely subjective. They relate only to the patient's condition on a previous day and are of little value to anyone reading the notes for information about the patient's present state of health. It is important to list problems logically and to pinpoint observations and reactions. A note such as "able to lift arm 6 inches from side" offers a better indication of a stroke patient's progress than "moves arm sideways."

The following are some pitfalls to be avoided:

1. *Wordiness.* Avoid repetition of words that do not add to the meaning of the communication or that do not help convey the thought.

2. *Redundancy.* Avoid repetition of the same thought or observation. New meaning, interpretation, or insight is not conveyed by repeating a statement.

3. *Observation* vs. *impression.* Differentiate between an interpretation and a verifiable fact.[10]

Knowing the pitfalls of poor nurses' notes does not necessarily make for good notes, but some of the important goals to consider are:

1. *Be specific.* If the patient is "weak," the chart should indicate whether he has trouble walking, or is so weak that he cannot hold a cup.

2. *Insist on proper spelling.* Medications that are spelled similarly can have vastly different effects.

3. *Relate observations to knowledge.* If the patient's pulse is thready, look for other warning signs and include them in the notes.

4. *Use common sense.* If the patient has stopped breathing, initiate treatment and/or notify the charge nurse, whichever is appropriate.[11]

Good nursing notes should reflect the patient's total care, his clinical status, the type and severity of his symptoms, the effects of medication and other therapeutic measures. The best test of all is for a nurse to read her notes and see if she is able to visualize the patient, his problems, and care by referring to those notes alone.

Abbreviations

The abbreviations used in medical reports should be commonly understood by all personnel. Otherwise, they obstruct communication rather than facilitate it.

The list of commonly used medical abbreviations often found in medical charts, as cited below, is only a partial one. Specialty areas will necessarily use abbreviations for terms common to that specialty. However, a familiarity with some of the more general terms will not only help save time in maintaining nursing notes but will help in improving communication.

---

[10]Judith T. Bloom et al. 1971. Problem-oriented charting. *American Journal of Nursing* 71:2148.
    [11]Ibid.

BP = blood pressure
BM = bowel movement
$\bar{c}$ = with
hct = hematocrit
h.r. = heart rate
h/o = history of
(L) = left
neg = negative
$\bar{o}$ = none, no
$\bar{p}$ = after

P.E. = physical examination
(R) = right
Rx = treatment
RR = respiratory rate
$\bar{s}$ = without
SOB = shortness of breath
Sx = symptoms
U/A = urinalysis
WNL = within normal limits

SUMMARY

Today, more and more people are becoming involved in patient care. The patient's psychological, social, and educational needs are being considered as well as his physical problems. As a result, nurses, doctors, physical and occupational therapists, social workers, lab technicians, and other health care workers are all making decisions affecting the patient.

In order to ensure that patient care is coordinated as well as comprehensive, there must be effective communication among all members of the health care team. An important part of this communication is the written patient record, or chart. By providing detailed information about the patient, the written record gives each member of the team an in-depth picture of the patient and the care he has been receiving. The chart also serves as a legal record of the patient's treatment and progress as well as a basis for audits of that treatment. In addition, the record provides data for research and for statistical records.

The medical record, however, is only as good as the efforts of those involved in maintaining and using the record make it. Ideally, all those involved in the patient's care should be able to read the chart easily and quickly. It should give them a complete briefing on the patient's total range of problems and the ways in which they are being handled. There are several methods of record keeping now in use.

The problem-oriented record (POR) is a type of charting that has been used with much success. This method itemizes the patient's problems and keys each treatment plan, progress report, and patient response to the particular problem with which it deals. In this way, the treatment progress of any given problem can be easily followed. The notes of all members of the team are organized according to the patient's problems, rather than according to who is treating them.

Less efficient and effective, but still used in many places, is the source-oriented record. This record itemizes the patient's progress notes according to the type of health care worker recording them. Thus, there are separate sections for nurses' notes, physicians' notes, lab reports, etc.

An abbreviated form of record keeping, the Kardex, provides basic patient information on a compact card for quick identification of the patient's problems.

While some charting systems have definite advantages over others, all are a means of describing the patient's experiences while undergoing professional health care. They are all intended to serve the basic goal of giving the patient the best possible care. Since the nurse has the closest and most continuous contact with the patient, her observations are vital for all members of the health team. The efficient and accurate charting of the nurse's observations, assessments, and plans will go far to ensure coordinated, thoughtful, and effective patient care.

STUDY QUESTIONS

1. Describe four aspects of nursing in which written records play an important role.
2. What is a problem-oriented record? What are its essential components? Compare the problem-oriented system with other record-keeping methods.
3. What does the acronym SOAP stand for? Define the terms represented by each letter.
4. How does the problem-oriented record relate to the nursing process? Describe its use during each phase of the process.
5. What are the characteristics of useful nurses' notes? Give examples.

SELECTED BIBLIOGRAPHY

Bloom, Judith T., et al. 1971. Problem-oriented charting. *American Journal of Nursing* 71:2144–48.

Easton, Richard E. 1974. *Problem-oriented medical record concepts.* New York: Appleton-Century-Crofts.

Weed, Lawrence L. 1971. *Medical records, medical education, and patient care: The problem-oriented record as a basic tool.* Cleveland: Case Western Reserve.

Woody, Mary, and Mallison, Mary. 1973. The problem-oriented system for patient-centered care. *American Journal of Nursing* 73:1168–75.

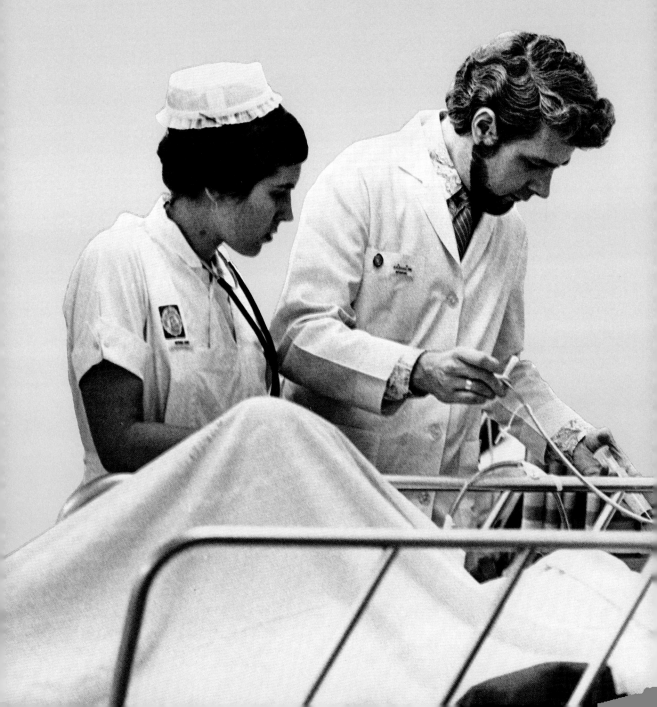

Part Three

Psychosocial and interpersonal concerns of the nurse

Some months ago, Anita was in the doctor's office, waiting for him to tell her the results of her annual gynecological examination. Although the examination had become routine for her, she felt a little nervous this time. Lately she had experienced occasional nausea and back pain. She had also noticed some swelling in her abdomen. It might just be the first signs of menopause, but Anita was worried that it could be something more serious.

She hardly felt prepared for the doctor's news, however—she was pregnant. Although she was relieved to

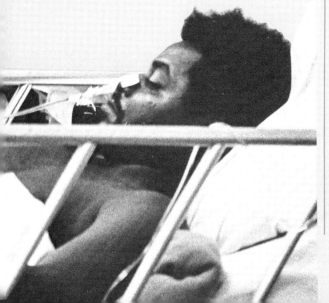

hear that she was not ill, she felt uneasy about the prospect of having a child at her age. She recalled articles she had read about the risk of retardation or abnormalities in babies born to mothers over 40. The doctor told her that the risk was indeed high among women who had never had a child before. But since Anita had already had three normal pregnancies, the outlook was good. He also told her about various tests that would be taken from time to time to monitor the baby's prenatal development and identify any potential problems.

Reassured by the doctor's attitude, Anita began to imagine what it would be like to have a baby around the house again. She would have to postpone certain plans for awhile, of course. Her return to work would have to wait, and she and Richard would not be able to take a long-planned-for trip to Europe in the near future. But she felt that they were still young enough to wait a few more years. At least this time around she could expect the older children to help out, taking some of the daily burden from her shoulders. Linda might actually enjoy having a real baby to observe up close for her child-care classes.

151

When she got home from the doctor she broke the news to Richard first. He was delighted at the prospect of having a little one around the house. He felt it would keep them young for a good while yet. The reactions of the children were not what Anita expected, however. With the exception of Steve, they were not at all happy. This left Anita feeling puzzled and not a little hurt.

Linda's reaction was the most unexpected. She seemed to be embarrassed, almost ashamed, by Anita's condition. Paul also seemed to feel that the whole idea was strange. He didn't really want his mother to be "different" from the mothers of all his friends.

Anita, who herself had not had time yet to come to grips with the changes her condition would bring, felt that the older children were almost accusing her of having done something wrong. Fortunately, Steve's attitude brought some relief. Anita had worried that he might resent having a rival for his parents' attentions. Far from being upset at the possibility, he was actually thrilled at the idea of no longer having to be called the baby of the family.

As Anita's pregnancy progressed, she felt more and more excited by the idea of having another baby. She and Richard decided to take a natural childbirth class conducted by a nurse at the local hospital. This made the baby seem more like a joint project, rather than Anita's responsibility alone, as had been the case with the others. Her pregnancy went well, but Anita worried about her stamina and still had some lingering fears that the baby would not be normal. As the doctor had predicted, however, her delivery was uncomplicated and the baby, a girl, was healthy.

After Anita and the baby came home, it seemed as though life would never return to "normal." Richard and Anita, although delighted that the baby was healthy, were finding that they had long since forgotten the strains and pressures of the first few months after childbirth. It was almost like having a first baby again. Linda and Paul felt that the baby was taking over the household and resented the intrusion. Even Steve's enthusiasm waned a bit when he realized the enormous shift in attention toward the baby.

Who is the focus of the nurse's concern in this situation?

What is the effect of the pregnancy on each member of the family? Consider each individual's stage in the life cycle, personal characteristics, and so forth.

How is the family unit altered by the baby's birth?

What are the needs for teaching/learning in this situation?

---

8 Psychosocial and emotional needs of the patient

What are man's basic needs?

As defined by Maslow (see p. 107), man's needs may be divided into five basic groups:

1. Physiological
2. Safety and security
3. Love or belonging
4. Self-esteem
5. Self-actualization

Maslow's theory emphasizes the automatic, inborn human drive for **homeostasis** (balance) over imbalance and chaos. This drive for balance extends to both the physiological and the psychological areas of functioning. According to this theory, man's needs arrange themselves in a definite order, or hierarchy, with basic bodily needs (e.g., hunger and thirst) being the first that man strives to meet. Once his physiological needs have been met, man's drive for homeostasis is directed to the more complicated psychological needs of love, security, self-esteem, and self-integration. The drive for balance involves the conscious or unconscious selection and manipulation of environmental factors (e.g., food, water, a mate) that fill man's perceived needs as well as prevent sickness and a general feeling of ill-being.

If all his needs are unsatisfied, man is dominated totally by his physiological needs. All other needs will seem nonexistent or are pushed into the background. "For the man who is extremely and dangerously hungry," Maslow says, "no other interests exist but food."[1] In this state, man's concept of the future tends to change. For the hungry man, the ideal future is one in which food is plentiful.

[1] Abraham H. Maslow. 1970. *Motivation and personality,* 2d ed., p. 37. New York: Harper & Row.

Upon completing this chapter, the reader should be able to:

1. Organize the importance of the five stages in Maslow's hierarchy of basic needs.

2. Explain the term "crisis" and the two specific types of crises, maturational and unexpected.

3. Describe the interrelatedness of problem solving, the nursing process, and crisis intervention.

4. Determine the impact of the individual's sociocultural and spiritual beliefs on his response to the health care system and acceptance of health care services.

5. Discuss the relationship between the behavior patterns found in the three stages of illness (transition, acceptance, and convalescence) and crisis resolution.

However, once basic physiological needs are satisfied to some degree, psychological needs emerge in order of strength and priority. The first and strongest psychological need that arises is the desire for *safety* (defined as security, stability, protection, dependency, and freedom from fear, anxiety, and chaos). Once that need is gratified somewhat, a quest for *belongingness and love* assumes priority. Physiological and safety needs no longer seem important or relevant, and the most pressing vital problem becomes a sense of loneliness, rootlessness, rejection, and friendlessness.

With his needs for love and belonging satisfied, the individual thinks that now he will be happy and content. But this gratification only gives way to another and higher need—the need for *self-esteem*. This is the need for achievement, mastery, competency, dominance, and status.

Satisfaction of these basic needs stimulates the individual toward *self-actualization* (self-realization, individuation, autonomy, creativity, and productivity). Self-actualization is the realization of man's full potential. ("What a man can be, he must be.")[2] The person no longer feels the constant need for esteem, love, or safety. He is primarily motivated by the need to develop his fullest potentialities and capabilities. He experiences joy or zest in living, and is confident of his ability to handle life's stresses, anxieties, feelings, and responsibilities. He feels further needs to know, to understand, and to have a pleasing environment. Spiritual needs become important.

Barriers to need-fulfillment

Certain conditions, such as freedom to express and defend oneself, freedom to seek information, fairness, justice, and honesty, must exist in order to satisfy these basic needs. Without these preconditions, basic need satisfaction is virtually impossible. The individual will then react acutely with an emergency response.

Anxiety

"Apprehension, uncertainty, waiting, expectation, fear or surprise, do a patient more harm than any exertion. Remember, he is face to face with his enemy all the time, internally wrestling with him, having long imaginary conversations with him. You are thinking of something else."—Florence Nightingale.[3]

We all experience **anxiety** (uneasiness, apprehension, nervousness) at some time. Virtually all patients experience feelings of anxiety when

[2]Ibid., p. 46.
[3]Florence Nightingale. 1859. *Notes on nursing: What it is and what it is not.* London: Harrison & Sons.

TABLE 8-1
Degrees of Anxiety and Their Effects

Degree of Anxiety	Effects	Learning Tasks of the Anxious Person
Mild anxiety	Alertness Noises seem louder; restlessness; irritability	Recognition of anxiety as a warning sign that something is not going as expected. This is done by 1. Observing what goes on 2. Describing what was observed 3. Analyzing what was expected 4. Analyzing how expectations and what went on in the event differed 5. Formulating what can be done to change the situation or change expectations 6. Validating with others
Moderate anxiety	Reduced ability to perceive or to communicate Concentration on a problem Someone talking may not be heard Part of the room may not be noticed Increased tension Muscular tension, pounding heart, perspiration, gastric discomfort	Recognition that in moderate and severe anxiety, the focus is reduced and connections may not be seen between details, and that anxiety provides energy that can be reduced to mild anxiety and then used to find out what went wrong
Severe anxiety	Only details are perceived. Connections between details are not seen. Physical discomforts Headache, nausea, trembling, dizziness	Moderate to severe anxiety may be reduced by 1. Working at a simple concrete task 2. Talking to someone who can listen 3. Playing a simple game 4. Walking 5. Crying
Panic	A detail perceived is elaborated and blown up. Inability to communicate or function	The person experiencing panic needs help in getting more comfortable. (In this stage, learning cannot be expected to take place.)

Adapted from Dorothea Hays, Teaching a concept of anxiety. *Nursing Research* 10 (Spring 1961): 109.

hospitalized, no matter what their general level of need-satisfaction has been up to that point. They are anxious about their condition, the new situation they find themselves in, and about possible future consequences of their illness and treatment. They are often overwhelmed by the number of diagnostic and treatment techniques (when the blood pressure cuff and the thermometer are often the only instruments the patient is familiar with). They are distressed by their confinement and isolation from family and everyday surroundings. Finally, they feel threatened by their dependency on others.

But anxiety is also a means of self-protection. The overall effect of anxiety is to prepare the body for **fight or flight** in an emergency situation.

Anxiety leads to a mobilization of the body's defenses and protective mechanisms. It can stimulate positive action, surprising physical strength, and constructive growth for many people. As long as the person is not "frozen" by anxiety, it increases alertness, helps him to focus his attention and respond to a perceived threat. For example, with mild anxiety, a student may find that his rate of learning is accelerated when preparing for a test. When a nurse is worried about her ability to care for a patient, her desire to prepare for that experience by gaining a complete understanding of the patient and his disease process is heightened.

A person may notice that certain bodily changes occur as he experiences anxiety feelings. Certain physiological changes occur that prepare the body for "fight" (dealing with the threat) or "flight" (avoiding the threat). When a person perceives danger, his body's blood supply is directed toward the brain and skeletal muscles, resulting in an increased pulse rate. With the change in the blood supply, the skin pales and becomes cool. Perspiration increases, causing clammy hands and skin. There is an increase in the elimination of feces and urine, and the mouth becomes dry.

Anxiety has been associated with three underlying states of mind: a sense of helplessness, a sense of insecurity (threat to identity), and a sense of isolation (alienation).

In the following statements, these states of mind are expressed by hospital patients:

People just keep coming over to me, jabbing me with needles; now I find out they're going to open me up tomorrow. (*Sense of helplessness*)

We both accept that the mastectomy was necessary, but can I expect my husband to ever really find me attractive again? (*Sense of insecurity*)

How can you really understand? You're not sick. Only someone who's got what I've got knows what it's really like. (*Sense of isolation*)[4]

These statements reflect the same underlying feelings that students of nursing may have:

If I don't pass this final examination in anatomy, I'll be dropped from school, and I don't know what I'll do if I can't become a nurse. (*Sense of insecurity*)

I don't know how they can expect us to learn so much material when we have other courses to study for, plus clinical experience in the hospital. It's just impossible. (*Sense of helplessness*)

I spent so much time studying for this test I feel I'm not part of the real world any more. They expect us to do nothing but study. (*Sense of isolation*)

[4] Anxiety—recognition and intervention (programmed instruction). 1965. *American Journal of Nursing* 65:132.

These states of mind threaten the self-image of the person who is experiencing anxiety. The person's image of himself is reflected in his ability to satisfy his wants, to control himself and, to a degree, his environment, and to communicate with others. He wants to belong, to be useful and productive, and to be able to meet the goals and expectations he has for himself. Anxiety is a reflection of his concern that something overwhelming is preventing or will prevent him from controlling these aspects of his life. The larger the threat appears to be, the more anxiety will be experienced.

Sometimes previous experience causes automatic reactions of anxiety. To one man, the presence of a policeman may provoke anxiety. To another, the same policeman elicits a feeling of protection and safety.[5]

Fear

There is a difference between **fear** and anxiety, however. Fear occurs in response to an observable external danger and is proportional to the danger. If a man is being chased by an enraged bear, we might infer that he feels fear. If he is not being chased by an enraged bear but feels and acts as if he were, we say he feels anxiety. Fear is the response to an observable external danger; anxiety is the response to an unobservable, unexplainable, unrecalled, or internal danger.[6] In both states, the physiological changes are similar.

It is obvious that some degree of anxiety will stimulate constructive action, while excess anxiety will prevent any action at all. With increasing levels of anxiety, one becomes less able to focus on the situation. Complete preoccupation with this state of distress results in **panic.** This is an acute episode, usually accompanied by somatic (physical) symptoms, and the person may even be rushed to the hospital as an acute medical emergency. He "shakes like a leaf, goes pale, sweats profusely, may vomit, have difficulty breathing, have vague aches, and be conscious of his heart thumping and racing. Invariably he has the fear that he is dying."[7] Anxiety is pathological (abnormal) when it is severe and persistent or when it seems to be triggered by some minor cause.

Nursing actions

Because attitudes and feelings can affect the course of a physical illness, nursing action is imperative in preventing or controlling patient anxiety.

[5]A. C. Burgess and A. Lazare. 1972. Nursing management of feelings, thoughts, and behavior. *Journal of Psychiatric Nursing and Mental Health Services* 10:8.
[6]M. H. Peterson. 1972. Understanding defense mechanisms (programmed instruction). *American Journal of Nursing* 72:1655.
[7]J. M. Hughes. 1971. Anxiety. *Nursing Mirror* 132:18.

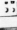

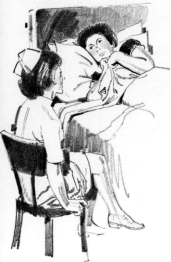

Preventing needless anxiety is perhaps the best way a nurse can assist patients.

Anxiety grows if it is not dealt with, and therefore nurses must be aware of early behavioral expressions of this state. The patient may express anger, numerous complaints, irritation, restlessness, sullenness, withdrawal, or tearfulness. His anxiety may be provoked by a realistic threat (in which the anxiety is normal) or an unrealistic threat **(neurotic anxiety).** In either case, the experienced anxiety is real and extremely distressing.

Preventing needless anxiety is perhaps the best way a nurse can assist patients. Simply explaining procedures and other mysteries of hospital life will help new patients adjust more easily to the routine. Brief explanations of illness and treatment will greatly alleviate often unrealistic fears. One patient, long after bedtime, sat up smoking cigarettes and staring into space. She said she had not been able to sleep since her admission to the hospital several days before. Why? She had no idea of what was wrong with her and why she still had complaints of abdominal pain. She did not ask her doctor—"I don't know who my doctor is, there are so many"—and no one had told her what was wrong. She was convinced that she had cancer, or "something worse," and that the doctors just did not want to tell her. When the nurse reviewed the chart and told her that the medical staff thought she had intestinal blockage due to adhesions (scars) from a previous surgery, she exclaimed happily, "Oh, is that all!" She went right to bed and slept soundly the entire night.

When the patient is experiencing mild to moderate anxiety, the nurse can alleviate the anxiety and assist the patient in finding constructive ways to deal with it. The nurse must first recognize that the patient is anxious. She should encourage him to face anxiety and gain insight into its cause. Then she can assist him to redirect the energy and strength sapped by anxiety into more positive thinking patterns and behavior.

Below is an example of a patient experiencing anxiety and appropriate nursing intervention.

Mrs. Brown entered a maternity hospital, had an uneventful delivery, and seemed very happy about the outcome until the time to go home approached. Shortly after being informed that the date had been set, she retired to her bed, maintaining that she was too weak even to sit up in a chair. She began to complain of intolerable pain being caused by her sutures. She stopped chatting with other patients in her room, responding to their conversational overtures with either listlessness or annoyance. Her physical condition was satisfactory.

Recognize the patient's anxiety

Mrs. Brown's nurse was busy, but she took note of Mrs. Brown's unusual behavior. She rearranged her schedule and sat down to listen to Mrs. Brown.

NURSE   Hello, Mrs. Brown, how are you feeling today?

MRS. BROWN   Just miserable. I feel so weak . . . I just haven't got the strength to do anything . . . I feel weak when I try to get out of bed. . . .

Assist the patient in gaining insight into anxiety

NURSE   You must feel pretty upset by all this.

MRS. BROWN   Yes, I do. The stitches are killing me, and I feel so weak. . . .

NURSE   It's too bad that you feel this way. You seemed to be feeling fine until a few days ago.

MRS. BROWN   Yes, that's true . . . I was feeling fine.

NURSE   Well, then, what happened that made you feel worse?

MRS. BROWN   Gee, I don't know.

NURSE   Well, before all this began to happen, do you remember being upset or concerned about anything?

MRS. BROWN   No . . . (then, with some surprise) yes . . . yes, maybe I was.

NURSE   You were worried?

MRS. BROWN   (hesitantly) About going home. . . .

NURSE   You felt anxious about going home?

MRS. BROWN   (with relief) Yes, yes I did.

NURSE   Do you think you might have been concentrating on your weakness and pain too much? Maybe just so you wouldn't have to think about going home?

MRS. BROWN   It's true I didn't want to think about going home.

NURSE   And maybe you've been so annoyed with everyone these last few days just because you were really upset about going home?

MRS. BROWN   Yes, that could be true.

NURSE   You must feel pretty concerned about going home.

MRS. BROWN   I just feel so helpless . . . having to take care of a baby and everything . . . I never had a baby before. . . .

NURSE   You're worried about how you'll manage?

MRS. BROWN   Yes.

NURSE   Most mothers are anxious about that, especially the first time. But you must feel particularly anxious. I wonder why?

MRS. BROWN   (beginning to cry) Oh, I never do anything right. . . . It's like my mother-in-law always says . . . I can't even take care of myself properly. And now with a baby, how will I ever manage?

NURSE   You sometimes think of yourself as less able to manage than most women?

MRS. BROWN   Yes, I do.

Help the patient cope with the threat

The nurse suggests to Mrs. Brown that perhaps she has an exaggerated idea of her own incompetence. She helps Mrs. Brown to consider the possibility that perhaps her image of herself has been influenced by her

The nurse should encourage the patient to face anxiety and assist him in finding constructive ways to deal with it.

mother-in-law's attitude toward her, and that her mother-in-law may have some personal need to see her as incompetent.

The nurse emphasizes that all mothers are anxious about caring for their infants, that babies are really much more hardy than they look, and that as long as Mrs. Brown is concerned for her baby's welfare she probably will manage to care for the baby quite adequately. She refers Mrs. Brown to sources that will help her learn how to care for the baby.[8]

Even in routine nursing care, the nurse can indirectly allay anxiety by gentleness of touch and voice and by providing expert nursing care. She should treat each individual as a worthwhile adult human being, respecting his privacy and giving him the dignity he is entitled to.

Defense mechanisms

If we assume that all human behavior is purposeful and goal-directed, we can conclude that all human actions are the result of meaningful desires and motivations. Sometimes we are aware of our motives **(conscious motivation),** and sometimes we are not **(unconscious motivation).** Sometimes behavior is unpredictable or appears irrational. This is usually the result of a conflict within the personality between a wish and a contradictory desire.

Defense mechanisms are unconscious processes in which anxieties that result from these conflicts are prevented or relieved. They are intellectual techniques used to avoid pain—the pain of recognizing emotionally troublesome feelings. Defense mechanisms are not necessarily pathological. Whether they are constructive or destructive depends upon the extent to which they are used and the manner and circumstances of their use.

Following are some of the more common defense mechanisms. They are described not for the purpose of stereotyping human behavior but to point out the variety of ways in which human beings ordinarily defend themselves against psychological threats.

Repression is thought to be the primary defense against anxiety, and it may function alone or in conjunction with other defenses. It is the unconscious exclusion from awareness of unacceptable, inappropriate thoughts, memories, or impulses. If this exclusion is conscious, it is termed **suppression.** For example, a woman misidentifies a purse snatcher and causes him much embarrassment. She consciously attempts to forget the incident. Her conscious attempt to forget illustrates suppression; if her forgetting had been unconscious, it would have illustrated repression.[9]

Denial is the mind's way of completely disregarding a disturbing reality situation. For example, a woman who has given birth to a deformed infant may simply deny that she has had a baby at all.

[8] Anxiety—recognition and intervention, pp. 142–43.
[9] Peterson, p. 1656.

Displacement is the transference of emotional components from one idea, object, or situation to another more acceptable one. In other words, the feelings remain the same but are shifted to another focus. A young man who has been rejected by his girlfriend immediately "falls in love" with another eligible young woman. We say that he has shifted, or displaced, his feelings about the first young woman to the second.

Projection is the attribution of one's own ideas and impulses to another. This frees the person from any association with the action. A driver who crashes into the rear of another car stops at a traffic light, jumps out of the car, and shouts, "You stupid idiot, look what you've done to my car!" He has projected his own mistake onto the other driver.[10]

Rationalization is a way of justifying behavior by stating motives (usually with an element of truth) other than the genuine ones. It justifies decisions that are not necessarily rational or logical. A student may rationalize failure on a test by attributing the failure to poor teaching methods.

Conversion is the attempt to resolve conflicts and prevent anxiety by the development of physical symptoms in areas of the body controlled by the sensory-motor system. A soldier who is afraid of war discovers that his right arm (and the hand that holds a gun) is paralyzed.

Somatization also involves the body, but the symptoms are produced in organs or viscera (internal organs) controlled by the autonomic nervous system. Since this mechanism does not really alleviate anxiety, and because its symptoms are the physical components of anxiety, this is not truly a defense mechanism in the same sense as the others.

Reaction formation involves the denying of real feelings and behaving as if the opposite were true. It means "bending over backwards" to avoid acting on inappropriate or unacceptable impulses. A man who is petrified at the thought of meeting strangers attends a party and becomes the "life of the party"—laughing, dancing, and engaging the more retiring people in lively conversation.

In **compensation,** an individual, either consciously or unconsciously, makes up for real or imagined handicaps by succeeding in other areas of functioning. A young woman who is extremely shy attempts to make up for it by taking a course in public speaking to become proficient in speaking before groups.

Dissociation is the splitting off of one portion of consciousness from the rest. The tendency is to compartmentalize activities so that they remain separate from each other. A woman talks calmly of the terrible tortures she experienced in a concentration camp and shows no emotional expression. In this case, her feelings have been split off from the memories of the experience.

Identification is the unconscious modeling or patterning of the self after another person or group. A young girl begins dressing and speaking

---

[10]Ibid., p. 1658.

The nurse herself will experience anxiety in many stressful patient situations. . . .

very much like her older, but disliked, sister. (When done in a conscious way, this is called imitation or copying.)

Idealization is the overestimation and exaggeration of valuable attributes or qualities. A high school student comes home and describes her new history teacher as the perfect man having no faults or problems.

Sublimation is the channeling of strong urges such as hunger or aggression into constructive purposes. A young man with intense competitive and aggressive drives becomes the star of a national basketball team.

In **symbolization,** an object, idea, or act represents a complex of objects, ideas, or acts. Or, one of them may represent another through some aspect they have in common. In the first case, a flag may represent patriotism and love of country. In the second, a person associates the characteristic of firmness as typical of tall people, based on some earlier experience with one tall person who was quite firm.

Undoing is the attempt to cancel a painful feeling state. It negates previous behavior, and it may be the basis for magic or compulsive rituals.

All of these defense mechanisms (also called mental mechanisms or ego defense mechanisms) reflect the unconscious attempt to avoid awareness of conflict rather than to confront it and make realistic attempts at resolution. These mechanisms may be harmful because they attempt to bury or disguise conflicts. And if a conflict is not really resolved, it continues to influence behavior.

The nurse herself will experience anxiety in many stressful patient situations and will use some of these mechanisms to lower her anxiety. Nurses may idealize doctors, sublimate aggressive drives in unit management, rationalize poor nursing care, project feelings onto patients of similar age and background, or dissociate their feelings from memories of patient deaths. If the nurse recognizes this, she can understand what is *really* happening and can attempt to resolve the conflict by using a problem-solving approach.

Using the problem-solving approach to overcome defense mechanisms

As was pointed out in chapter 4, the problem-solving approach is a conscious, rational, and methodical process whereby one accurately assesses problems and seeks solutions. This approach minimizes the need to use defense mechanisms. Moreover, the decisions that are made by this conscious process are more open to reevaluation and inspection than unconsciously determined ones.

To review the problem-solving process:

1. The individual must accurately perceive the problem and its possible cause.

2. He then searches for a workable solution, evaluating the possible consequences of each alternative and choosing the most appropriate one.
3. Finally, he must test the effectiveness of the chosen solution.

The goal of the nurse is to translate the patient's defensive thinking into nondefensive, direct thinking.[11] But this is not to be done without offering the patient an acceptable substitute when interfering with a mechanism.

What is a crisis?

We progress in a more or less steady state through life, and then something unexpected turns up, something shocking, frightening, threatening, and disastrous—a **crisis.** A crisis creates tremendous emotional upheaval, disruption, disorganization, disequilibrium, and confusion. Solutions that worked for us in the past are no longer effective. Our existing repertoire of responses proves hopelessly inadequate for the problem. We are tense and frustrated. Anxiety increases and our coping powers decrease. We feel helpless and are completely unable either to escape the problem or to resolve it successfully.

Crises are generally of two types. First, there are the expected, maturational crises that occur at times of life change and development. For example, the 5-year-old's entrance to school may create a crisis—both for the parents and for the youngster. Adolescence is another time of expected crisis.

The second type is the unexpected, accidental crisis. This crisis may arise with the loss of a job or the loss of a body part. It is important to remember that a crisis can occur with any change, even when it is generally considered a happy event, e.g., the birth of a child or a personal achievement.

The onset of illness or physical trauma often creates a crisis—not only for the individual but for his family as well. On the other hand, illness may itself be precipitated by an emotional crisis, such as the death of a spouse, offspring, or sibling.[12] In one attitude study, investigators compiled a list of 43 life events which seemed to precede illness most often. Assigning an arbitrary value of 500 to the event of marriage, they asked 394 persons to rate each event in light of the following:

As you complete each of the remaining events, think to yourself, "Is this event indicative of more or less readjustment than marriage?" "Would the re-

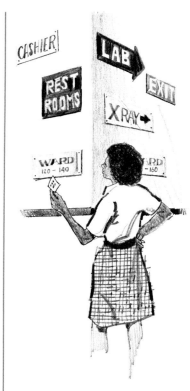

The onset of illness or physical trauma often creates a crisis—not only for the individual but for his family as well.

---

[11]Burgess and Lazare, p. 10.
[12]T. H. Holmes and M. Masuda. 1972. Psychosomatic syndrome. *Psychology Today,* April 1972, p. 106.

adjustment take longer or shorter to accomplish?" If you decide the readjustment is more intense and protracted, choose a *proportionately* larger number for the event. If you decide the readjustment required is less than marriage, then choose a *proportionately* smaller number for the event.

The results of the study showed that the three most stressful life events were death of spouse, divorce, and marital separation.[13] (A complete ranking of events is given in Table 8-2.)

Of course, listings such as these alone will not allow us to predict how an individual will react to any one occurrence. They do, however, provide us with guidelines for recognizing potential crisis situations.

Reactions to crises

A person's reaction to a crisis appears to depend largely on three major factors:

1. *His perception of the event as a crisis.* The same life situation may be a crisis for one individual and his family but not for another.
2. *His (and his family's) emotional resources.* Since an individual does not usually face a crisis completely alone, his family and friends will usually participate in the search for a solution. The individual tends to be more dependent on these personal relationships at a time of crisis. Those around him can either facilitate the search for a solution or add to the problem.
3. *His success in coping with similar problems in the past.* Some people have much to call upon at such times, while others "seem to have the dice so loaded against them by their idiosyncratic situation and experience" that no amount of assistance will help.[14]

What is crisis intervention?

The principle that should organize **crisis intervention** is the problem-solving process.[15] Its goal is to restore the person to his precrisis level of functioning or to improve his level of functioning once the crisis is past by teaching him more effective coping techniques. It begins in a logical way with an assessment of the person and the factors influencing his disequilibrium—usually through discussion in order to clarify the problem. The next step is planning specific therapeutic intervention. Can the nurse assist him alone, or is psychiatric referral indicated? What sources of support are available to the patient within his own family and circle of friends?

[13]Ibid.
[14]G. Caplan. 1964. *Principles of preventive psychiatry,* p. 30. New York: Basic Books.
[15]J. M. Hitchcock. 1973. Crisis intervention. *American Journal of Nursing* 73:1388.

TABLE 8-2
Social Readjustment Rating Scale

Rank	Life Event	Life Crisis Units	Rank	Life Event	Life Crisis Units
1	Death of spouse	100	23	Son or daughter leaving home	29
2	Divorce	73	24	Trouble with in-laws	29
3	Marital separation	65	25	Outstanding personal achievement	28
4	Jail term	63	26	Wife begins or stops work	26
5	Death of close family member	63	27	Begin or end school	26
6	Personal injury or illness	53	28	Change in living conditions	25
7	Marriage	50	29	Revision of personal habits	24
8	Fired at work	47	30	Trouble with boss	23
9	Marital reconciliation	45	31	Change in work hours or conditions	20
10	Retirement	45	32	Change in residence	20
11	Change in health of family member	44	33	Change in school	20
12	Pregnancy	40	34	Change in recreation	19
13	Sex difficulties	39	35	Change in church activities	19
14	Gain of new family member	39	36	Change in social activities	18
15	Business readjustment	39	37	Mortgage or loan less than $10,000	17
16	Change in financial state	38	38	Change in sleeping habits	16
17	Death of close friend	37	39	Change in number of family get-togethers	15
18	Change to different line of work	36	40	Change in eating habits	15
19	Change in number of arguments with spouse	35	41	Vacation	13
20	Mortgage over $10,000	31	42	Christmas	12
21	Foreclosure of mortgage or loan	30	43	Minor violations of the law	11
22	Change in responsibilities at work	29			

Nursing intervention can continue by drawing out the person's feelings about the crisis and by helping him to devise alternative solutions. Such solutions may involve changes in housing, employment, etc. Referral to community agencies may be necessary at this point if such solutions are to be realistic. Such changes alone may lessen the event's impact on the individual and help him to mobilize his own resources.

The final aspect of crisis intervention is evaluation and anticipatory planning. Is the plan of problem solving working? Has the person made plans for the future to resolve the crisis? Does he wish to help in dealing with other issues this crisis may have uncovered?[16]

When the crisis passes and the person's equilibrium is restored, hopefully he will be better equipped to deal effectively with future crises. At this time the individual may either be more mentally healthy or less mentally healthy than he was before the crisis, depending on the solution that has been reached. If a problem is evaded, rather than faced, it will continue to influence the individual and interfere with his psychological functioning.

Is the nurse sufficiently equipped to assist a person in crisis?

In many ways, nurses routinely function in the area of "advance" crisis intervention. Preoperative teaching of hospitalized patients is an example of such intervention. But when the person is already experiencing a crisis, the intervener's actual effectiveness stems from his own humanity combined with a positive attitude toward the strengths of the person in crisis. The responses that the intervener is called upon to make—activity, concern, action, and involvement—are all components of nursing. Since crisis intervention is not depth therapy but assistance in dealing with here-and-now issues, the nurse should be able to adequately work with the person in resolving the crisis in most cases. (Crisis intervention is sometimes called partnership in problem solving.) At a time of crisis, the usual problems of psychological resistance and motivation do not exist. A person in crisis is highly motivated toward change and new opportunities for growth. "Any nurse with warm feelings toward patients, ability to express her belief in another human being, and sufficient interest to learn simple steps can offer effective crisis intervention."[17]

The crisis of personal vulnerability

With repeated exposure to illness and death, the nursing student herself may experience a crisis of personal vulnerability when confronted with the obvious vulnerability of others around her. The manner in which she changes in response to these situations will profoundly affect her ability to respond to and care for ill, suffering, and dying human beings.

One good way to deal with such a crisis is to utilize the problem-solving approach previously described. If her reactions are not acknowledged and examined, the nursing student may attempt to deny or control

[16]Ibid.
[17]Ibid., p. 1390.

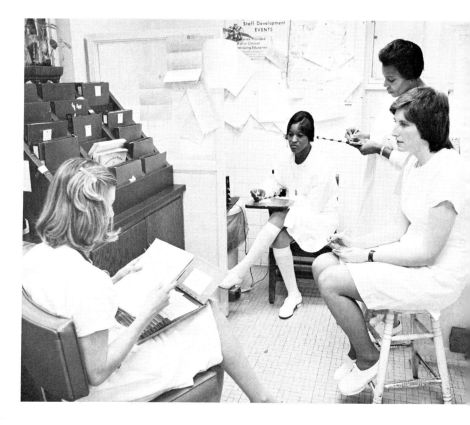

Conferences with other nurses can be of great value in working out problems with patients.

[Photo courtesy Medical College of Virginia, Virginia Commonwealth University]

her feelings. Such denial commonly results in anxiety and causes the nurse to withdraw. She becomes detached and indifferent. The nurse also may deny the importance of her feelings and handle anxiety by reacting to patients in a casual, facetious manner.

The nursing student can begin by discussing her reactions to the sick or dying patient with instructors, other nurses, and classmates. This will help her to clarify her feelings and understand what they mean in terms of her background, family expectations, and life experiences. Through these discussions she can realize more fully what it means to be human and that she shares this common humanity with every patient. An acceptance of her own humanity will facilitate the nurse's ability to reach out to others in a way not possible before.[18]

Stages of illness

The psychological impact of the illness experience is complex, but its progress is predictable and uniquely human. The "sick" person progresses through three main stages, each with its own particular behavioral patterns.

[18]J. Travelbee. 1971. *Interpersonal aspects of nursing,* 2d ed., p. 40. Philadelphia: Davis.

Transition

The first stage, that of **transition** from health to illness, is characterized by the onset of noticeable symptoms and signs. A variety of reactions follow. Some individuals attempt to convince themselves that they are really healthy through a flurry of activity—a "plunge into health."[19] Others minimize the importance of their symptoms. Some respond with aggressive anxiety (and become irascible, ill-humored, and querulous), while still others react with compliance and passivity. And not all react negatively to signs of impending illness.

Acceptance

When illness begins to develop, the individual eventually accepts the fact of illness. Then he becomes less concerned with others and the world around him and becomes more centered on himself. Day-to-day routines that previously provided some satisfaction prove painful and tiring. He is beginning the **acceptance** stage of illness. He abandons the pretense of health and assumes the sick role. He temporarily withdraws from the world of adult responsibilities, and society frees him of his ordinary obligations.

He becomes dependent, impatient, complains of minor irritations, and, in general, reverts to earlier ways of behaving **(regression).** And the more he regresses, the less interested he is in the outside world.

Some of these changes are illustrated in this excerpt from Leo Tolstoy's story, "The Death of Ivan Ilyich":

From the time of his visit to the doctor Ivan Ilyich's principal occupation became the exact observance of the doctor's prescriptions regarding hygiene and the taking of medicine, and watching the symptoms of his malady and the general functioning of his body. His chief interests came to be people's ailments and people's health.

The pain did not grow less but Ivan Ilyich made great efforts to force himself to believe that he was better. And he was able to deceive himself so long as nothing happened to excite him. But the moment there was any unpleasantness with his wife, or he suffered any rebuff in court or held bad cards at bridge he was at once acutely sensible of his illness.[20]

The world of the sick is simple and constricted. The patient is allowed to be childlike in behavior. Few demands are made. Although he may still have fears, he delegates some of his concerns to others. The behavioral features of this period are egocentricity, constriction of interests, emotional dependency, and hypochondriasis.

---

[19]Henry D. Lederer. 1952. How the sick view their world. *Journal of Social Issues* 8:5.
[20]Leo Tolstoy. 1960. The death of Ivan Ilyich. In *The Cossacks,* pp. 128–29. Baltimore: Penguin.

Convalescence

The third stage is either **convalescence** from illness to health, or death. (Dying and its nursing implications will be discussed in chapter 28.) The convalescent period begins when medical therapy has reversed or arrested the pathogenic process. It involves the return of physical strength and reintegration of a healthy personality. This means returning to maturity from feeling and thinking in a regressed way.

This is not always the easiest thing to do even though the patient is physically feeling much better. Many times the reintegration of social and psychological functioning lags behind the resolution of physical illness. The person has had a difficult time accepting illness and has just as hard a time accepting that he is well.[21]

This stage is in many ways similar to adolescence. The patient has conflicting desires. He wishes to remain within the comfortable environment where demands are few and self-satisfaction is a major concern. But he also desires to "grow up" and once again become a responsible, independent adult. He longs for health but is afraid of it.[22]

It is apparent that the stages of illness are similar to the stages of problem solving and crisis intervention. Illness proceeds from confusion and denial to understanding and acceptance. The illness (crisis) is resolved once an adequate solution has been found.

The nurse should expect regression in the early stages of sickness and not interpret demanding behavior personally. She should remember also the variety of meanings that sickness may have for various individuals (e.g., punishment, loss of masculinity, weakness, family shame).

In acceptance, once the patient has regressed to a degree, he may have fewer available psychological responses. Thus, he may react in a more stereotyped manner. He may see doctors and nurses as either omnipotent or as total incompetents. This also should not be taken personally.

When the patient has accepted his illness, there is the danger that he may become "stuck" in this stage. Nurses and doctors are comfortable with sick patients and may tend to keep treating them that way. If the patient's dependency needs were not well satisfied prior to his illness, he may need extra assistance to move out of the sick role.

Convalescence requires a program of graded challenges so that the patient is not overwhelmed and exhausted when he is just beginning to regain strength.

An essential element of recovery is hope. Nurses can convey this through their own attitudes about the patient in many ways. Without hope, patients are not able to utilize their remaining resources.

---

[21]H. W. Martin and A. J. Prange. 1962. The stages of illness—psychosocial approach. *Nursing Outlook* 10. In *Nursing fundamentals,* ed. Mary E. Meyers, p. 39. Dubuque, Iowa: Brown, 1967.

[22]Lederer, p. 14.

Problem patients

"Problem patients do exist, but it is the nurse's responsibility, not the patient's, to cope with and understand the difficulty."[23]

"Problem" patients are not those requiring complicated nursing procedures, but those unpredictable, demanding, complaining, intransigent, and uncooperative patients who arouse anger and exasperate the staff.

Nursing and medicine perhaps have a simplistic idea of illness. The staff usually assumes that the patient's values regarding illness are similar to their own. But, as we have seen in earlier discussions, this is not always the case. For example, the common reaction of health personnel to a relapsed alcoholic illustrates their simple solution to his problem: stop drinking. This ignores the complicated metabolic, psychological, and social processes involved in alcoholism.

Rejection of a patient who fails to subscribe to the medical treatment model is common. If it is the patient who has failed, the nurse can write him off her conscience.[24] Nurses often cannot accept patient unwillingness to follow instructions "for his own good." However, the assumption that patients can be taught obedience to a medical regimen is just unrealistic. The nurse needs to accept the fact that the patient may never adapt as she would like. She also needs to realize why such patients bother her so much: they inconvenience her and prevent her from functioning in the way she expects to function; that is, they frustrate her.

What happens when the nurse is frustrated? She may find herself very angry at the patient and attempt to coerce him into cooperation, or she may blame the hospital for not letting her function as she would like. Sometimes she blames herself for not being able to help her patient. She feels inadequate and incompetent. Carried to extremes, these reactions may prove harmful to the patient and to the nurse.[25]

The uncooperative patient

This is the patient who seems to willfully disobey medical orders. He cheats on his diet. He refuses medications and treatments. He gets out of bed when he is not allowed.[26]

How does the uncooperative patient affect the nurse? The uncooperative patient puts the nurse in a bad light. He demonstrates to others that she is unable to control her own patients. She is frustrated in her goal of helping him. He represents a threat to her authority as a nurse and as a representative of the system that says medical orders are "law."

Rejection of a patient who fails to subscribe to the medical treatment model is common.

[23]G. B. Ujhely. 1967. *The nurse and her "problem" patients*, p. 1. New York: Springer.
[24]M. E. Levine. 1970. The intransigent patient. *American Journal of Nursing* 70:2111.
[25]Ujhely, p. 8.
[26]Ibid., p. 30.

In order to deal effectively with the uncooperative patient, the nurse must first find out whether the patient's lack of cooperation disturbs her because of what it does to *her* or because of its consequences for *him*. Once she has a more realistic understanding of this process within herself, she can more easily (and less defensively) explore the problem with the patient. By working together they can come to some constructive conclusion about the problem.[27]

It is important to demonstrate to the patient that he is considered to be important and worthwhile.

The overly dependent patient

This patient seems to act more helpless than he really is, and nurses feel irritated when he refuses to help himself. Many times the nurse's anger at such patients can be traced to her own experiences and the part that such dependency and self-sufficiency played in her own upbringing. It is important that the nurse explore this part of herself if she finds that she becomes angry with and contemptuous of the dependent patient.[28]

One way to help the overly dependent patient is to accept him at his current level of functioning and support him in the dependency stage until he has enough strength to move ahead. It may only be a small move, but each additional step that is supported by the nurse will encourage further independence.

The demanding patient

Nurses frequently become angry when faced with complaining and demanding patients. This may be because the nurse does not expect to receive orders from anyone except doctors and supervisors. She expects that the patient will take orders from her. She does not expect that he will issue them.[29]

There are multiple explanations that can be given for the behavior of a demanding patient. One reason may be that he feels he is not receiving enough sympathy and recognition from other people. This often happens with patients who are hospitalized for long periods of time. For these patients the outside world has faded somewhat, and relations within the hospital world have become more important.

The nurse can help the demanding patient by responding to his underlying pleas for care and attention in addition to responding to his overt requests. Anticipating and meeting needs *before* the patient announces them can also be quite effective in reducing demands. It is important to demonstrate to the patient that he is considered to be important and worthwhile.

---

[27] Ibid., pp. 30–34.
[28] Ibid., p. 49.
[29] Ibid., p. 60.

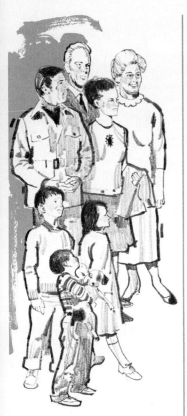

Where families exist in tight-knit groups . . .

Sociocultural factors and attitudes toward illness

As was discussed in chapter 1, when a person encounters the health system, he brings with him a lot of "baggage." This baggage is his life experience in a particular community, culture, and family that influences his attitudes and reactions to health and medical care.

These sociocultural influences are the customs and values of the cultural and social structure to which he belongs. They revolve around the expectations of behavior that a group places on an individual. They can be the major determinant of the way he perceives reality, and they modify his psychological and physical needs to fit a prescribed place in the social structure.

The family is the basic unit in most societies. The family socializes and orients the young to meet the major emotional needs of its members. It is a "closed corporation,"[30] and as such is only selectively open to outside influences. It may be more open to members of the extended family, friends, and neighbors than it is to medical professionals—although the family doctor often has high accessibility to the family. It is thought that the more open the community (such as the modern city), the more closed in form the family is likely to be. The more closed the community (such as an isolated rural community), the more open the family is to nonfamily members. And where families exist in tight-knit groups that resist intrusion, outside agencies may find it impossible to effect change.

The family is situated in some cultural matrix; that is, it identifies with some specific cultural or religious group. The beliefs and attitudes of that group determine what the health needs of its individual members are and what treatment is appropriate.

When the sick individual and his family are confronted by medical care, these cultural beliefs can negate, retard, or support the regimen that is prescribed by the health professional. Here are some examples of factors that may operate in particular cultures and influence the way health services are received.

Chinese culture

Chinese culture was evaluated by students at Russell Sage College during a course (in New York's Chinatown) entitled "Chinatown—Culture and Health."[31]

Close family and kin relationships were observed. When a family member is hospitalized, the Chinese family is in constant attendance. This is viewed as an essential family responsibility.

[30]R. Hill. 1958. Generic features of families under stress. *Social Casework* 39:33.
[31]R. M. Wang and L. Moore. Chinatown is the classroom. *American Journal of Nursing* 74:1113–14.

The Chinese people who were hospitalized seemed to accept Western medicine, but many of them employed Chinese and Western methods simultaneously.

The process of aging is accepted without distress. One student said: "The old men in Chinatown are not ashamed of being old and do not see any problems in it."

"The Chinese believe that good eating will promote virtue in body and mind and assure one's good health and fortune." Harmony is the principle involved in food selection—a balancing of opposites to achieve a harmonious whole.

Gypsy culture

Gypsy culture was studied by a team of nurses, sociologists, an anthropologist, and a medical student.[32]

The method of communication is word of mouth within the Gypsy culture and extends beyond the local community.

Medicines are seen as solely curative, not preventive. Thus, crisis care was used predominantly; prevention and follow-up were neglected.

Gypsy culture is highly family-centered and resistant to extrafamily intrusion.

Gypsies are wary of medical personnel and facilities; they change doctors as a result of unfavorable experiences or recommendations of fellow Gypsies.

Health is highly valued and many Gypsies were aggressively inquisitive about the health care being rendered to family members.

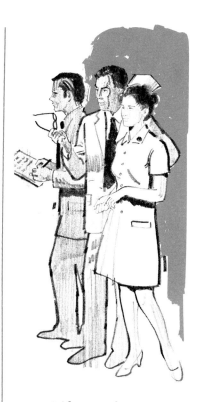

. . . outside agencies may find it impossible to effect change.

Puerto Rican culture

Puerto Rican culture was evaluated in an unsuccessful family planning program, and the conclusion was that the following cultural factors prevented women from securing family planning advice:[33]

Some men from the lower socioeconomic class in Puerto Rico object to their wives' using contraception because it undermines male authority. "They hold that control in the sexual sphere belongs exclusively to the husband."

The husband feels that if the wife controls conception, this will give her freedom to be unfaithful.

The most frequently cited objection is that birth control measures might impair health. Both men and women fear that birth control methods cause cancer and other dread diseases.

[32]G. Anderson and B. Tighe. 1973. Gypsy culture and health care. *American Journal of Nursing* 73:282–85.
[33]Benjamin D. Paul, ed. 1955. *Health, culture, and community*, pp. 196–98. New York: Russell Sage.

It is thus possible that sociocultural factors may prevent the acceptance of medical services. They may also interfere when a member of one sociocultural group plans services for a member of another group. In the health field, most program planners have middle-class backgrounds and values—definite plans towards goals, and mechanisms and motivations to achieve these goals.[34] What is planned by this class is very often at odds with the values of the group planned for, which is usually the lower economic classes.

It is known that all individuals evaluate advice given from the "outside" according to their own culturally conditioned understanding.[35] Health care innovations will be accepted only if they "fit" with existing patterns in the group. If new material is presented in ways that violate established patterns, it is likely to be rejected.

The nurse, who is also part of a class, culture, and program of professional "socialization," should remember several factors when implementing or planning care in situations where sociocultural differences exist:

1. Many persons (including the health professional) fear and suspect anything new.
2. Many suspect any program supported by the government. (Lower economic groups are inclined to view authority with suspicion and will seek their help only as a last resort.)
3. Religion may be a barrier to acceptance of a medical program.
4. Medical personnel are often unable to translate medical descriptions into instructions that are meaningful for the patient.
5. Health expectations differ between the population affected and the medical personnel involved.

Religion

Patients cannot be lumped into categories of religious beliefs by the religious denominations listed on their chart. The designations "Jewish," "Protestant," and "Roman Catholic" can mean anything from orthodox practice and profound belief in a particular faith to a nominal belief and a perfunctory belonging "in name only" to a religious group. A patient who states he has no religion may be a highly spiritual person.

This means that there are all kinds of beliefs and spiritual needs. With the sick person, these needs may arise more often than in ordinary circumstances. The spiritual person examines his current illness in a religious framework: What is the meaning of life? What is the meaning of sickness?

Patients cannot be lumped into categories of religious beliefs by the religious denominations listed on their charts.

[34]G. M. Foster. 1958. *Problems in intercultural health programs,* p. 230. New York: Park Avenue.

[35]M. C. Dougherty. 1972. A cultural approach to the nurse's role in health-care planning. *Nursing Forum* 11:313.

What is his relationship with a higher being? What does he want it to be? From where shall he draw strength in this time of stress? And for these patients, although physical care and emotional support are essential for their recovery, spiritual assistance may be what they need most.

The perceptive nurse, whether she is religious or not, can recognize requests from patients for spiritual help. Spiritual assistance is indicated:

1. Whenever a patient indicates his need by mentioning the subject casually, thus opening the door for discussion.
2. Whenever a patient who is able to cope with such discussion gives off emotional cues that the nurse recognizes as a request for spiritual help.
3. Whenever a patient who has indicated a belief is faced with a condition that has an undesirable outcome, e.g., amputation of a limb or other disfigurement.
4. Whenever a patient who is a believer is faced with a predicament that he cannot resolve—unemployment, alcoholism in a family member, or being sent to a nursing home.
5. Whenever an adolescent who is a believer is questioning his own self-confidence and ability to build a meaningful future.[36]

Some nurses, by virtue of their own beliefs, may be able to assist a patient in spiritual difficulty, but usually a referral is made to the appropriate spiritual adviser. Consultation with the appropriate clergyman may be quite helpful in planning the patient's care.

The Jewish patient

The Jewish patient who follows the dictates of his religion will have difficulties adjusting to many of the customs in a nonsectarian hospital or hospital of another affiliation. In many cases, the patient will prefer to enter a hospital affiliated with the Jewish religion.

In everyday matters, the patient will have special preferences in relation to food, Sabbath observances, fast days, and visitation by relatives.

Food. Customs regarding dietary restrictions are found in the Talmud (the authoritative body of Jewish tradition) and the Torah (the five books of Moses). These requirements allow the eating of only those animals that are ruminants (cud-chewing) and have divided hooves, and only fowl that are not birds of prey. Only fish that have both fins *and* scales may be eaten. Animals must be healthy and free of defects and must be slaughtered in a prescribed way and treated to remove all blood. Foods manufactured

Consultation with the appropriate clergyman may be quite helpful in planning the patient's care.

[36]R. Piepgras. 1968. The other dimension: Spiritual help. *American Journal of Nursing* 68:2612.

in accordance with Jewish dietary standards are then considered "kosher." The eating of meat and milk together is prohibited. (In the non-Jewish hospital, disposable utensils and dishes should be used because the non-disposable dishware has been previously used for nonkosher meats or fish.)

Sabbath. This is observed from Friday at sundown through Saturday evening. During this time the religious Jew may refuse to ride in a wheelchair, write, use the telephone, eat any freshly cooked food, or allow diagnostic tests or surgery. Holy days may impose other restrictions.

Visitation. An essential feature of Judaism is the religious duty of visiting the sick. Orthodox Judaism forbids the family of a person near death to leave his bedside. At this time, religious readings may be performed by family members and the rabbi. Allowances should be made in hospital visiting rules to provide for this.[37]

The Roman Catholic patient

Baptism. In emergency situations, the nurse, or any other person available, may be called upon to baptize a patient. It is required in the Roman Catholic faith that all persons (including products of conception) should be duly baptized prior to death or as close after death as possible. The patient may be an adult near death who is requesting baptism, or baptism may be requested for a dying infant. The procedure should be performed as follows: While pouring a small amount of plain water over the forehead of the person to be baptized, the nurse says, "I baptize you in the name of the Father, and of the Son, and of the Holy Spirit, Amen." This is all that is necessary, and even in emergency situations, it should only take a few moments. If the patient is an infant, the wishes of the parents regarding baptism should be respected, and when the baptism is performed, they should, of course, be informed.

Holy Communion. Regulations about fasting prior to Communion are relaxed for hospitalized patients, and necessary medications may be taken prior to receiving Communion. If a priest is distributing Communion, the nurse should inform the patient of the approximate time of his arrival, to allow time for spiritual reflection or to allow the patient to see the priest for Confession prior to receiving Communion. After Communion, allow the patient a few minutes alone, undisturbed by hospital routine. (This also applies to Protestant patients who receive Communion from their ministers.)

In modern hospitals it is usually impossible for work to cease while

---

[37]P. Berkowitz and N. S. Berkowitz. 1967. The Jewish patient in the hospital. *American Journal of Nursing* 67:2335–37.

Communion is being administered, but it is desirable that loud conversations and unnecessary noise be curtailed.[38]

The Protestant patient

It is especially difficult to make generalizations about "Protestant" patients since there are many denominations with varying customs. For Protestants of strict or fundamentalist sects, as well as for patients of other religions, there may be problems adjusting to the typical hospital routine and diet. There may also be people, such as Jehovah's Witnesses, whose religious beliefs prohibit medical or surgical care.

SUMMARY

Patients with physical illnesses have needs other than those for medical treatment and skilled technical nursing care. An individual enters the health system with an entire range of psychological, social, and emotional needs. If these factors are not taken into account when developing plans for care, the medical or nursing regimen may be hampered or totally disregarded.

Needs range from the most basic drives for food and water to sophisticated desires for productivity and creativity. When certain needs are frustrated or threatened, the human organism reacts in a variety of self-protective ways. These include psychological defense mechanisms as well as anxiety and panic reactions.

A change in an individual's life can precipitate a crisis—an overwhelming situation for which no easy solution can be found. This change can be the death of a spouse, sickness, or marital separation. The assistance of another person who helps find a solution and helps the patient return to a state of basic emotional equilibrium is called crisis intervention. The successful outcome of this experience can enable the individual to face future crises in more constructive ways.

The method that is used to find a crisis solution is the problem-solving method. It is a rational, step-by-step method for discovering and clarifying the cause of the crisis, finding acceptable solutions, and evaluating their effectiveness.

Sociocultural factors play a large part in determining behavior and attitudes about health, illness, and health services. In addition, religious beliefs can determine whether a medical treatment is effective or useless.

The stages of illness—transition, acceptance, and convalescence—progress from disorder to recovery in a way similar to crisis resolution. At each stage of illness, the patient has particular needs that the nurse must be aware of.

---

[38]J. W. Griffiths. 1971. The patient and holy communion. *Nursing Mirror* 132:18.

Patients become "problem patients" when they do not conform to hospital regulations and when they create inconvenience for the staff. Their demanding, uncooperative, overdependent, and intransigent behavior frustrates and angers the nursing staff. It is the nurse's responsibility to discover the reasons behind this persistent behavior—to find the patient's real need hiding behind his overt actions and to plan appropriate methods of intervening.

STUDY QUESTIONS

1. List man's basic needs as theorized by Abraham Maslow. Briefly define each need.
2. What is anxiety? How can the nurse recognize and help the anxious patient?
3. Define five common psychological defense mechanisms. Give examples of each.
4. What is a crisis? Describe a recent crisis of your own, the sources of support you found, and your resolution of the situation.
5. Referring to the chart on p. 165, add up your own score in life crisis units over the past 12 months.
6. With another classmate playing the role of the nurse, role-play the most difficult type of patient you can imagine (or the patient you would be most reluctant or afraid to care for). Analyze your own feelings as the patient and give possible reasons for your behavior.

SELECTED BIBLIOGRAPHY

Anxiety—recognition and intervention (programmed instruction). 1965. *American Journal of Nursing* 65:129–52.

Johnson, Mae M.; Davis, Mary Lou C.; and Bilitch, Mary Jo. 1970. *Problem-solving in nursing practice.* Dubuque, Iowa: Brown.

Martin, Harry W., and Prange, Arthur J. 1962. The stages of illness—psychosocial approach. *Nursing Outlook* 10. In *Nursing fundamentals,* ed. Mary E. Meyers, pp. 33–44. Dubuque, Iowa: Brown, 1967.

Maslow, Abraham H. 1970. *Motivation and personality,* 2d ed. New York: Harper & Row.

Peterson, Margaret H. 1972. Understanding defense mechanisms (programmed instruction). *American Journal of Nursing* 72:1651–74.

Ujhely, Gertrud B. 1963. *The nurse and her "problem" patients.* New York: Springer.

9 Nursing throughout the life cycle

A patient's age can be as important a guide to his special needs as the more obvious factors of health condition and cultural background. The nurse must be as aware of the range and complexity of distinctions between **infancy** and **adolescence** and **maturity** and **senescence** as of the differences between an accident victim and a child with a hearing disability.

The significance of age distinctions is most obvious in the patient's physical condition, but bodily change is only one aspect of the growth process. It is accompanied by a variety of other changes, notably those involving motor activity and emotional, intellectual, and social development.

Development

Maturation, the growth of bodily functions, progresses at a more or less steady pace in man as in all animals. **Development,** the growth of personality functions, is a progress by phases that occurs only in man. Man is the most adaptable creature ever to have evolved. He is unique in his ability to cope with his environment, changing it to suit his needs and modifying himself to survive its hazards. This adaptiveness is at the core of his ability to evolve intellectually and emotionally. It takes him beyond **instinct** into **cognition.**

Adaptability is not simply an inherited, individual quality; it is also a social one. It is made necessary by the expectations and restrictions society imposes upon the developing individual. It begins with the demands made by parents and family.

No development is possible in a cultural vacuum. The human-to-be cannot live without parental care, both physical and emotional. He cannot exist as a separate identity without a society to set boundaries, develop communications, and help him create a self-image. The search for identity that plays such a role in contemporary life arises in part from the gradual vanishing of the extended kinship family. This type of family provided

Upon completing this chapter, the reader should be able to:

1. Describe the relationship between age groupings and the individual's response to himself, illness, and the health care system.

2. Analyze each stage of development according to specific related theorists and/or human functions, such as psychological, physical, cognitive, sexual, and social.

3. Explain the need for mastery of the developmental tasks at each level before the individual can progress to the next stage of development.

4. Identify the specific developmental tasks and the related implication for nursing intervention within each of the six stages in the life cycle.

179

many possible definitions from which to formulate a self-definition. It is now being replaced by the isolated nuclear family, with only one or two parents against whom to measure identity.

Development through phases—the **epigenetic principle**—is the result of five primary circumstances:

1. Physical maturation
2. Expectations imposed by society
3. Time itself—as awareness of its passing affects the person
4. Development and decline of cognition
5. Internalization of parental characteristics[1]

The process of development has been categorized into stages according to a variety of approaches—physical, sexual, emotional, intellectual, social, and moral. The flaw found in too many of these systems is that they end with adolescence, as if no further human development were possible beyond that point. This is a legitimate stopping point in a cognitive system, such as that of Jean Piaget (see page 183). In this system, the final intellectual step of which man is presently capable—conceptualizing—first becomes possible in early adolescence. It is less valid in a consideration of man as a psychological and social, even sexual, creature.

The **psychosocial** development system of Erik Erikson (see page 182) takes the infant through maturity into old age. This system shows how development is an integral part of life, no matter what form it takes or at what age it takes place. According to Erikson, the cognizant human does not reach a peak and then stagnate during the remaining decades.

The concept of the developmental task

A phase of development is not a stopping point at which the individual is momentarily allowed to rest before being swept passively toward maturity, decline, and death. It is, rather, a point of balance accomplished as the individual moves into a new situation and learns to cope with its demands. Defenses, compensations, mastery techniques, and understandings may need to be created or strengthened. The self may even need to be redefined in terms of new roles.

Each phase includes its own **developmental tasks.** These tasks must be accomplished and the personality reoriented to accommodate them before further development is possible. No stage may be bypassed, since the overall movement is toward the achievement of an integrated identity that is the sum and resolution of each preparatory phase.

[1]Theodore Lidz. 1968. *The person: His development throughout the life cycle,* pp. 72–73. New York: Basic Books.

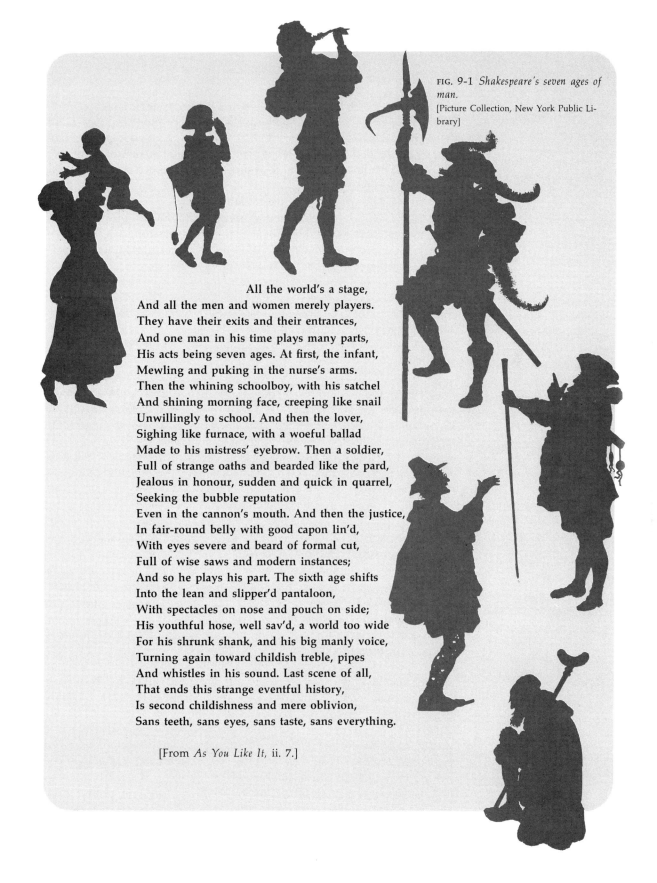

FIG. 9-1 *Shakespeare's seven ages of man.*
[Picture Collection, New York Public Library]

All the world's a stage,
And all the men and women merely players.
They have their exits and their entrances,
And one man in his time plays many parts,
His acts being seven ages. At first, the infant,
Mewling and puking in the nurse's arms.
Then the whining schoolboy, with his satchel
And shining morning face, creeping like snail
Unwillingly to school. And then the lover,
Sighing like furnace, with a woeful ballad
Made to his mistress' eyebrow. Then a soldier,
Full of strange oaths and bearded like the pard,
Jealous in honour, sudden and quick in quarrel,
Seeking the bubble reputation
Even in the cannon's mouth. And then the justice,
In fair-round belly with good capon lin'd,
With eyes severe and beard of formal cut,
Full of wise saws and modern instances;
And so he plays his part. The sixth age shifts
Into the lean and slipper'd pantaloon,
With spectacles on nose and pouch on side;
His youthful hose, well sav'd, a world too wide
For his shrunk shank, and his big manly voice,
Turning again toward childish treble, pipes
And whistles in his sound. Last scene of all,
That ends this strange eventful history,
Is second childishness and mere oblivion,
Sans teeth, sans eyes, sans taste, sans everything.

[From *As You Like It,* ii. 7.]

The rate of development is limited by the need for emotional security. Inability to handle a new situation can cause anxiety and frustration. Until these are overcome, the individual is not prepared to move ahead and face further challenges. Failure to cope with the developmental tasks of any given phase can result either in **fixation** at the unresolved stage or **regression** to an earlier one.

The task left undone, or less than satisfactorily accomplished, becomes a handicap to future development. A sense of frustration, of incompleteness, makes mastery of subsequent tasks more difficult and less satisfactory. This also means that the end result—the mature, integrated personality—will be harder, if not impossible, to achieve.

This is not to say that progress through any developmental phase can or ought to be easy. The very fact that these tasks are difficult to accomplish is a positive factor. The individual learns to be strong, to defend himself, and to survive.

Psychological development

Freud. Sigmund Freud theorized that there are five stages of **psychosexual** development between birth and maturity. These are the **oral, anal, phallic** (or **oedipal**), **latency,** and **genital** stages. His theory stresses the overriding importance of the early childhood years in the formation of the adult. As a result, the last of the five stages coincides with the onset of **puberty.** Achievement of this final stage, genital sexuality, he equated with emotional maturity.

Erikson. Upon this foundation, Erik Erikson has built his psychosocial theory of personality development.[2] He has expanded and extended Freud's basic ideas to cover the whole person as an individual seeking for his identity rather than as a sexual extension of the child he was. Erikson's psychosocial system will provide the framework for this chapter's discussion of the various kinds of developmental tasks and their implications for the nurse. His first five phases roughly parallel Freud's psychosexual stages; the final three are postadolescent. (See Fig. 9-2 for a brief overview of the eight stages of development.)

In each phase of psychosocial development, two extremes of attitude are present. In infancy, for example, the individual develops both basic trust and basic mistrust attitudes. He must find a way to strike a balance between them. This is not accomplished simply by learning a "good" quality and conquering a "bad" one. The negative aspects must also be present to allow the individual to function in society. A person who had developed only the basic trust attitude would lack some of the defenses needed to permit growth to final maturity.

[2]Erik H. Erikson. 1963. *Childhood and society*, 2d ed., pp. 247–74. New York: Norton.

Trust vs. mistrust (birth to about 1 year): The mother's reaction to the infant's needs helps to form this attitude.

Autonomy vs. shame, doubt (between 2 and 4 years): The child is pulled between his own newly discovered will and his need to remain dependent.

Initiative vs. guilt (about 4 and 5 years): The child's first real social (play) contacts bring him into contact with society's expectations.

Industry vs. inferiority (about 6 to 11 years): The child learns the difference between work and play and finds himself measured against his peers.

Identity vs. identity diffusion (about 12 to 18 years): The adolescent tries to define himself in terms of his peer group and the roles it and society expect of him; his newly sexual body must be reevaluated as part of his self-image.

Intimacy and solidarity vs. isolation (young adulthood): He tries to come to terms with the relationships expected of the mature individual—sexual, love, friendly, leadership, combative.

Generativity vs. stagnation (the middle years): The adult's concern moves toward the establishment and guiding of the next generation.

Integrity vs. despair (old age): The individual must either accept himself as he is and for what he has been or despair at what it is too late to change.

FIG. 9-2 *Erikson's eight stages of development.*

Most important, the developing individual is learning through extended social experience, not merely through coming to terms with his own body and those it relates to. As Sutterley and Donnelly summarize:

> The key concept in Erikson's psychosocial scheme is that of "identity." The developing individual pursues his identity throughout the life cycle as it is attained, maintained, lost, and regained through complex feedback processes as the individual interacts with significant "others" in multiple environments.[3]

Cognitive development

Piaget. A completely different, but equally important, theory of development is the cognitive approach of Jean Piaget.[4] This system makes little reference to emotional and social development and concentrates on the child's development of cognitive, or intellectual, capacities. These include intelligence, reasoning, language, and concepts of nature and of time, space, and causality.

Piaget outlines a very active process in which new experiences are continually being assimilated and used to reorganize and expand existing

---

[3]Doris C. Sutterley and Gloria F. Donnelly. 1973. *Perspectives in human development: Nursing throughout the life cycle,* p. 73. Philadelphia: Lippincott.

[4]A basic understanding of Piaget's theories is presented in Alfred L. Baldwin. 1967. *Theories of child development,* pp. 190–220. New York: Wiley.

FIG. 9-3 *Piaget's developmental stages.*

Sensorimotor (birth to 18/24 months): Preverbal intellectual development.

Preoperational (preschool): Development of ability to use symbols and language.

Concrete operations (prepuberty): Acquisition of a workable system for understanding and dealing with the world and using the experiences it provides.

Formal operations (beginning in early adolescence): Development of ability to conceptualize, to reason in abstractions. (Since formal education can play a part here, not all individuals necessarily reach this fourth stage.)

FIG. 9-3 *Piaget's developmental stages.*

capabilities. These, in turn, prepare the way for the individual to absorb increasingly complex experiences. The individual seeks to repeat the situations that produce new experiences until such time as they have been completely assimilated. Figure 9-3 outlines the major stages of development according to Piaget.

Paralleling this purely cognitive development, Piaget covers also what he calls the "decentering" process. This occurs as the **egocentric** infant learns, little by little, to move and think outside the framework of self. The end result of this process is for the individual to see himself objectively in relation to his world and time and their abstractions.

Motor development

The developmental systems outlined above cover the intellectual, **affective** (emotional), and social growth of the individual. They do not take into account his somatic (physical) development. Bodily development, too, can be broken down into a variety of subcategories. Among these are growth and **motor activity.**

As is true for the other systems, each age period has its motor tasks to accomplish before the child can move on to the next. An infant, for example, must learn to coordinate eye movements before he can learn to reach and grasp. The developmental span of the motor skills, however, is very short. A child starting school normally has acquired sufficient neuromuscular control to make possible the learning of any general skill he will ever be able to master. The degree of facility and strength will not be that of the adult, but the ability will be present.

From birth to roughly $6\frac{1}{2}$ years, the child must learn to handle the whole universe of his body and his senses. His eyes must learn to focus; his hands to grasp and release; and his arms and legs to help him roll over, sit up, crawl, and walk. Before he enters school, he will probably be able to ride a bicycle, throw overhand, print his name, and tie knots in his shoestrings. After that point, he is simply learning variations of skills already acquired.

The nurse's influence on the patient's growth and development

Today's nurse must be prepared to deal with all aspects of human life without exception, whether or not the patient is communicating directly about them. Especially important are her efforts to act calmly, constructively, and compassionately in situations where sex or death is involved.

Sex and death are, in a sense, the positive and negative forces that define the life cycle. They exist at any point along it. As a result, the nurse has to be as much aware of sexuality in the elderly as of the possibility of death for the infant. Man balances between these two forces throughout his life. At each stage of his development, the balance is different—and he is different. The nurse must act with the understanding that the 8-year-old girl who was in the hospital 5 years ago is not the same person when she returns at the age of 13.

The nurse's awareness of this special kind of difference and its effects on psychological and emotional health can be a significant factor in the effectiveness of patient care. It is not a solution simply to maintain an equal, impersonal regard for all. Aside from anything else, the nurse is a human being and as such belongs to a particular sex and age group. If the nurse giving a sponge bath happens to be a pretty young woman, it is unreasonable to expect the same response from a middle-aged man who fears losing his attractiveness to women and from a 15-year-old boy who feels he is about to die of embarrassment.

If the whole patient is to be helped, then the whole patient must be understood. He must be accepted in the context of not just his racial, religious, and ethnic group but also of his age group—his stage in the life cycle.

Infancy (birth to approximately 1½ years of age)

Infancy as a stage in the life cycle is distinguished from the following stage, childhood, by its characteristic of dependence. During most of infancy, the child is virtually helpless, dependent upon others to supply his primary needs. These needs include:

1. The adequate food and bodily care that keep him well and help him grow
2. The security that comes from a combination of affectionate attention and freedom from tensions he cannot handle
3. The stimulation of exposure to new experiences that forms the basis of his cognitive development

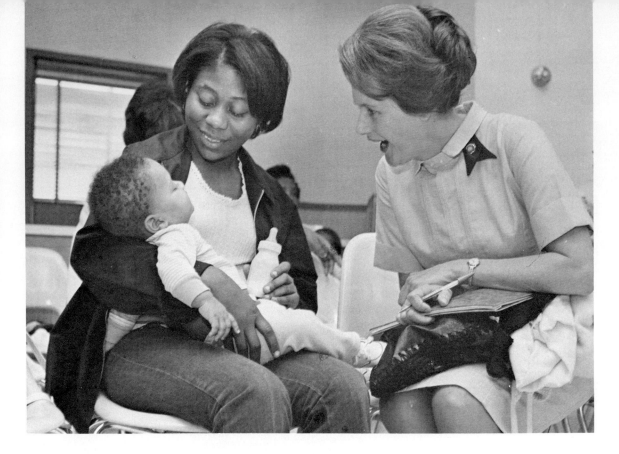

Developmental tasks

The various developmental areas are too closely related to make possible any division into sharply separate categories. Some cognitive activities are not possible until a certain stage of neurological growth is reached. Some social reactions are a direct result of sensory stimulation. The list given below, therefore, simply follows the normal progress from purely physical through the intellectual and into the psychological and social tasks. During infancy, the individual must learn to:

Stabilize newly independent physiological processes. The physiological system of the **neonate** (the newborn infant during his first few weeks) must adjust to the shock of birth. He must also adjust to operating independently, without help from his mother's surrounding, nourishing body. The infant does not even provide his own antibodies against illness until he first becomes ill, when he has used up the small reserve provided by his mother.

Develop control. Muscular development begins with the head (focusing the eyes) and extends past the shoulders and arms to the fingers. Coordination between eyes and movement develops by the end of the first year. The nervous system matures around the fifteenth month. This allows the infant to handle objects, talk, walk, and control his sphincter.

Learn to understand and control the physical world through exploration.
During his first month, the infant is capable only of reflexive action—
sucking, grasping, and eye movements. These earliest experiences are
involved with his own bodily sensations. The infant then moves on to
experiences involving his surroundings, often introducing new objects into
old patterns. He is moving out into a world that is separate from him,
a world that he can now affect by experimenting upon new objects with
old actions.

Begin to acquire language. The infant's birth cry is his first preverbal
communication. By about 6 months, he can sense the meaning of words
and phrases addressed to him by the intonation given them. By the time
he is ready to cross the line into childhood, he is learning to assign meaning
to a specific sound and getting ready to say his first word.

Establish himself as a separate entity. Not until the infant can be aware
of himself as a distinct person can he begin to establish relationships
outside himself. This awareness develops at about 7 months, when he
recognizes his mother as a being separate from himself. He also becomes
aware of how vital his mother's presence is to his security. Extended
separation from her results in reactions ranging from depression and crying
to extremes of apathy and withdrawal. It may even lead to retardation.
He may need to cling to his mother more than usual during this period
and should not be discouraged from doing so.

Develop independent emotional relationships with others. By the tenth
month, the infant usually is able to react with confidence to other familiar
people. Each increase in the circle of people to whom he can relate contributes to his social, intellectual, and emotional development.

Learn to trust. This is the significant first developmental task in Erikson's
psychosocial system. Failure to develop this trust may result in various
personality problems during later years. These problems range from pes-
simism, lack of self-confidence, bitterness, and antagonism, through withdrawal or dependency or bullying to pathological optimism or even schizophrenia. Trust in self cannot develop, however, without trust in others.

Parents create trust in the infant through the consistency and prompt-
ness of their response to his needs, not just by their demonstrations of
affection. Prompt answering of an infant's cry of distress, instead of spoiling
him, teaches him that he can always count on his needs being taken care
of. This confidence later enables him to learn to wait for satisfaction and
to develop a degree of patience and self-control. He can then do without
his mother for short periods of time without fear or anger.

Another factor that builds a child's trust is a healthy balance between
freedom and discipline. There is security in the consistency of firm but

By listening attentively and uncritically, the nurse creates an atmosphere of encouragement and understanding.

pleasant restraints. The infant must also have the freedom to explore and exercise.

Sensory stimulation and sexuality

One especially important effect of the mother's expression of affection is its sensory stimulation of the infant. His use of his senses—responding to his mother's rocking, cuddling, talking, etc.—prepares him for later intellectual development. Lack of such stimulation can lead to impaired body-image and ego development. This stimulation, or lack of it, also plays a significant part in the development of sexuality.

In infancy, one of the first experiences of a sexual nature is the quality of the mother's touching and handling as she responds to the infant's clinging and searching. If these experiences are warm and consistent, the child will learn to be comfortable with his body and regard it as a source of pleasure. If this experience is harsh or disorganized, he may not find this pleasure. This may drastically reduce his ability either to give or receive pleasure in later years.

Implications for nursing

One of the nurse's first responsibilities is to understand two basic kinds of information. She must be aware of (1) normal behavior and developmental tasks for the infant and the mother, and (2) the mother's background and how it will affect the mother and her response to the infant. It is important to realize that the patient here is not just the infant, but the infant/mother or infant/parents unit. Having adequate information about the family will prevent the nurse from offering useless and often resented advice. For example, the nurse would not tell a working mother to take a nap every afternoon.

The mother in particular may have to play several conflicting roles in her daily life. If she cannot coordinate them, she may find it difficult to relate to the infant, who is the symbol of a new conflict. She may be upset to find that her maternal instincts are not as strong as she has been taught to believe they should be. The mother of a sick infant may exhibit an unconscious feeling of guilt through a misleading display of anger toward the child.

By listening attentively and uncritically, the nurse creates an atmosphere of encouragement and understanding. The mother must know that she can talk to the nurse, that her questions and problems are important. The nurse who scolds or cuts off an anxious mother with a "Cheer up" or "Let us worry about that" is telling the mother she is not competent to care for her child. Parents are also helped to gain self-confidence by hearing praise for their new baby and having his progress pointed out to them.

Some mothers are ready to take over caring for their new infant sooner than others, and each must be allowed to set her own pace. The nurse should also avoid imposing her personal beliefs in such matters as, for example, breast-feeding vs. bottle-feeding. Once all available information has been offered, the nurse's responsibility is to help the mother make her own decisions.

The father should also be encouraged in his new role. He or some other close person should become familiar to the infant as a mother substitute. In this way, the mother can occasionally get away without the infant feeling a loss of security.

The sick infant is benefited by his mother's presence, especially during treatment that causes pain or discomfort. The nurse should also find out about familiar routines, foods, toys, names of brothers and sisters, or pets. All of this information can be used to lessen the infant's feeling of loss of security. If possible, the initial contacts with the infant should be made in the mother's presence.

Childhood (approximately 1½ to 9 years of age)

> The childhood years are a time of extraordinary intellectual and physical activity.

The childhood years are a time of extraordinary intellectual and physical activity. Bodily growth slows down as nourishment is increasingly converted into the fuel needed to sustain this activity. Physically, the child develops from a **biped,** only newly able to grasp things and stand erect, into a tool user with sufficient neuromuscular coordination to acquire many skills. Intellectually, he performs incredible feats in these few years. He acquires symbols and concepts of language, numbers, physical and social reality, and even ethical values. His need to learn during this period is insatiable. Psychologically, the child develops from a helpless, egocentric little animal into an independent, reasonable, social being.

Developmental tasks

Develop the neuromuscular skills needed for socialization. Neither the child's bodily control nor his understanding of his own capabilities is at first able to cope with his activeness. Play becomes the means of developing the strength, skill, and understanding needed to enable him to explore his world and learn from it. Because children have no sense of what is dangerous, they need constant supervision. Accidents are the leading cause of death in 2- to 4-year-olds.[5]

Develop improved cognitive capacities. At the beginning of this period, the child's intellectual and verbal abilities lag far behind his motor devel-

[5] Alice L. Price. 1965. *The art, science, and spirit of nursing,* p. 103. Philadelphia: Saunders.

opment. Now, however, his extraordinary need to learn pushes him ahead at a speed he will never again achieve. He learns to organize his sensations and build them into perceptions. He moves from the very beginning of symbol use to the ability to extract and organize general concepts.

Language is his means of expressing his symbolic and conceptual understandings. He learns that differences in sounds are significant and useful. Soon he can assign a specific meaning to a specific sound and join words together. He talks incessantly and acquires a vital trust in the reliability of verbal communication.

Develop self-acceptance and self-trust. The child's sense of satisfaction with his ability to meet the demands made upon him encourages him to trust his ability to meet future demands. He eventually discovers the rational purposes behind long-accepted, unquestioned parental directives (for health care, for example). He compares his behavior with that of other children and gains the confidence he needs to be free to express and assert himself in relations with them.

Learn the appropriate sex role. During the critical period between 18 months and the third or fourth year, the child learns to identify with a parent of the same sex. He also acquires the goals expected of that sex.

It is natural for the child to be interested in the differences between the sexes and where babies come from. The manner of the parents' answer, even more than the information they give, will influence the child's future attitudes. Above all, answers to questions and reactions to situations must be calm and accepting.

Establish autonomy. The toddler must be encouraged to develop a sense of his own ability to control himself and deal with his environment. His own orientation now expands from the self-centered to the world-centered. His ability to be concerned about the feelings of others slowly develops at the same time. Through identification with his peers and his perception of himself as a person separate from home and mother, he finally achieves independence. Failure to achieve this independence, which is the second stage of Erikson's cycle, can lead to a sense of shame or doubt.

Establish a sense of initiative and develop a conscience. The child who has a certain amount of faith in himself is now ready to act on his own initiative and adapt to new situations.

Fantasy plays a large part in the child's life at this point. The preschooler often will have difficulty in separating his fantasy from reality. His first efforts to achieve new tasks often are acted out in fantasy. His imagined success encourages him to make a genuine effort.

His fantasy life, as it extends into his sexual life, brings developing oedipal conflicts into sharp focus. He resents the parent of his own sex, seeing him as a rival for the affections of the other parent. His fantasies toward both parents create feelings of guilt. His mastery of these basic psychological impulses forms the core of his emerging conscience. His resentment toward the same-sex parent is replaced by the desire to be like him and retain the affection of the other parent in this more acceptable manner. The personality integration reached at the end of this period strengthens the child to meet the emotional demands of puberty.

This conflict of initiative vs. guilt is the third stage in Erikson's system of development.

Establish a sense of industry and adapt to the world of peers. Erikson's fourth stage, the conflict of industry vs. inferiority, crosses the border between childhood and adolescence, covering the sixth through twelfth years. This is the stage in which the child develops a sense of competence.

The idea of industry is a fairly specific one. At this stage, the child needs to know about things. He wants to know how they work, how they are made, and what they do. It is important that he succeed in dealing both with things and with his peers. Failure to gain a sense of industry may leave him with a lasting sense of inferiority.

As he grows closer to his peers, he becomes gang-oriented. He develops a concern for his friends' welfare that he cannot yet feel for adults. At one and the same time, he is ready to cooperate with his peers in work and to compete with them.

Implications for nursing

The nurse must realize that the child's imagination is still far ahead of his reasoning ability and his emotional control. He must be given a strong sense of security and reasoned reassurance. "Everything will be just fine" is not enough. He needs to be told—clearly, confidently, and truthfully—just what is to happen. When possible, he should be shown instruments, pill containers, tongue depressors, and so on, and allowed to play with them. What he imagines they can do to him may be much worse than the truth.

Emotional reactions need to be handled understandingly. The child often blames himself for his illness. Perhaps his mother once said, "If you don't eat your cereal, you'll get sick," and here he is in the hospital. Or he may feel he is being punished for being angry at one of his parents. He may have a very real fear of death. He should be encouraged to express himself, both to make clear what is troubling him and so that he can get rid of his fear or hostility by acting it out. Puppets are useful in stimulating this kind of expression.

The child's anxieties are heightened by the strangeness of his surroundings. He may never have been served a meal in bed before. Every effort should be made to keep his daily routine consistent and familiar.

The hospitalized child does not lose the need for exposure to new experiences.

He will be reassured by having his own clothing to wear, and the more colorful the better. The toddler is most secure when cared for by only one or two people. If it is not possible to arrange for a parent to live in, parents should understand how vital it is that their visits be as regular as possible. The child should know exactly when to expect them in terms of his routine. He needs to know that his mother will always come just before lunch or just after his favorite television program. When visiting time is over, the parent should leave quickly, but the nurse should stay on for at least a few minutes.

The hospitalized child does not lose the need for exposure to new experiences. Skill-building toys and activities and safe play areas, if the child is ambulatory, should be provided. The older child may be encouraged to collect something.

Adolescence (approximately 9 to 18 years of age)

The years between childhood and adulthood are those in which the individual attains his full physical and sexual growth. During this period, he makes his first approach to psychological and ethical maturity. The **adolescent** survives an upsurge of sexual pressures that thoroughly disrupt the pattern of his life. The resulting personality dislocations can keep him and his parents in a state of emotional turmoil for several years. Eventually, however, the dependent child, with his unshaped future, develops into a responsible, independent individual. He now has a coherent identity and a plan for his life.

Developmental tasks

Attain physical maturity. The upsurge in growth that marks the onset of puberty usually occurs at around 10 or 11 in girls and 12 or 13 in boys. For the boy, bodily growth and development of the sexual organs extend over some 4 years. These are virtually complete before the final appearance of full body hair and beard and the deepening of his voice. The girl progresses more rapidly from the development of her breasts and the growth of pubic hair to the **menarche** (the initial menstruation).

Develop the ability to use logic and abstract concepts. The adolescent's intellectual development is basically more a change in kind than an increase in capability. He learns to use both logic and imagination in his reasoning. For the first time, he is capable of making logical use of nonreality. He can, for example, imagine the existence of a thousand-mile-an-hour train if necessary to solve a problem in mathematics.

He learns to evaluate the quality of his own thinking and to think objectively about himself and how his decisions will affect his future. He learns also to see himself and his family and their values in the broader context of society and its values.

Reorganize the superego for independent functioning. The adolescent, moving into society, becomes interested in ideals and ideologies and begins to apply them in evaluating his own behavior. The **superego** (the operating conscience) acquires new functions. The adolescent now moves from outer-imposed discipline to self-discipline, and his sexual impulses are redirected. His superego now is further modified by the incorporation of the adolescent's new ego ideals and his acceptance of society's frequently arbitrary standards.

Achieve new ego identity. In a sense, this task is a culmination of the others. It is the task of Erikson's fifth stage, identity vs. role confusion. While his earlier stages involved reorganization of the personality, this stage is one of reintegration. The achievement of ego identity involves the forming of new relationships and the consolidating and strengthening of the sex role. Independence is achieved, and the individual prepares for the sharing of intimacy and the choice of a career.

The alternative to the achievement of **ego identity** is **role confusion.** The adolescent who overidentifies with his gang may be using this in place of the career he cannot decide upon.

Implications for nursing

Much of the approach to the child is still valid in dealing with the adolescent. Needed are patience and acceptance, honesty, empathy, and appreciation of his strengths. Questions should be encouraged and answered clearly, bearing in mind that there may be some questions the patient is embarrassed to ask. The outward appearance of physical maturity frequently covers a surprising ignorance about the human body, especially where sexual matters are concerned. It should be made clear that discussions with the nurse are in confidence. If the adolescent is told ahead of time about any special problems connected with his condition, he will be better prepared to cope with and accept them. He will be most responsive when treated as an individual, mature person and when he understands all necessary routines and rules.

A nurse of any age should keep in mind that an adolescent needs a stable, supporting professional, not a buddy. Personnel of nearly the same age sometimes tend to identify too closely and uncritically with adolescent patients.

Rebellion is to be expected, as are negativism, criticism, and frustration at enforced bed rest. Rebellion is often a sign of anxiety and probably represents an identification of hospital rules with parental authority. The anxious adolescent may also regress. The nurse needs to discover what

Rebellion is often a sign of anxiety and probably represents an identification of hospital rules with parental authority.

fears he is hiding. These can range from unadmitted homesickness to fear of pain and the unknown. The adolescent may be embarrassed at frequent examinations and physical procedures. He may fear losing body control under anesthesia or the possible results of surgery. Appearance is very important. The hospitalized adolescent may be more worried about overweight or acne than his medical condition.

Arrangements should be made to provide as much independence and physical activity as possible. Visits with other teen-agers, group activities, and opportunities to plan his own routine are all important to his self-esteem. Food is also important, as it symbolizes security and affection, not just nutrition.

Plans for continuing education should be discussed in cases of long-term confinement. The student who feels he is losing ground scholastically has to cope with an extra, unneeded load of strain, anxiety, and loss of self-confidence.

Young adulthood (approximately 18 to 30 years of age)

These are the years of full physical and mental vigor. Bodily growth will have ceased sometime between 18 and 20, and regressive physiological changes will not begin until around 30. The **young adult** now finds himself at the point of selectiveness. His capacity for intimacy comes to focus on one person, and career possibilities are narrowed down to a final choice.

This is the time of Erikson's sixth stage, intimacy vs. isolation. This stage is primarily concerned with the developmental task of choosing a mate. It is also relevant to the task of choosing a career, since inability to work with others is as isolating as inability to form a one-to-one relationship. The choices of an occupation and a mate arise out of a wide variety of psychological factors. These two choices are the primary shapers of the pattern of the years that follow.

Developmental tasks

Choose a career. There are four kinds of traits that shape career choice:

1. Genetic (the tone-deaf are unlikely to be drawn to music)
2. Psychosocial (an anal type of person is often attracted to meticulous fields, such as accounting)
3. Personality (the extrovert is drawn more to people-oriented fields, such as sales)
4. Intelligence

In choosing a career, the young adult finds himself choosing a way of life as well. Certain traits he brings to his job will be developed or reinforced. Social roles and patterns will be imposed and his status in the community will be determined. His ethical standards will be influenced by contacts with his co-workers. Even his physical environment will be determined by his choice of career.

There is still a tendency for women, except highly educated ones, to look for jobs that are supportive in nature. Work itself is apt to be divided into the period before marriage and that after the children are grown. This pattern is slowly changing, however. Women are moving more and more into previously male dominated areas. There is also less of a tendency for them to think of the home as the only significant career.

Choose a mate. Both sexual and emotional drives push the young adult toward marriage, or whatever equivalent serves the same purpose for him. Social pressure and the desire for children also play their part.

The young adult will be drawn to one particular mate by a wide range of factors. Most of these are the result of his development within a family structure. The classic factor in choosing a mate is the recognition that the other person possesses traits also found in the parental love model. Personal attraction must be present and is often influenced by the judgments of others.

The need for love is not the only factor that can compel an individual to marry. Also vital may be the need for sexual outlet, status, security, children, companionship, or even escape from parents.

Form a coherent personal ethical structure. In adapting to the needs of a marital partner and those of employers and co-workers, the young adult must move outward from his own ego center. Value judgments now can be made on the basis of both social and ideological standards. The individual has learned what society expects of him and what he expects of himself. He also has learned to accept the fact that, although society's rules are not always reasonable, they are necessary to keep society functioning. This tolerance extends to individual people as well. Being able to accept others' capabilities and limitations realistically, the young adult is less apt to be hurt or disillusioned by their behavior.

Implications for nursing

The young adult needs to find in the nurse the same qualities of acceptance, encouragement, and empathy that the adolescent does. Clear explanations about medical and surgical procedures he will undergo are important to his peace of mind. Worries can range from concerns about constipation to fear of death. Loneliness and loss of self-confidence are to be expected. Also common is anxiety about business and household matters, and about the cost of health care itself. Possible change in body-image is a special cause for alarm.

A great variety of anxieties and emotional problems express themselves in the form of migraine headaches, changes in gastrointestinal functions, backache, etc. An abnormally high or low anxiety level may be a sign of exaggerated emotional reactions to follow.

The patient should retain all possible independence and should participate in the planning of his own routine. A hospital is less depersonalizing if he has some of his own belongings around him. Unnecessary assaults upon his dignity should be avoided. His sense of helplessness may be increased by the nurse who presumes to call him by his first name or an artificial endearment without having been asked to. Where advisable, his environment should be kept free from pressure, and he should be encouraged to be active and to socialize with other patients. A careful choice of roommates can be of real value here. A sense of continuity with family should be maintained with the help of a regular visiting pattern. Family members should understand clearly what the situation is and how they can contribute usefully.

This age group has its own questions about sexual matters. These are apt to center around what their expectations should be of their own performance. The nurse should be able to answer all such questions frankly and informatively.

Middle years (approximately 30 to 60 years of age)

The "over-the-hill" years have been turning into the "prime-of-life" years during the last few decades, thanks to better nutrition and improved health awareness. Currently, four out of five American adults live to be 60, and the age of the average worker is 45.

These are the years that see the children leave home and the parents seek new means of fulfillment. They are years of assessment and adjustment. Bodily processes usually will not slow down perceptibly until the second half of the period and the intelligence remains unimpaired. Successfully traveled, these are the years of fulfillment.

Developmental tasks

Invest in a new generation. Erikson's seventh stage, **generativity,** is the desire to establish and guide a new generation, to create something worthwhile and lasting. Having children is not the only way in which the urge toward generativity can be fulfilled. This urge may express itself in other areas in the form of creativity or productivity. The individual then finds satisfaction through recognition in work.

Failure to achieve generativity results in stagnation and is characterized by a sense of impoverishment or boredom. The stagnating adult tends to

Successfully traveled, the middle years are the years of fulfillment.

regress to a point where he himself acts like a child. He turns inward and becomes absorbed in himself. Such self-concern often expresses itself in the form of early invalidism. This invalidism may be either physical or psychological.

Adjust to the circumstances of middle age. Middle age requires adjustments in many areas: the body, marriage, sex life, career, leisure patterns. These adjustments can be helped by feelings of dignity and respect. Also important are contacts with other members of the same age group. The process of adjustment must also take into account basic physiological, psychological, social, and aesthetic needs.

The particular crises of the middle years are the end of child-raising responsibilities and retirement from a job. Such crises need not necessarily be destructive. They can provide the individual with the opportunity to redirect his life.

Reevaluate life's accomplishments and goals. This may be the most difficult task of all. It requires total honesty with oneself and the ability to give up dreams that may have been a lifetime in the making.

During this period, the adult comes to realize that his life is half over. He sees that some goals toward which he has worked for many years are not obtainable in the time remaining to him. He may have to give up hopes of fame, wealth, romance, and high adventures. If his ego functions maturely, he will be able to adjust his self-concept to match his actual self. He will be able to modify his goals to correspond with what he can actually accomplish. These can be satisfying years if the individual has previously set realistic goals and has not expected more of himself or life than can be provided.

Implications for nursing

The middle-aged patient is treated as is the young adult, with only those differences that result from the nurse's awareness of his special needs and concerns.

The danger of loss of self-esteem is of particular concern for members of this age group. The middle-aged adult already feels threatened by actual or possible loss of physical power and attractiveness. The additional threat posed by one of the illnesses common at this period (cardiovascular disease, cancer, diabetes, etc.) can send him into severe depression. It can also cause him to make dangerous demands upon his physical reserves in an attempt to deny the aging process.

Sexuality is an additional source of anxiety. The individual may fear the permanence of diabetes-caused impotence. He may feel that his heart attack will prevent him from enjoying a normal sex life. The menopause may leave a woman feeling elderly and empty. If an illness or accident

Middle age requires adjustments in many areas: the body, marriage, sex life, career, leisure patterns.

leaves the individual with any kind of handicap, he may feel that his role and status in his family, work, and community will be diminished. The nurse can help the patient make the necessary adjustments by providing information about rehabilitation, job training, economic help, self-care, and so on.

The patient's hospital life should be as normal as possible. He should have the opportunity for socializing and for interesting activities in addition to recreational therapy. Newspapers and regular family visits can help him feel less isolated from the rest of the world. Moderate physical activity should be encouraged when possible. Care should be taken not to let the patient get too involved in activities that are difficult to accomplish before becoming overtired.

An important part of the nurse's task is to educate the patient in preventive measures. Routine medical, dental, and eye examinations; tests for cancer and diabetes; and rectal and gynecological checks should be encouraged. He should know the value of moderate physical activity and should be shown techniques for tension reduction. Erect posture, weight watching, proper dental care, and the need for moderation (if not abstinence) in smoking and drinking should also be stressed. He needs help in setting goals that are realistic in terms of his physical ability.

Old age (approximately 60 years of age to death)

Whether the declining years are bleak or golden depends upon a combination of factors. These include personality development, physiological heredity, and the expectations of society. This period is marked by the need to cope with retirement, lessened physical ability, and the prospect of death. The individual may have to adjust to life without a familiar partner and with increasing dependency upon others. He must find a way to accept life as it has been, without bitterness or despair.

The U.S. Census Bureau has estimated that by 1980 there will be some 25 million people over 65 in the United States.[6] Interestingly, those who survive into old age tend to have the hardiness to survive even longer. At 65, an individual may anticipate another 12 years of life. At 80, he still finds 10 years before him. As he grows older, his body's decline seems to slow down.[7]

Theodore Lidz has separated this period into three parts: **elderly, senescent,** and **senile.** These correspond roughly to **independence, de-**

[6]United States Bureau of the Census. 1962. Current population reports, series 25, no. 241. Interim revised projections of the population of the United States by age and sex, 1965 and 1970. Washington, D.C.: U.S. Government Printing Office. In Lidz, p. 490.
[7]Lidz, p. 477.

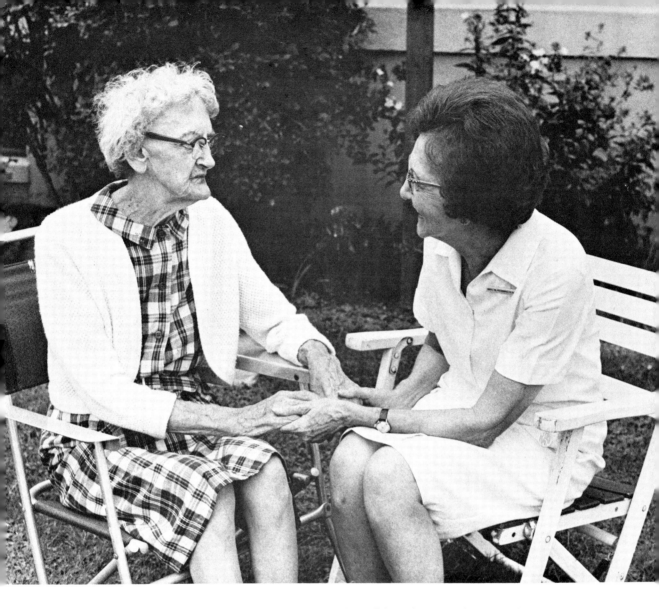

pendence, and **second childhood.** He points out that although some individuals become senescent, even senile, by 65, others are still clear-minded and independent at 90.[8]

Developmental tasks

Accept life with serenity. The culmination of Erikson's seven stages is this final phase, in which the individual emerges with either ego identity or despair. The fulfilled ego is a caring, adapting, generative one. It knows its own worth and recognizes the integrity of other egos. It has a sense of kinship with the whole of life.

[8]Ibid., pp. 478, 486.

FIG. 9-4 *Developmental tasks throughout the life cycle.*

Infancy (birth to 1½ years)
Stabilize newly independent physio-
    logical processes
Develop control
Learn to understand and control the
    physical world through exploration
Begin to acquire language
Establish himself as a separate entity
Develop independent emotional rela-
    tionships with others
Learn to trust

Childhood (1½ to 9 years)
Develop the neuromuscular skills
    needed for socialization
Develop improved cognitive capaci-
    ties
Develop self-acceptance and self-
    trust
Learn the appropriate sex role
Establish autonomy
Establish a sense of initiative and de-
    velop a conscience
Establish a sense of industry and
    adapt to the world of peers

Adolescence (9 to 18 years)
Attain physical maturity
Develop the ability to use logic and
    abstract concepts
Reorganize the superego for inde-
    pendent functioning
Achieve new ego identity

Young adulthood (18 to 30 years)
Choose a career
Choose a mate
Form a coherent personal ethical
    structure

Middle years (30 to 60 years)
Invest in a new generation
Adjust to the circumstances of middle
    age
Reevaluate life's accomplishments
    and goals

Old age (60 years to death)
Accept life with serenity
Adjust to new limitations
Adjust to retirement
Adjust to reorganized family patterns
Accept death with serenity

FIG. 9-4 *Developmental tasks throughout the life cycle.*

The self-accepting ego is not afraid to follow another's leadership because it is not afraid to trust. The final expression of this trust is the ability to accept death. The individual who has not achieved an integrated ego fears death. In some sense, the achievement of this trust brings the individual full circle back to Erikson's first stage.

Adjust to new limitations. As the physical state of the body declines, intellectual capacity may also be lessened. At this point, society tends to impose its own limitations upon the elderly person.

Pride and confidence may lessen as a result of the decrease in physical strength. Ego control may fade along with the ability to conceptualize. A decline in the energy level may make new situations more difficult to deal with, but adjustment to change is far from impossible.

Only now is society learning that its old people need dignity and security as much as health care assistance. Eyeglasses, dentures, hearing aids, and nursing homes cannot help the person whose spirit is being torn down faster than his body can be built up.

Adjust to retirement. Retirement may be greeted with a variety of emotions—a sense of accomplishment, relief, or resentment. Its arrival throws the once-busy person back on his own resources with many hours to fill. He needs a new focus for his life, but will probably find himself with less money with which to create new interests or expand old ones. This can be a period for enjoying things for which there was never time before. The person who cannot develop outside interests frequently concentrates on his bodily condition. His health becomes all-important. Many of his medical complaints are actually the result of his loneliness and feeling that he is being neglected.

The person in old age needs to find absorbing and worthwhile interests. He should also have an organized schedule to provide a shape to his days. Ideally, he will be able to use this time to develop new ties of friendship with his peers.

Adjust to reorganized family patterns. Advancing years frequently pose a double threat. The death of the spouse can be like losing a part of the self. In addition, it is often accompanied by the need to move to an environment where the survivor can be cared for. This often represents a loss of both independence and dignity.

Approximately 13 percent of those over 65 are cared for in their children's homes.[9] Individuals in these situations worry about being useless and emotional and financial burdens. They fear lack of respect and the possibility of becoming senile before dying. These fears may be expressed in depression, aggression, resentment, and sensitivity. If, earlier, the individual helped his adolescent children gain their independence, he will probably find himself in a warm, supportive atmosphere. His dignity will be respected and his companionship sought. In such an environment he can be a profound influence for good upon both his children and grandchildren. He can teach them much about a successful attitude toward life.

Accept death with serenity. The individual who has learned to accept his life for what it was and who accepts the inevitability of death can meet death with less fear. Also important is the feeling that he has provided for the future, either of his children or of the world. If life has become unacceptable through pain, loneliness, or despair, death can be an escape. Death can also be the final, terrible barrier across the road to achievement of a lifetime's goal. The individual's whole life prepares him to meet death. (See chapter 28 for a discussion of loss, death, and grief.)

Implications for nursing

There is no qualitative difference between the approach to the adult patient and the elderly one. The nurse must be especially conscious of

[9]Lawrence H. Schwartz and Jane Linker Schwartz. 1972. *The psychodynamics of patient care,* p. 336. Englewood Cliffs, N.J.: Prentice-Hall.

the need to preserve his dignity and independence. Physical or mental disability may make the patient appear somewhat more childlike, but *he is not a child* and should not be treated as one.

If hearing is impaired or comprehension is slow, it is important to speak clearly and make sure the patient has understood. (Embarrassment may keep him from asking a second time.) Instructions may be both written out and demonstrated to make sure.

Both routines and surroundings can be modified for a slower pace and limited ability. Needs can be anticipated. This may simply mean ensuring that water, tissues, eyeglasses, and call bell are all close at hand. A nightlight can be left on or a door left open to prevent darkness, which can be confusing to an older, partially disoriented person.

One very real need of the elderly patient is the need to talk to someone. The nurse who fills this need demonstrates an appreciation of his past and helps him find hope for the future. She also shows that she cares enough to listen.

SUMMARY

The nurse must understand the significance of the patient's age as a factor in his ability to handle himself, his illness, and his involvement with the health care system. At different ages, different things are threatening. The young child fears loss of the person upon whom he is dependent; the elderly person fears losing his independence. Each developmental stage has its own needs in terms of attitude, environment, and program.

Humans not only mature bodily but also develop intellectually, sexually, psychologically, and socially. Bodily growth is a fairly steady process. Development is a process of experimenting, adjusting, absorbing, stabilizing, and then going on to new experiments. It is made possible by man's ability to adapt himself to his environment and to change his environment to suit his own needs.

If the individual cannot cope with a developmental task of a certain phase, he may either fixate at that stage or regress to an earlier one. His development as an integrated, productive human depends upon his successful accomplishment of each stage.

Throughout all these stages the individual is struggling toward the creation of an integrated ego identity. He does this through interactions with both his internal and external worlds. In adjusting to his body, feelings, and conscience, he is also adjusting to society's expectations and demands upon him.

The life cycle falls into six basic stages, each with its own developmental tasks. The stages of the life cycle are:

1. Infancy (birth to $1\frac{1}{2}$ years)
2. Childhood ($1\frac{1}{2}$ to 9 years)

3. Adolescence (9 to 18 years)
4. Young adulthood (18 to 30 years)
5. Middle years (30 to 60 years)
6. Old age (60 years to death)

During these years the development of ego identity advances. The child becomes a separate person, with a gender role, a conscience, and a system for acquiring information. His growing sexuality in adolescence thrusts him out of the nest of the home and into independence. By now, his ability to conceptualize and use logic has equipped him for a career. He is sure enough of himself to entrust his ego to another person in an intimate relationship. His growing need to create for the future brings him into parenthood or to seek satisfaction through creativity in his work. A life of successfully accomplished tasks brings the individual to the end of life with acceptance and serenity.

STUDY QUESTIONS

1. What is a developmental task? List and briefly define four of the developmental tasks in Erikson's system of psychosocial development.
2. What is meant by the term "identity"?
3. Compare and contrast Erikson's developmental theory with that of Piaget.
4. Using your own clinical experience, analyze the behavior and treatment of a particular patient in terms of his place in the life cycle.
5. Using Erikson's theory as an organizing principle, write an autobiographical analysis of your own development.

SELECTED BIBLIOGRAPHY

Erikson, Erik H. 1963. *Childhood and society,* 2d ed. New York: Norton.

Lidz, Theodore. 1968. *The person: His development throughout the life cycle.* New York: Basic Books.

Murray, Ruth, and Zentner, Judith. 1975. *Nursing assessment and health promotion through the life span.* Englewood Cliffs, N.J.: Prentice-Hall.

Schwartz, Lawrence H., and Schwartz, Jane Linker. 1972. *The psychodynamics of patient care.* Englewood Cliffs, N.J.: Prentice-Hall.

Sutterley, Doris C., and Donnelly, Gloria F. 1973. *Perspectives in human development: Nursing throughout the life cycle.* Philadelphia: Lippincott.

10 Communication aspects of nursing

What is the communication process?

Characteristics of interpersonal communication

Before beginning an examination of what **communication** means, it will be helpful to explore briefly what it does *not* mean.

First, communication does not refer to just any transfer of information from one person to another. A mother who is lecturing her son is not necessarily communicating with him, even though he is sitting in the same room and perfectly capable of receiving the information. Communication is not exclusively a verbal undertaking. It is more than the mere sum of what passes between people—more than a mechanical process of action and reaction.

Now let us consider what communication is.

In the many definitions that have been offered for the word, two features are prominent. Two people must share an idea before they can communicate, and communication is a social process, not a mechanical one. One author proposes the following definition: Communication is a **transactional** process involving a **cognitive** sorting, selecting, and sending of symbols in such a way as to help a listener elicit from his own mind a meaning or response similar to that intended by the communicator.[1]

We as individuals are complete, self-contained communication systems, capable of receiving messages from within or without. No one can exist for any significant length of time without interacting with other people. The quality of this interaction depends greatly upon the skills a person develops in **interpersonal communication.** If we are to understand and improve our ability to function in social situations, we must first explore the makeup of the communication system.

Three qualities can be named immediately in reference to interpersonal

[1] As quoted by Raymond S. Ross. 1974. *Speech communication: Fundamentals and practice,* 3d ed., p. 10. Englewood Cliffs, N.J.: Prentice-Hall.

communication. The process is mutual; it is transactional in nature; and it is dynamic and ongoing.

Communication is mutual

It may seem obvious to state that interpersonal communication is mutual, but consider the fact that one part in the system—for instance, the son being lectured to—is often reluctant to receive the message of the other. As Carl Rogers points out in *On Becoming a Person,* "I have found it of enormous value when I can *permit* myself to understand another person."[2]

Many people are hesitant to try to understand another point of view, fearing that by so doing they will jeopardize their own position. Underneath lies the suspicion that the other person might be right; as a consequence, the listener might change his own opinions.

For example, Howard is explaining to George how much he liked the people in a country he has just visited. George answers with only a grunt. He has a lifelong prejudice against these people. Although he respects his friend and suspects he may be right, he does not want to change his opinion. Are the two men communicating?

Communication is transactional and dynamic

The word "transactional" refers to the fact that interpersonal communication is a process involving a common experience and mutual influence. If George had ever been to the country Howard had visited, he could have communicated with Howard. Transactional means that each side is trying to influence the other to change. The transactional process is ongoing and dynamic, not just an interchange of meanings with a beginning and an end. It is a continuing psychological event that involves both parties.

Transactional communication is concerned with what might be called **relationship communication,** in which meanings are largely born out of the ideas we construct about other people while actively interacting with them. Consider the example offered by Oliver Wendell Holmes.[3] Naming two characters John and Thomas, he points out that there are three Johns: (1) the real John, known only to his maker; (2) John's concept of himself; (3) Thomas's concept of John, often quite different from John's concept. One might also add a fourth: John's concept of Thomas's concept of John.

Interpersonal communication, then, is a mutual, transactional, and dynamic process. It refers not to the response itself but essentially to the relationship set up by the transmission of signs and the evocation of responses.

[2]Ibid., p. 8.
[3]Ibid., p. 9.

Perception

Crucial to communication is **perception,** the process by which particular signals—**verbal** or **nonverbal**—strike the receiver's sensory end organs (ears, eyes, etc.). Perception falls into two phases, **sensation** and **interpretation.** The process is identical to the process of communication, but the emphasis is on receiving. It is primarily through our knowledge and experience that we interpret or attach meaning to a **symbol.**

If an inkblot or a cloud formation is shown to two people and they are asked what it looks like, they will give two different answers. The two individuals are receiving the same visual stimuli, yet they are perceiving them differently. The sensations—in this case, sight—are the input to the sensory system, and perception is the process by which incoming data are organized.

The perceptual process allows us to organize our sensations and to screen out those which are nonessential. For example, when we hear, we screen out a number of sound waves that are hitting our eardrums but that are of no interest to us. We may be standing on a corner where truck traffic is roaring by, but if the conversation of the people next to us is interesting, we pay no attention to the trucks. Likewise, a woman may be looking out a window to see when her husband will arrive home; snow is falling heavily against the windowpane, but she is nevertheless able to "see through" it.

Perception includes not only sensory stimuli but situations. For example, a young couple is going through a difficult period in their marriage. When the wife's mother analyzes the situation, she screens out elements that would reflect unfavorably upon her daughter and perceives the situation as one in which her daughter has been wronged.

Or, a patient complains that he is hot at night. The nurse thinks this is because he is using too many blankets; the aide is convinced that the temperature in the room is too high.

Our perceptions are also very much influenced by our expectations. For example, we are used to the idea that a wall and a ceiling meet at a right angle. Thus, when we look into the room from the doorway, we "see" a right angle, even though optically the wall and ceiling are at odd angles from our position.

Expectation has a great deal to do with a person's level of perception as well as his individual acceptance of a stimulus. A person who thinks he dislikes fish will turn his nose up at the most elegantly prepared fish dinner; a person who is deeply religious may find it impossible to entertain negative (even if warranted) thoughts about the local clergyman. This tendency to hear, see, and think according to one's own desires—known as **autistic thinking**—is one of the greatest barriers to good communication.

Perception, then, depends not only on facts, which are universally accepted, but on ways of perceiving those facts, which vary widely with the individual. First, a person's perceptions of the world are affected by his physiological condition: the sharpness of his hearing, vision, etc. An even more important influence is a person's family, whose attitudes have often been passed from one generation to the next. Although we may resent or challenge our upbringing, the values, goals, and beliefs instilled in us during childhood remain a reference point for life.

The prevailing attitudes of our social groups also strongly influence perception. What is considered immoral or even a crime in one country may be an honorable act in another. A food held as a delicacy in certain places may be repulsive in others. And within the same country, different groups have different standards and attitudes. A father may be a strong nationalist who believes in the necessity of war, while his son considers military service the least of his duties in life.

Our perceptions, then, are limited by our own environment and our own heredity. Complete self-knowledge is beyond the attainment of most, and like the Scottish poet Robert Burns, we can only hope:

O wad some power the giftie gie us
To see oursels as ithers see us!

A person's ability to communicate closely depends on the validity of his self-image, or self-concept. To a large degree, this self-image is shaped by interactions with people we consider significant. A realistic self-image can be crucial to the accuracy of a person's perceptions, the nature of his communications, and his motivations.

When a self-image is unrealistic and frustration results, a person may resort to various forms of compensatory behavior. For example, Helen's image of herself is of a woman who is always correct. One day she makes a mistake at work that has major repercussions. Instead of accepting the blame, thus endangering her self-image, she places the responsibility on her subordinate.

A communication model

Experts in communication have devised verbal-pictorial models to try to give us a better understanding of the communication process. Although a model runs the risk of being too simplified, it provides a frame of reference in understanding a concept. Symbolic language is often more expressive than verbal language.

Several models have been proposed for the communication process. Essential to them all is the following sequence:

source ⟶ encoder ⟶ message ⟶ decoder ⟶ interpretation

Communication de-
pends heavily upon
what a person already
knows.

Encoding means putting the information or feeling into a form that can be transmitted; **decoding** means relating the message to the "picture in the mind" of the receiver. The **encoder,** who is sending the message, and the **decoder,** who is receiving the message, are each limited by their own experience. Between the two must be an overlap of information or a common experience that makes the process meaningful to both. Without this overlap the intended message cannot be communicated.

Once the message has been decoded by the receiver, he in turn reverses the process and becomes the encoder. His encoding may or may not result in overt communication; much depends on barriers that may exist. Nevertheless, the process is constant and continuing, and one individual communication is only a part of a greater network. In the process of communication, each person is both encoder and decoder.

Examine the model presented here (Figure 10-1), keeping in mind the definition of communication suggested at the beginning of this chapter. Assume that the person whose head is represented on the left side of the model wishes to communicate the concept of love to the person whose head is represented on the right. The fan projecting from each brain represents the sum of each person's knowledge, experience, feelings, attitudes, emotions, and the other elements that make him an individual.

From this storehouse the sender selects the items that help him define what he is trying to say. In this process his brain serves as a sort of computer into which a program is fed. This program must include three instructions: What do I have stored under love? What do I know about the other person? What do I have filed for this particular situation and context? The brain goes to work sorting and selecting the appropriate knowledge, past experience, and so on.

Then follows the process of encoding by which the sender chooses his codes and emits the signs or symbols to transmit those codes. In the case of love, the language will probably be verbal: the first person says "I love you." However, his message can be modified by the words he chooses **(arrangement)** and his tone of voice **(voice action).** The process can also be affected by any of the situations noted in the borders around the process model; noise may distract the listener, for instance, or he may be sitting in a crowded room and not want to discuss personal matters.

Within a matter of seconds, the stimuli (in this case, words) strike the sensory end organs (in this case, ears) of the receiver. This part of the perception process is called **sensation;** it is followed by the part called **interpretation.**

The receiver now proceeds to decode the message, drawing upon his own storehouse of knowledge and experience. In the process he sorts out those meanings that allow him to create a message concerning love. Communication depends on the extent to which this recreation is similar to the sender's intended message. In other words, it depends heavily upon what a person already knows.

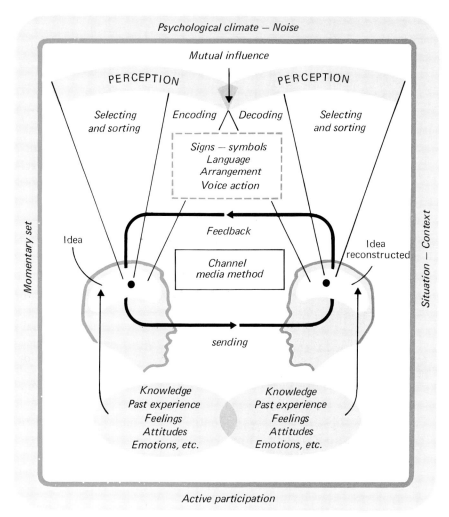

FIG. 10-1 *Ross Transactional Communication Model*

[From Raymond S. Ross, *Speech communication: Fundamentals and practice,* 3d ed., p. 15. Englewood Cliffs, N.J.: Prentice-Hall, 1974. © 1974. Reprinted by permission of Prentice-Hall, Inc.]

Notice the word **feedback.** In engineering this term refers to the return of some of the transmitted energy to the source. However, in communication it refers more to a process of self-correction. As our transmitted signal is bounced off the receiver, it feeds back information that allows us to correct and refine our signal. For example, if our message is met with a yawn, we may begin to reevaluate and recode our emitted signals.

Feedback is a process that allows us to control our signals by incorporating information about their effects. It can be either positive or negative; either way, it can be made to work for us.

Although the model we have been examining includes only two people, the same general principles of communication apply in a modified form to small groups and even to large audiences.

Kinds of communication

Conversation between a nurse and patient is not like conversation between a nurse and one of her friends. The difference is that her conversation with the patient is essentially **therapeutic;** that is, it is intended to bring about a change in his behavior.

Like a psychotherapist, the nurse steers communication in such a way that the patient is exposed to situations and message exchanges that will eventually bring about more gratifying social relations and personal fulfillment. From the outside, this therapeutic communication appears no different from ordinary communication. It is only the purpose that is not the same.

Of course, the nurse cannot and must not attempt to be purposeful/ therapeutic at all times; neither she nor the patient would be able to tolerate such a continuous and intensive interaction. Socializing keeps the lines of communication open and assures the patient that he can change the level of interaction if he wishes. The crucial task for the nurse is to recognize the difference between purposeful/goal-directed and superficial/social interactions and to be able to use each appropriately.

In order to do so, she must learn to distinguish the following types of communication: verbal and nonverbal, purposeful and nonpurposeful, directive and nondirective. None of these categories is mutually exclusive; they tend to overlap.

Nonverbal communication

While we commonly think of words as the standard means of communication, much more is happening at a deeper level in response to tone of voice, inflection, pauses, hesitations, and omissions. Even more is expressed through facial expressions, bodily gestures, and touch.

When we look at a patient while he is talking, we show our interest in him as a person and our desire to understand what he is saying. If we turn away or look elsewhere, the patient will conclude we are not interested. Reaching out a hand to touch the patient may convey the message, "I am here with you; I care about you." The strokes a nurse uses when bathing a patient, rubbing his back, or touching him to change his position reflect how she feels. Is she rough or gentle, distracted or attentive? Does she wrinkle up her nose at the smell of the drainage from a colostomy bag?

Listening

Although we readily acknowledge the importance of the ear in verbal interchange, its function in nonverbal communication is not generally recognized. The ear listens not only to words, but to the tone in which they are conveyed. The ear is also the organ through which such emotionally charged words as "bad" and "naughty" are transmitted to the child's psyche. In other words, the ear is a perceiver of attitudes associated with words as well as a receptor of sound.

To use our ears for communication, we must learn to listen, to pay attention to the patient's voice. This means concentrating to remove distractions and wearing the expression of someone who believes that something interesting is being said. The nurse who is "too busy to listen" reveals her attitude through many nonverbal clues.

Along with being able to listen, we must know when to be silent. Many people look upon silence as something negative to be avoided. However, well-chosen silences can convey an attitude of calmness, warmth, approval, or humility. Through the constructive use of silence, we can weave stronger ties with others and develop deeper feelings than words can achieve.

Touch

Touch is perhaps the most obvious and readily understood means of nonverbal communication. In many interpersonal relations, tactile language communicates more fully than vocal language. It is through touch that we become oriented to the spatial dimensions of the world and people. In the United States, for instance, we measure the warmth or sincerity of a person by his handshake; a "limp" handshake is generally taken as the sign of a cool reception or a cold personality.

People do not respond in the same way to touch. One man may jump if someone comes up from behind and touches his shoulders; another may respond with warmth. Because touch is potentially the most meaningful form of communication, it is important for the nurse to understand it and to learn how to use it. Often the difficulty nursing students experience when touching patients relates to their own discomfort at being touched.

Smell

Smell is another one of the senses that is subject to much nonverbal interpretation. Since our society has great concern about odors, nurses must become aware of how they verbally and nonverbally deal with various odors associated with their patients. Physical deterioration of bodily tissue is frequently accompanied by a disagreeable odor, of which the patient may be well aware. His embarrassment will only be intensified when the nurse reacts to the odor.

Often it is almost impossible not to react, of course. When this happens, the nurse can alleviate the situation by commenting to the patient that the odor must be distressing to him. This gives the impression that the nurse is more concerned with the patient's reaction than with her own.

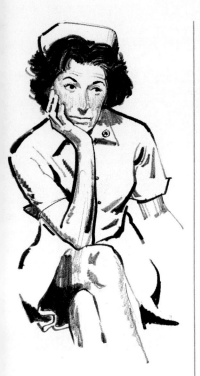

A nurse who is frowning while listening may only be concentrating; however, perhaps in the patient's opinion she is disapproving of what he says.

Body language

We also communicate a great deal through the way we move and the way we speak. Patients, like anyone else, are more likely to put faith in actions than words. A nurse who is frowning while listening may only be concentrating; however, perhaps in the patient's opinion she is disapproving of what he says. It is vitally important for the nurse to understand what she is conveying through her **body language** or "bedside manner" if she is to work in the interests of the patient.

Verbal communication

Verbal communication can be manipulated in different ways to serve different functions. In order to communicate effectively, it is necessary to first identify the aim of talking to the patient, to find out not only about his immediate symptoms, but about himself. What have been his experiences in life and his reactions to them? What events led up to his present situation?

It is not enough to ask about the specifics of his health history; it is essential to learn how he reacted to each incident and how it affected him. One illness often predisposes a patient to another by weakening his defenses. In many chronic illnesses, such as heart disease, the handicap plays a major role in the patient's life, and the nurse must understand how the illness affects him in order to help him deal with it.

Another general aim when speaking with a patient is to learn the pattern of his illness in order to predict, and possibly prevent, events in the future. For example, a patient may reveal that his peptic ulcer always "kicks up" during Christmas. Although the patient attributes this fact to the general stress of the holiday season, the nurse may be able to discover something out of the ordinary in his eating habits that may be causing problems.

Purposeful conversation is necessary to disclose the true nature of the patient's problems. But in addition to being purposeful, it must be directive. In other words, it must be aimed at producing specific positive changes in the patient's behavior.

In maintaining the professional attitude needed to bring about change, the nurse must learn to beware of two pitfalls. The patient is not her personal friend, nor is the patient the "living example" of a particular disease. Some nurses seek from patients the friendships they should be developing outside their professional arenas. This tendency is as fraught with hazard for the patient as is the opposite—impersonal treatment. The professional nurse has a limited time in which to offer direct and specialized experience. If the patient is to learn anything from her, he must be allowed to concentrate on her as a professional.

Nursing students learn a number of techniques that make conversation with a patient as purposeful and directive as possible and that obtain maximum interest and cooperation. For example, if the patient becomes silent, one may try an open-ended question: "And then what happened?" Or an imprecise question: "How did it feel?" rather than "Was the pain sharp?" Questions such as these allow the patient more freedom and prevent him from being forced into a single line of thought. Questions that can be answered with a simple yes or no should be avoided.

Again the point should be stressed that all conversation is not directive or purposeful; both patient and nurse need the relief of small talk. However, the nurse should guard against burdening the patient with details of her personal life. Otherwise she runs the risk of shifting the major focus onto herself and away from the patient.

Interviewing

What is the role of interviewing?

Interviewing is a goal-directed method of questioning that involves effective interaction between two people. In communication between professional and patient, the professional focuses attention on the patient and directs communication so that specific goals can be reached. Although social conversation is sometimes meaningful, purposeful, and goal-directed, the professional interview is *always* this way.

During the interview the nurse applies her knowledge of interviewing principles. Throughout the interview she is aware of what she wants to accomplish and how she is progressing. Interviewing is a specific nursing action that the nurse uses in formulating her plan of nursing care.

The specific actions that the nurse performs include observation, listening, verbal and nonverbal responses, interpretation of data, and recording of data. Each of these actions can be deliberately formulated from scientific facts and principles. The nurse interviewer learns these principles, then practices, evaluates, practices again, and evaluates again—until she improves her ability to apply them.

Although friends may assist each other to verbalize feelings and work out problems, in the interview with a patient the nurse is deliberately focusing on the patient. She is encouraging him to express feelings and to identify needs and goals. The exchange of information is relative not to the nurse's feelings about the patient, but to his own needs and feelings as identified by her.

What is the rationale for use of the interview within the therapeutic process? First, patients frequently communicate their needs and feelings in ways that are devious. Only through careful probing will the nurse be able to identify what problems they—and she—have to look forward to.

The nurse encourages the patient to express feelings and to identify needs and goals.

For example, a patient is upset about the fact that his family has not visited him. Instead of stating the fact to the nurse, he begins to have chest pains. Through interviewing this patient, the nurse learns that he, like many people, frequently communicates his problems through physical symptoms.

People behave in this manner because they do not want to face feelings of anxiety, guilt, uncertainty, or embarrassment that would accompany open admission. Such defensive behavior is a form of self-protection—of hiding an emotionally charged area from scrutiny. Yet these feelings do manage to surface, in disguised form, because the afflicted person does want help.

The nurse can be of most help to the patient by approaching his problems in the same indirect manner, and by not scaring him off with point-blank questions such as, "What's the matter with you?" This need for indirection is the reason for several interviewing principles.

It should be noted that many of the problems of dependency and hostility, which one encounters in patients, stem from the fact that they feel isolated in their illness. Through interviewing techniques, they can be drawn out of their unaccustomed isolation.

Essentially, the interview has seven major purposes:

1. Initiating and maintaining a positive nurse-patient relationship
2. Determining the nurse's own role in caring for the patient
3. Collecting information on emotional crises in the patient's life
4. Influencing the patient's ability to cope with immediate crises
5. Channeling the patient's feelings directly
6. Channeling communication between patient and professional personnel
7. Preparing the patient for health instruction[4]

However the patient chooses to express himself, the nurse should bear in mind that he is expressing need and that he is motivated by unconscious forces over which he has little control. Interviewing is a vehicle through which the nurse can determine this need.

Principles of interviewing

The skills of interviewing are very specific; they can be learned no matter how little "intuition" the nurse thinks she has. Basic guidelines have been offered by psychiatrist Maurice H. Greenhill of the University of Miami:[5]

1. *The patient is given the initiative.* This does not mean that the patient manages, controls, or regulates the interview himself. However, it does

[4]M. Greenhill. 1956. Interviewing with a purpose. *American Journal of Nursing* 56:n.p.
[5]Ibid.

mean that the interviewer prompts him to begin the discussion, is careful not to interrupt, and gives the patient plenty of room to bring up his own subjects for discussion. On the other hand, the interviewer is not required to sit across from the patient like a statue but is free to interject remarks that further the conversation.

2. *The approach to the patient is indirect.* The interviewer must think in terms of starting at the outer edge of a circle and gradually moving toward the center; she must not aim directly for the center. A patient may make a casual remark such as, "Well, there have been some problems with the business." The interviewer knows that this touches on a subject important to the patient.

Instead of asking, "Oh, is your company in financial trouble?" she might merely repeat the patient's comment, "Oh, you've had some problems with the business?" More often than not, the patient will continue on his own. Although this indirect approach may appear to be more time-consuming, ultimately it takes less time. The patient will open up and reveal the core of his problems more quickly.

3. *Interviewing should be as open-ended as possible.* The nurse must beware of squelching conversation unintentionally—a particular hazard when she is trying to be reassuring. A patient may suggest hesitantly that he fears his vision will be permanently affected as a result of a stroke he has suffered. The nurse, trying to comfort him, comments, "You shouldn't worry about such things, you're in good hands." The patient may be momentarily reassured, but he will be reluctant to voice further doubts about his condition. The nurse might better have made a comment such as, "It's upsetting to think of having problems with your vision."

An excellent technique for keeping an interview going is to use an incomplete form of statement, inviting the patient to fill it in. For example: "You say that your leg has been. . . ." "It's been giving me pain at night, and I hate to take a lot of sleeping pills just for that," the patient may reply.

4. *The interviewer uses minimal verbal activity.* First, the patient should not feel that he cannot get a word in edgewise; essentially, the interview is his show. Often a patient will throw a test question at the nurse. For example, he may try to draw her out about her personal life, essentially in an effort to find out whether she is more interested in her own life or his. In such instances, a minimal response is all that is necessary.

Many nurses interview effectively up to the point of discussing health education—then, they suddenly begin to overwhelm the patient with information. In order to make sure the information is getting across, they go into needlessly detailed explanations, descriptions, and interpretations. As a result, the patient absorbs very little, although he may appreciate the nurse's apparently excessive concern for his condition. Small, properly timed doses of information will be swallowed much more easily.

5. *Spontaneity should be encouraged.* By assuming a relaxed attitude and

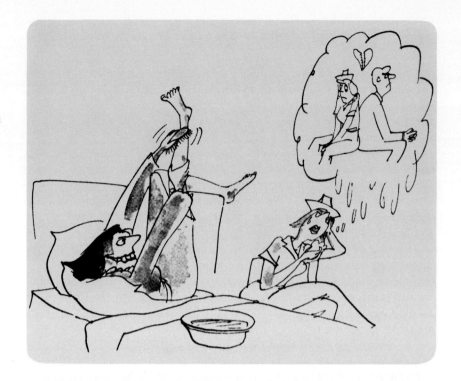

making a minimum number of comments, the interviewer encourages the patient to make the kind of spontaneous remarks that can provide a gold mine of information. The patient may start off talking spontaneously about something that seems irrelevant to his hospital situation; however, the wise interviewer will allow him to follow out his train of thought.

For example, Mr. Evans starts talking enthusiastically about his 10-year-old daughter and the new kitten she has just brought home. Suddenly the nurse is struck with the suspicion that the mysterious sinus inflammation with which Mr. Evans came to the hospital may be caused by an allergic reaction to the cat.

6. *Interviewing should facilitate expression of feelings.* When a patient is allowed to vent his feelings about particular people or events, he often supplies useful information as well. For example, Mrs. Lopez is very dissatisfied with the way the President of the United States is doing his job. She is particularly upset that he is neglecting the unemployed. Further discussion brings out the fact that her husband is unemployed and that he greatly resents the fact that her illness is keeping her away from her job—the only source of family income. Suddenly the nurse understands why Mrs. Lopez is her most impatient patient.

7. *The interview must focus on areas that are emotionally charged.* Because patients are reluctant to discuss such areas, which may evoke painful associations, it is up to the interviewer to bring the conversation around to these points. She must learn to bring out into the open personal or social problems that may have a great deal of meaning to the patient. If such areas are not probed, the interview will yield diminishing returns. By

focusing on subjects close to the patient's heart, the interviewer lets the patient know that they are on the same wavelength.

8. *Movement in interviewing depends on picking up verbal leads, clues, or signals from the patient.* Sensitive areas are not always obvious, and the nurse must be closely attuned to lightly dropped clues. For example, if the patient refers to her husband in a hurt tone of voice, the interviewer might gently raise the subject of her home life. If she mentions her mother several times, it may be because some problem exists between the two women.

9. *The data must come from the content of the interview itself.* It is of no use for the nurse to depend completely on a prepared list of questions. Although she may use a set of standard questions from a nursing history form as a guide, she must let the interview develop from what the patient says. Otherwise the patient may feel he is being cross-examined and become very closemouthed.

These nine principles cover the essentials of the interview, but other measures can enhance its effectiveness. For example, the patient should be made as physically comfortable as possible, and the nurse should try to make sure that the interview will be free of interruptions from telephone or staff.

The traditional therapeutic interview takes place in an office, with patient facing therapist, and usually lasts 45 minutes to an hour. The nurse can try to make the setting as formal as possible, a factor that has been found to improve results. If the patient is well enough, he can be taken to a room and seated opposite the nurse. Otherwise, a curtain can be drawn around his bed.

Any goal-directed contact between patient and nurse constitutes an interview, however, and a formal setting is not necessary. The skilled nurse can interview her patient while standing at his bedside for a few minutes, wheeling him to the sundeck, giving him a massage, or making a home visit. Often the physical contact of such situations acts as a powerful catalyst to the process of communication.

If the nurse keeps her focus on the specific objective of interviewing as applied to nursing care, she cannot go "too far." In discussing emotionally charged areas, her purpose is merely to provoke a response, not to expose deep-seated psychological problems.

Communication and the nurse-patient relationship

The relationship between nurse and patient can be thought of as unfolding in three phases: **orientation, working,** and **termination.**[6]

---

[6]G. B. Ujhely. 1968. *Determinants of the nurse-patient relationship,* p. 103. New York: Springer.

> Any goal-directed contact between patient and nurse constitutes an interview.

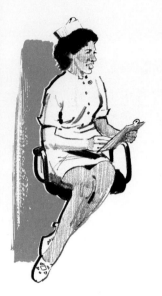

If the nurse lets the patient take the lead in conversation during the orientation phase . . .

The orientation phase

During the orientation phase, the patient reveals—directly or indirectly—where he needs help. The orientation phase also serves largely as a model for the later phases.

If the nurse lets the patient take the lead in conversation during the orientation phase, listening not only to what he says but to how he says it, she will soon get an idea of the key concepts or ideas that underlie his statements and bind them together. She will then become aware of three kinds of underlying key ideas or themes, which will continue throughout all phases of the relationship.

1. The **content** theme (the "what" of the patient's story)
2. The **mood** theme (how he tells his story)
3. The **interaction** theme (the way he relates to the nurse and indicates how he would like her to relate to him)

Content refers to subject matter, implicit or expressed. If a patient tells the nurse that he is quite worried about having to undergo an additional diagnostic procedure, he may be implying that he does not think his insurance will cover it. In this case the content theme might be termed financial insecurity.

How does the patient express his thoughts—with fear? With anxiety? If he seems defiant, the mood theme might be termed frustration or anger. How does he behave toward the nurse? Does he ignore her comments and behave as if she were not there? Does he ask her for specific instructions? Their behavior toward each other constitutes the third communication theme, interaction.

As the nurse listens, she will be able to either confirm or modify her initial hunches about the themes that will develop. She must beware of trying to discover the cause of the patient's problem too early in the relationship. This will become apparent only after all the facts are in.

The advice to let the patient develop his themes during the orientation phase is not as easy to follow as might appear. Often the nurse will interfere quite unwittingly. For example, she may pounce eagerly on the patient's first statement and pursue it in detail, eager to hear the whole story. Or she may say nothing at all, hoping the patient will be carried on his own steam. Instead, she finds that he has run out of conversational material. She must learn to listen not passively but in such a way as to help the patient mark out his concerns.

The working phase

During the working phase, the patient fills in the territory he has outlined and begins to come to grips with his experience. At first, he still needs considerable help in learning to gain fuller awareness of what really bothers him about the episodes he has related. The nurse at this point actively steers his self-questioning so that she can obtain as complete a picture as possible. The patient will have touched on many topics during orientation, and it is up to the nurse to steer him first toward "content" topics. For instance, she may ask for a blow-by-blow description of a particular incident the patient is focusing on.

Once the patient is aware of content, he should be directed to analyze the mood theme associated with his story. Frequently this process requires much assistance from the nurse, who may be aware of feelings that the patient himself is unaware of. Yet she cannot jump directly to a discussion of feelings but must begin with a discussion of the content themes. People find it easier to discuss events and actions than emotions, especially with someone they do not know. Also, the mood theme usually depends heavily on the content theme. In other words, if a patient is unhappy, it is usually because of some particular event. The event should be discussed before the unhappiness.

The interaction theme is the nurse's concern, but not the patient's. She must be aware at all times of the relationship between herself and the patient and must not fall unwittingly into a complementary role that is detrimental to the patient's growth.

For example, the patient may begin to reminisce about his trip to Paris; the nurse has also been to Paris, but it is not her function to start reminiscing too. She must keep her mind on a possible connection between the patient's memories and his present state.

The nurse should not challenge the patient's way of interacting with her as long as he is able to present material for discussion. This will prevent the development of a relationship that becomes so involved the nurse cannot handle it. According to one psychiatric nurse,[7] the only times a nurse should deal with the interaction process are: (1) when it blocks the problem-solving process (for example, if the patient is maintaining a stubborn silence), or (2) when the patient's behavior with the nurse is the same as the behavior he describes in problem situations.

As the working phase progresses, the nurse helps the patient to sort out the themes most significant to his situation and to examine the component parts. She further shows him how to manipulate these parts to bring about a solution appropriate to his own life. With patience and encouragement, she urges him to try out his new insights.

Of course, progress is very slow with some patients. There are those who are severely lacking in intelligence or insight; others have a very low tolerance for anxiety. However, the nurse should not give in to disappointment nor should she attempt shortcuts. As long as she has built a

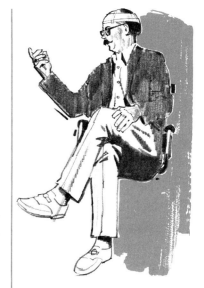

. . . she will soon get an idea of the key concepts or ideas that underlie his statements and bind them together.

[7]G. B. Ujhely. 1968. What is *realistic* emotional support? *American Journal of Nursing* 68:761.

solid foundation, her relationship with the patient can be allowed to come to a temporary standstill and resumed at a later time when the patient is ready to move forward.

It takes time to put insights into practice, and patience is required. A patient may come to realize that his frequent outbursts of anger at his wife really reflect dissatisfaction with himself. This does not mean that he will be able to cease yelling at his wife all at once. Of course, the nurse cannot "cure" a deep-seated problem that may exist between the man and his wife. However, she can help him to identify and deal with this one aspect of his experience.

The termination phase

The termination phase of the nurse-patient relationship should not arrive suddenly one day as a surprise but should be built into the relationship from the beginning. The patient should be reminded of how long he and the nurse will be together—if this can be determined—so that he can gauge how much he wants to share with her in the time they are together.

Some nurses find the termination phase especially difficult because they fear the patient is incapable of adjusting to it. Often this fear reflects the nurse's own need to be needed. Patients will get over the separation in due time, especially if they have been adequately prepared.

Approaches that facilitate or clarify communication

Earlier in this chapter it was stated that one of the principles of interviewing is that the interviewer uses minimal verbal activity in order to encourage the patient to express himself. Greenhill distinguishes three degrees of verbal activity: low, moderate, and marked.[8] The latter is not appropriate in any communication between nurse and patient.

Low verbal activity

Low verbal activity can range from complete silence to an occasional comment or two. It is often accompanied by moderate nonverbal activity, such as leaning forward or nodding the head. Frequently, effective communication combines low verbal and moderate nonverbal activity.

There are two reasons for using low verbal activity. First, it encourages the patient to speak up and to act spontaneously; and second, it provides

---

[8]Greenhill, op. cit.

the interviewer with an occasion to search for verbal leads from the patient's comments. Sometimes the interviewer will find his purpose served by repeating the patient's last word, with rising vocal inflection, or by repeating a significant word or phrase. Other times she will provoke the desired response with a mild directive to "tell me more about that."

Moderate verbal activity

Moderate verbal activity is appropriate when the patient is not communicating well or is saying nothing. Often moderate activity is needed to focus on a certain topic and explore the patient's leads. It is also helpful at the beginning of a discussion of feelings when the patient may be hesitant to take the initiative. For example, the nurse might ask, "How did you feel when you heard you would need surgery?"

Another occasion when the interviewer uses moderate verbal activity is in responding to patients' test questions. A patient may query the nurse, "Where did you go to school?" or "How do you like working here?" In such cases, the temptation to respond at length must be resisted for the most part. However, a short factual answer is perfectly appropriate, followed by refocusing on the patient. The nurse might follow up with, "Why do you ask me that?" Usually the patient has some purpose in seeking the information, of which the nurse should be aware. If the nurse absolutely refuses to reveal any personal information about herself, however, she may appear rude or unduly secretive. This can be most upsetting to a patient who, after all, may be revealing very personal data about himself. In return, the patient deserves to know something about the human being with whom he is interacting.

Marked verbal activity

Marked verbal activity, always to be avoided, is activity on behalf of the nurse's own purpose. Silence can represent much more than the absence of conversation; it can serve a therapeutic purpose. Many students find difficulty in using silence as a therapeutic tool. When they are concerned about how the interview is progressing, they almost always err on the side of excess verbalization.

As the nurse becomes accustomed to the interview situation, she will no longer be driven by feelings of anxiety into an excess of talk or questioning. A good practical guideline is, when in doubt say nothing. Continue to look interested in what the patient has to say, and do not be distressed if his comments seem to be grinding to a halt.

If the patient is taking the opposite route and asking too many questions, one should remember that it is not the nurse's responsibility to supply answers to all of them. She can be supportive without reassuring him on every point.

Establishing the nurse-patient relationship

A major part of the nurse's responsibility is to establish a relationship that is human to human, not salesman to customer. Only when each individual in the interaction perceives the other as a human being is a good relationship possible.

Through the human-to-human relationship, the nurse accomplishes her purpose: to assist an individual or family to prevent, or cope with, the experience of illness and suffering; and to help him or his family find meaning in these experiences.[9] Such a relationship does not develop overnight. Rather, it is built up gradually each day as the nurse interacts with the patient. She purposefully establishes and cultivates this rapport.

Another point is that the relationship is meaningful to both nurse and patient. We have already cautioned against allowing the interaction between nurse and patient to serve the nurse's individual needs; essentially, the patient is the focus of attention. This does not mean that the nurse ceases to be a human being while interacting with patients.

Not all nursing authorities would agree with this statement. Many feel that the nurse should not meet any of her own needs in the relationship with her patient. However, others point out that some of her needs must be met if she is to experience job satisfaction and if she is not to completely dehumanize the nursing experience. If the nurse puts herself totally into the background, she will be less able to meet the patient's demands.

Although the relationship is a mutual one, established through a sequence of phases, it is up to the nurse to initiate and maintain it. This she does by consciously moving through four interlocking phases: the **initial encounter, emerging identities, empathy,** and **sympathy.**

The initial encounter

During the **initial encounter,** both nurse and patient form ideas about each other. These first impressions are based on the perception of interpersonal cues and on verbal and nonverbal communication. Usually the patient sees the nurse as a nurse, and the nurse sees the patient as a patient. Only later, when they come to know each other as human beings, are these stereotypes shattered. It is up to the nurse to be aware of her own stereotypes and to try to look upon the patient as an individual.

Emerging identities

Once this has been done, she is ready for the next phase, **emerging identities.** At this point, both nurse and patient begin to establish a bond and to view each other less as categories and more as human beings.

[9]Joyce Travelbee. 1971. *Interpersonal aspects of nursing,* 2d ed., p. 119. Philadelphia: Davis.

A major part of the nurse's responsibility is to establish a relationship that is human to human, not salesman to customer.

The inability to perceive the patient as a separate and unique human being is the starting point of many difficulties in the nursing situation. Often the fault lies in what is termed overidentification. Instead of responding to the patient as an individual, the nurse responds to something of herself that she sees in the patient's problems. "I know how I would feel in his place," she might reflect. However, her feelings may have nothing in common with the patient's. Similarities of experience are important in building mutual understanding, but separation of experience and identity is crucial to the therapeutic relationship.

> Empathy is the ability to momentarily enter the psychological state of another individual.

Empathy

Empathy, as was discussed in chapter 1, is the ability to momentarily enter the psychological state of another individual. The goal of the empathetic phase is to gain comprehension and thus be able to predict behavior. Once empathy has occurred in the nurse-patient interaction, the pattern of the interaction is irrevocably changed. Even if the individuals involved later grow to dislike each other, the dislike is apt to have a more violent character if the empathy had never occurred.

It cannot be expected that the nurse will empathize equally with all patients. However, it is possible to expand one's empathetic boundaries; it is not necessary to like a person in order to empathize with him. The ability to intellectually comprehend another person and to predict his behavior does not seem to rest on liking or disliking him but on the similarity of experience between him and the nurse.

Sympathy

The ability to sympathize grows out of the empathetic process. Sympathy differs from empathy in that it denotes desire to alleviate the distress of the other person. When the nurse sympathizes with the patient, she enters into and shares his distress, thus relieving him of the burden of carrying it alone. The presence or absence of sympathy can affect the patient not only psychologically but physiologically.

During the sympathy phase, it is the nurse's task to translate her feelings into helpful nursing actions. This requires a combination of the disciplined intellectual approach and the therapeutic use of self.

Rapport

All of these phases culminate in a final phase called **rapport,** which is another term for the human-to-human relationship. During any one of these phases, progress may cease temporarily or even permanently. It is the nurse's responsibility to identify reasons for failure and to intervene in a manner that reactivates progress.

Approaches that hinder or distort communication

Despite the best of intentions, a nurse may find that she is failing to communicate with her patient. Often she has conversational habits that the patient finds upsetting. For example, she may abruptly change the subject or may respond to an insignificant aspect of the patient's conversation. Look at the following commonplace nurse-patient interactions:[10]

NURSE It looks like you've had some bad news, Joan.
JOAN (suppressing a sob) Yes, my mother finally died last night; she was so sick.
NURSE (flustered) Oh, I'm so sorry. . . . Would you like me to help you get started with your bath now?

The nurse is obviously uncomfortable in a discussion of death; instead of pursuing a discussion, she tries to change the subject. Yet a verbal response was not even called for. She could have made Joan feel better simply by remaining with her sympathetically for some time.

Another way of limiting communication is to give opinions about the patient and his concerns in a moralizing tone:

MR. SILVERSTEIN I sure am tired of fish and chicken for dinner, and everything is overcooked here.
NURSE I know, Mr. Silverstein, but you should be thankful that the doctors have prescribed a special diet that will help you lose weight as well as lower your cholesterol.

First, Mr. Silverstein is entitled to express his opinions about hospital food, and he does not have to be reminded that it is "good for him" or that the staff is working on his behalf. If he has anything else to say, he will certainly withhold it once he has decided that the nurse does not want to hear his opinions.

A third form of verbal error is inappropriate reassurance. When a patient has an honest concern about his condition, he should be given as honest an answer as possible and not be put off by an empty promise:

NURSE How do you feel, Mr. Murphy?
MR. MURPHY Fine, but I'd love to know when they'll be taking my legs out of these casts. They're so uncomfortable.
NURSE Oh, I wouldn't worry about that, Mr. Murphy; you'll be up playing golf again in no time.

[10] Adapted from Helon E. Hewitt and Betty L. Pesznecker. 1964. Blocks to communicating with patients. *American Journal of Nursing* 64:101–103.

The patient has been involved in a very serious accident, and he does not really believe that he will be playing golf again very soon. The nurse probably wants to relieve his anxiety, but instead she merely cuts off communication when Mr. Murphy sees there is no hope of a reasonable response to his question.

Perhaps the nurse knows that Mr. Murphy is in for a long hospital stay and she does not want to be the bearer of bad news. Her hesitation is understandable, but she would be better to make a comment that would draw Mr. Murphy out and allow him to express himself, such as, "It's hard to be so tied down, isn't it?"

Another way to cut off communication with a patient is to jump to conclusions or offer premature solutions to his problems. Roger has suffered a fracture of the left forearm and right side of the pelvis, and his back is causing him a great deal of pain:

NURSE Here, let me help you turn on your side; your back will feel much better.

ROGER (yelping with pain) Please don't touch me; it hurts when you turn me sideways!

NURSE (with some irritation) But you must get off your back so that I can give it a rub.

The nurse seems to be more interested in completing a particular nursing task than in exploring the problem of Roger's unexplained pain. Perhaps the location of his fractures is preventing him from being comfortable when turned on his side. In any case, the nurse should avoid speaking in aggressive or impatient tones and cutting Roger off from verbalizing his feelings.

Frequently, if the patient is allowed to express himself freely, he will clarify his thoughts and feelings by himself and, as a result, modify his attitudes and behavior.

The inappropriate use of medical facts or nursing knowledge is another error common to nurses who are trying to change the attitude or behavior of a patient. Since she may be directly opposing or ignoring the patient's views or feelings, she may adopt an argumentative tone of voice. Consider this example of a conversation between a nurse and a patient recovering from tuberculosis:

MR. PAPPAS I'm getting too fat; I need more exercise, and I'm tired of lying in bed all the time when I feel all right.

NURSE Don't worry about getting fat now. Rest is probably the most important treatment for tuberculosis patients. You see, when you rest, your lungs are also at rest, and that way, healing takes place more rapidly.

MR. PAPPAS I don't care, I don't need that much rest.

If the nurse allows the patient to express his feelings rather than opposing his ideas, she creates a more positive climate and a more therapeutic relationship.

Although the nurse's presentation of facts is logical, it does not convince the patient. Also, note that the nurse does not address herself to the original complaint—"I'm getting fat"—but merely offers a summary of treatment for TB patients. This mode of interaction tends to weaken the relationship between nurse and patient. If the nurse would allow the patient to express his feelings rather than opposing his ideas, she would create a more positive climate and a more therapeutic relationship.

Another hindrance to communication, mentioned in the last section, is excessive verbal activity, which the nurse indulges in for her own ends. For example, she may want to make as complete a record as possible, or to interject her own ideas into a conversation with a patient. She may want to share an experience with the patient, socialize with him, or give him advice. Excessive verbal activity may take the form of overexplaining something, probing too deeply for information, or prematurely discussing the relationship between nurse and patient. In all cases, communication is hindered.

Specific communication handicaps

Language barrier. The importance of nonverbal communication is perhaps most apparent in the case of patients who cannot speak English. Sometimes a nurse is tempted to avoid these patients because she feels unable to give them adequate care, due to the communication barrier. However, she should bear in mind that with foreigners, as well as natives, communication between nurse and patient is essential if the nurse is to carry out her tasks of observation and understanding. If the language barrier is seen as insurmountable, it will become a barrier to all communication and will perhaps result in both nurse and patient feeling angry and frustrated.

If the nurse speaks a few words of the patient's language, she should speak them no matter how inadequate they seem. From the patient's viewpoint, the nurse's efforts mean that she cares about him. Also, foreign language dictionaries are available in every bookstore and library.

Three basic rules apply to the problem of language differences. The nurse should:

1. Observe the patient with her five senses to pick up his message. A person cannot avoid communicating in some ways when he is with another person.
2. Direct her responses to the cues she receives from the patient. By trying to match her response to his cue, she can find out if his message means the same thing to him that it does to her.
3. Emphasize her own gestures and focus on the patient's nonverbal behavior. In this way she demonstrates what she would be saying if she could speak the patient's language and helps him do the same with her.

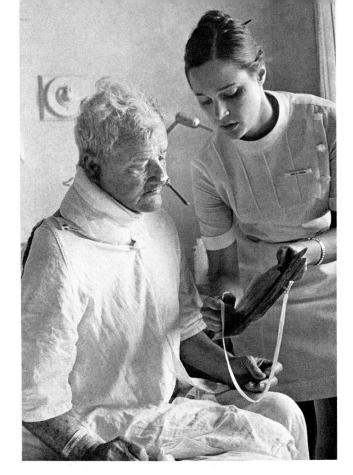

The use of a "magic slate" enables the tracheotomy patient to communicate.
[Courtesy the American Cancer Society]

When the patient does not speak English, it is particularly important to check out his eating, sleeping, and elimination habits. Members of the patient's family, his friends, or bilingual members of the health team can provide interpretation. Also, if the nurse cannot talk with the patient, she should at least talk *to* him. A person who cannot talk for whatever reason is severely handicapped; one can help assuage his discomfort and frustration to some degree by providing aural stimulation.

One word of warning: The nurse should never yield to the common temptation to talk loudly to these patients or to others who cannot understand the spoken word. Raising one's voice will not make words more intelligible and can create an expression of hostility.

Sensory-motor deficit. Communication with people whose senses are impaired or who have motor deficits affecting speech is less difficult than one might suppose. Two qualities that are needed in abundance are patience and empathy.

For example, most deaf people have lived with their handicap long enough that their other sense organs are well developed. Many are entirely fluent in oral language and can understand most conversation by means of lip reading. In talking to a deaf person who has this capability, use short phrases and sentences rather than single words. This provides him with more clues, and the normal rhythm and accent patterns of speech become part of the speech picture. However, do not use sentences that are too complex.

Unfortunately, many deaf people do not read lips but must rely on sign language to communicate with each other. Often these people are limited in their ability to read and write as well, so that writing notes to them is not very productive. Gestures that come naturally to nurse and patient will usually serve to supplement demonstrations and convey meaning. Sometimes it helps to illustrate actions with stick figures.

It is important that one person spend time communicating with the deaf patient every day. Otherwise he may be thrust further into himself and become confused and apprehensive.

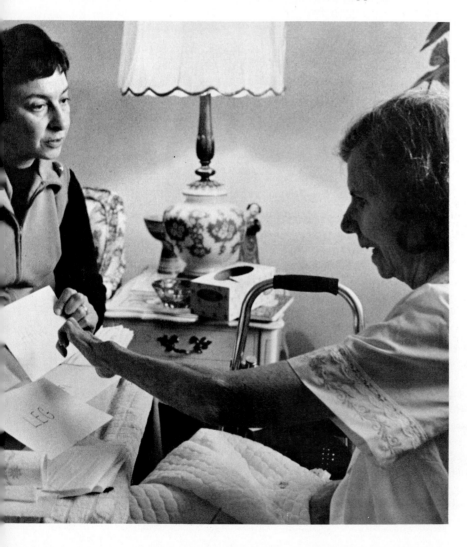

The use of cards with words and pictures of familiar objects can aid in reestablishing verbal communication with an aphasic stroke patient.
[Courtesy the Visiting Nurse Service of New York]

Cancer of the larynx is a disease in which loss of the voice is inevitable, either because the tumor metastasizes to the vocal cords or because the patient's larynx is removed. One way of helping these patients to communicate is to provide them with a "magic slate" on which to write notes. If paper is used, it should be destroyed after the conversation to protect the patient's privacy.

The nurse should resist the urge to finish the patient's sentences for him, which may cause him great frustration. Also, she should try to avoid situations where visitors and staff are chattering excessively in front of the patient, which often distresses him.

Intellectual impairment. Stroke, or cerebral hemorrhage, can occur in any of the brain areas that control use of spoken or written words. Fortunately, 50 to 70 percent of stroke victims recover speech spontaneously.

Speechlessness can be caused by the inability to hear, limitations in understanding, lack of word memory, or paralysis of the muscles of speech. Whatever the cause, the solution is the same: Find some means to start communicating, and keep working until all possible progress has been achieved. Here are some suggestions:

1. Speak slowly and simply, using short sentences. Do not try to talk over loud noises.
2. Give the patient plenty of time to respond to your questions.
3. Listen patiently to labored or slurred pronunciation, and try as hard as possible to understand the meaning.
4. Anticipate the patient's needs for care.
5. Explain and demonstrate the use of the call button as many times as necessary. Be sure it is placed near the functioning hand.

Word finding is one of the most frequent difficulties that besets the aphasic patient. The nurse can help him in his word search by waiting calmly while he tries to think and by not talking for him. If he is unsuccessful after a few attempts, she should supply him with a few words in multiple-choice fashion. This helps him maintain the feeling that he is communicating.

SUMMARY

A definition of communication was offered at the beginning of this chapter. Communication is a cognitive sorting, selecting, and sending of symbols in such a way as to help a listener elicit from his own mind a meaning or response similar to that intended by the communicator.

Communication is a mutual, ongoing, and transactional process that is based on common experience. The process of communication is closely bound to the process of perception—how we receive the signals sent to us and how we interpret them. Many influences color our perception, from the sharpness of our eyesight to the attitudes of our family.

The communication process has been put into the form of various verbal-pictorial models. Essentially, the following sequence of events takes place:

$$\text{source} \longrightarrow \text{encoder} \longrightarrow \text{message} \longrightarrow \text{decoder} \longrightarrow \text{interpretation}$$

The model presented in this chapter illustrates the above definition. The diagram on p. 209 illustrates how two people communicate; however, the same general principles apply to groups as well.

The communication between nurse and patient differs from her interchange with friends in one essential—purpose. In establishing verbal and nonverbal lines of communication with a patient, the nurse is seeking to influence his behavior in the interest of his health. Of course, not all of her conversation is goal-oriented; nurses and patients may indulge in small talk as long as the nurse is aware of the actual level and purpose of any given conversation.

The essential tool in the establishment of a nurse-patient relationship is the interview. The nurse observes, listens, responds verbally and nonverbally, and records data. She focuses on the patient and subtly draws out his feelings so that she can become aware of his needs.

Basically, the patient does the talking in an interview. Although the nurse prompts him with questions, she does not usually take the lead. The good interviewer is aware of a number of rules:

1. Approach the patient directly
2. Use minimal verbal activity
3. Encourage spontaneity
4. Focus on emotionally charged areas
5. Be sensitive to subtle clues

In these interviews, which may occur in a formal setting or be a sequence of impromptu conversations, the nurse looks for three types of theme: content (the "what" of the patient's story), mood (how he tells his story), and interaction (his relationship with the nurse). By being aware of the different themes and their progression, she is drawn closer to an understanding of problems that are bothering the patient. She helps him decide which themes are most significant to him and how they can be dealt with.

One of the main principles of effective interviewing is that verbal activity should be kept to a minimum; even complete silence can serve a therapeutic purpose. But while the focus of the nurse-patient relationship is on the patient, the nurse must put something of herself into the relationship or there will be no interaction. She can learn to establish rapport even if she dislikes the patient.

The nurse can also learn to avoid the many pitfalls to meaningful communication by being aware of them. Among the major stumbling blocks are: changing the subject abruptly; giving unwanted opinions; inappropriate reassurance; jumping to conclusions; and inappropriate use of medical facts.

Establishing rapport is particularly difficult when a patient is handicapped in his ability to communicate, but the task is not impossible if the nurse has patience and is sympathetic. With a non-English-speaking patient or one who has suffered a stroke, gestures, touch, and tone of voice assume added importance. With the deaf, who can often read lips, clear and slow speech is required. In all of these cases, the nurse must find some means of communicating if she is to carry out her essential tasks of observation and understanding.

STUDY QUESTIONS

1. What is transactional communication?
2. Using the Ross communicational model given on p. 209, briefly define the following terms: source, encoder, message, decoder, interpretation.
3. What is nonverbal communication? Give examples of ways in which we communicate nonverbally.
4. What is the difference between a conversation and an interview? Briefly list the characteristics and goals of the interviewing process.
5. Interview an acquaintance who has a hearing loss in order to determine his feelings and suggestions regarding communication.
6. Analyze a television news interview and identify the techniques presented in this chapter. Why were some of the interviewer's questions and nonverbal approaches more effective than others in eliciting a response from the individual being interviewed?

SELECTED BIBLIOGRAPHY

Bernstein, Lewis; Bernstein, Rosalyn S.; and Dana, Richard H. 1974. *Interviewing: A guide for health professionals,* 2d ed. New York: Appleton-Century-Crofts.

Greenhill, Maurice H. 1956. Interviewing with a purpose. *American Journal of Nursing* 56:n.p.

Hewitt, Helon E., and Pesznecker, Betty L. 1964. Blocks to communicating with patients. *American Journal of Nursing* 64:101–03.

Ross, Raymond S. 1974. *Speech communication: Fundamentals and practice,* 3d ed. Englewood Cliffs, N.J.: Prentice-Hall.

Sutterley, Doris Cook, and Donnelly, Gloria Ferraro. 1973. *Perspectives in human development: Nursing throughout the life cycle,* pp. 104–26. Philadelphia: Lippincott.

Ujhely, Gertrud B. 1968. *Determinants of the nurse-patient relationship.* New York: Springer.

11 Teaching-learning aspects of nursing

Upon completing this chapter, the reader should be able to:

1. Explain the concept of teaching as an integral part of nursing, organized to produce a change in patient behavior.

2. Discuss the organization of effective teaching as a number of planned steps, including evaluation of learning needs, evaluation of the patient's learning readiness, and involvement of the patient in constructing the teaching plan.

3. Describe techniques used in individualized teaching, such as the use of audiovisual materials, discussion, and demonstration.

4. Identify the parallel relationship between the steps in the teaching process and those in the nursing process.

What is learning?

Learning is the discovery of meaning. According to modern psychologists, learning involves two steps. The first is the acquisition of new information or experience. The second is the individual's discovery of the meaning that information holds for him.

Information can come from many sources. It may, for example, be provided by a book or a professor. The discovery of meaning, on the other hand, is an inner experience. It demands the involvement of the learner. Real learning—learning that produces a change in behavior—means finding the relationship between events and oneself.

As John Dewey pointed out, information by itself is unlikely to affect a learner in any important way unless he does something with it.[1] This may mean relating it to an event in his own experience or acting upon it. For example, a person may be aware that hunger is a problem for millions of people all over the world. This information may not become really significant, however, unless he deliberately fasts for 24 hours to feel the effects of going without food.

Learning is more effective when a person is ready to learn, in terms of both experience and desire. In order to maintain the desire to learn, he must receive satisfaction from learning. A teacher helps her student by setting realistic goals for him. If the learning steps are too easy, desire lags. If they are too difficult, the learner becomes discouraged. The teacher must constantly evaluate the student's progress so that she can change the established goals if necessary.

In order to learn a particular skill, a person must have a mental image of how it is performed. This mental image is best provided by demonstration. "The less mature an individual—whether child or adult—the more

---

[1] Arthur W. Combs, Donald L. Avila, and William W. Purkey. 1971. *Helping relationships: Basic concepts for the helping professions*, p. 113. Boston: Allyn and Bacon.

he needs concepts presented in concrete ways rather than abstractly. He must see, touch, smell, hear, and taste whenever possible rather than discussing something or reading about it."[2]

Teaching is the art of helping people learn.

What is teaching?

Teaching may be described as communication arranged in a certain order and directed by principles of learning.[3] More simply, it is the art of helping people learn.

Entering into a teaching relationship with a patient requires a definite commitment on the part of the nurse. She must see to it that the process is continued until specific goals are reached or until instruction is no longer profitable. In committing herself to this goal, the nurse must overcome possible fears that she is inferior in knowledge or social status to the patient. For example, a young single nurse may hesitate to adopt the role of teacher with a woman who has just had her fourth child. Or she may be uncomfortable teaching a middle-aged man how to care for his colostomy. A thorough knowledge of the subject matter will go a long way in helping to overcome these problems. The nurse must also realize that she has information or insight that will be useful to the patient in promoting or maintaining a high level of health. Experience in dealing with these situations also lends poise.

What are some of the principles of teaching in nursing settings? One author suggests the following:

1. *Good nurse-learner rapport is important.* By establishing a positive, constructive relationship with the patient, the nurse will encourage his cooperation.
2. *Teaching requires effective communication.* It is not enough to tell a patient to do something "frequently." Two different people may attach different meanings to the word. Communication must be as clear and specific as possible. The nurse must check often to make sure she is being understood.
3. *Learning needs of clients must be determined.* The nurse must find out how much the patient knows about health principles so that she does not try to teach him what he already knows.
4. *Objectives should serve as guides in planning and evaluating teaching.* There are three major reasons for formulating objectives: to make clear what is to be accomplished, to give direction, and to provide a means of evaluation.

[2] Ibid.
[3] Barbara K. Redman. 1968. *The process of patient teaching in nursing,* p. 61. St. Louis: Mosby.

5. *Time for teaching must be carefully and deliberately worked into the nurse's schedule.* Much teaching can be done while she is also doing something else, such as changing a dressing.
6. *Control of the environment is an aspect of teaching.* People learn better in a room that is well lit, free of noise, not too hot, and well furnished.[4]

What are the teaching responsibilities of the nurse?

The nurse provides the patient with anything from general health information to material related to his specific problems.

The nurse's best opportunities for teaching often arise informally. In such informal situations, teaching and learning may go on while other tasks are being performed. For example, the nurse who washes her hands in the patient's bathroom before and after changing his dressing is teaching him something about **asepsis.** She might also explain the reason for her handwashing, thus reinforcing the patient's learning from her example.

The patient may signal his learning needs in several ways. First, he may ask a direct question: "How can I keep the swelling in my legs down?" Or he may seek information indirectly, through a comment: "I can't seem to feel anything in my feet any more." In this case, the nurse would seize the opportunity to explore his comment more fully. Depending on what she knows his learning needs to be, she might then teach the patient how to elevate his legs properly when sitting down. In some cases, she might briefly explain the physiological reasons for the lack of feeling.

The patient may also show the need for teaching through his behavior. For example, a man who has just had a heart attack pulls his bedside stand closer to him. He then reaches for the bottom drawer. The nurse now has the ideal opportunity to teach him the importance of restricting his activities and what such restriction should include. However, she must also recognize and provide for his need to maintain independence at a threatening and anxiety-producing time.

The nurse must also be able to foresee the need for teaching. For example, a patient about to undergo cataract surgery must be prepared for the restrictions that will be placed on him after the operation. He must be ready for the inevitable period of adjustment before his vision improves. With preparation, his recovery period will be made easier.

Times for informal teaching occur at every point in the nurse's daily cycle of activities. They may occur while making home visits, giving immunizations in a clinic, bathing patients, or giving medications. Family members should be included in this informal teaching whenever possible.

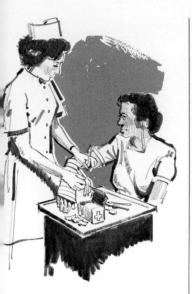

Times for informal teaching occur at every point in the nurse's daily cycle of activities.

[4]Margaret L. Pohl. 1973. *The teaching function of the nursing practitioner,* 2d ed., pp. 27 ff. Dubuque, Iowa: Brown.

Teaching and the nursing process

Assessment

Obtaining data. Teaching for a hospital patient should be based upon data obtained throughout the patient's illness. Such data will provide meaningful information about how he is coping with his condition.

The assessment plan contains four types of information:

1. *Preadmission and admission items.* These include admission and referral information, previous hospital care, age, sex, race, religion, marital status, family profile, living quarters, income, insurance, education, disablement, daily living habits, and diet.
2. *In-hospital data.* This information involves a physical assessment according to the primary disease. It also includes a judgment as to how the patient will respond to his disease. Also important are the patient's physiological and psychological reactions.
3. *A judgment as to how the patient will be cared for after he leaves the hospital.* Will he receive home care, hospital-based home care, or community-based home care? Will he go to an extended-care facility, a nursing home, or an ambulatory-care facility?
4. *Follow-up evaluation.* How did the patient respond to being in the hospital? What has been his behavior pattern following release? What are his current learning needs?

Identifying learning needs and problems. Once the necessary data have been collected, the nurse turns to an assessment of the specific needs of her patient. She must always keep in mind that each patient is an individual, whose feelings, concerns, and perceptions may vary from time to time in the course of his illness or disability.

Before the nurse decides on a teaching plan, she must take into consideration the patient's learning needs as he sees them. Then she must decide how to acquaint him with any other learning needs of which he may not be aware. It is usually best to deal first with those needs that the patient recognizes, including any which the nurse herself may not have been aware of previously.

Successful collaboration with patients is based on the belief that most are rational people who can understand all but the most complex aspects of their care. The nurse acts on this belief by assuring each patient that he has the right to know what is being done to, for, and about him and his illness.

One nurse has described the case of a 16-year-old boy who was discovered to be diabetic.[5] Her knowledge of his background and present status led her to decide that he should:

---

[5]Sheila H. Huang. 1971. Nursing assessment in planning care for a diabetic patient. *Nursing Clinics of North America* 6:140.

1. Take insulin daily
2. Learn to give himself his own insulin shots
3. Be able to perform a urine test
4. Learn to select the proper food and to change his diet according to his physical activity
5. Learn how to recognize **insulin reaction** and how to prevent or lessen it
6. Know that a diabetic is more prone to infection
7. Understand the need for long-term follow-up and regular physical checkups

In coming to these conclusions, the nurse made use of the patient's own reactions to his condition. He showed some of his concerns through asking questions. For example, he asked for an explanation of the nature of his illness. Besides the obvious desire for information, this question also implied a need for assurance that he could still lead a normal life. Other aspects of his behavior showed a need for confidence in his ability to learn self-care as well as a certain dependence upon his mother.

Observation of the patient's readiness and capabilities for learning. The patient's ability to absorb new knowledge is based partly on his level of awareness. His behavior will be a direct result of this awareness.

The patient who is well-informed about his condition will be ahead of other patients in the speed with which he will learn. Also, the more intelligent patient usually will have a head start on the patient of limited intelligence.

Yet even people with severely limited abilities can be taught effectively. One nurse tells of a 67-year-old patient admitted to the hospital with a diagnosis of malignant rectal mass.[6] She eventually underwent a sigmoid colostomy. This woman had spent over 20 years in a state mental hospital due to **paranoid schizophrenia** and mild mental deficiency. The nursing staff at first despaired of teaching her to care for her colostomy bag. However, they soon learned that she had been bathing and dressing herself for years. Although able to focus on only one task at a time, she was very thorough and learned to care for the bag after only 3 days of training.

Psychological factors are also important. As was discussed in chapter 8, severe anxiety often accompanies changes in health status. For example, patients who are about to undergo surgery are particularly subject to both specific fears and "free-floating" anxiety about what will happen to them. Many patients fear that they will never wake up from anesthesia. They worry that spinal anesthesia will paralyze them. The best thing a nurse can do in this situation is to create an atmosphere in which the patient

[6]Linda Harman Aiken. 1970. Patient problems are problems in learning. *American Journal of Nursing* 70:1916.

feels free to voice these concerns. The nurse can then explain to the patient what is going to happen to him. She should answer his questions as fully as is necessary to help relieve his fears.

The nurse should also remember that patients go through different psychological stages in the course of their illness. Briefly, these psychological stages are:

1. *Disbelief,* including hostility and denial of illness
2. *Awareness* of illness and a feeling of loss of identity
3. *Acceptance* of illness and resumption of some control
4. *Adaptation* to illness and reaffirmation of identity

A patient's desire and ability to learn will be related to the stage he has reached. For example, while he feels powerless or lacking in control, he will not be an effective learner.

Like psychological stress, the physiological stress of acute illness also affects the patient's ability to learn. Because most of his energy is at first directed toward survival, he is unable to deal with the details of his therapy. In the beginning, the nurse's teaching role is mainly supportive. She helps the patient through his crisis and attempts to relieve his anxiety so that learning can take place.

What about the elderly patient? While his ability to learn may be lessened in some cases, he can usually take some part in planning his own care. A teaching plan that allows him to make decisions and participate in caring for himself helps the older patient recognize his own abilities. In this way he can regain much-needed self-esteem. However, being pushed beyond the limits of his abilities will increase his feelings of inadequacy and should be avoided.

Older people sometimes have shorter attention spans and do not always grasp ideas as easily as younger people. Often they learn better when materials are presented in a concise and concrete manner. Because the older patient's sight is often impaired, good lighting is essential during a teaching session.

Planning and implementation

Setting goals in collaboration with a patient. Nursing goals can be divided into short-term and long-term goals. They are determined by the patient's immediate and long-range needs. A single need of a patient may result in several nursing goals. On the other hand, one nursing goal may meet several of the patient's needs.

While the patient is acutely ill, he will not have much of a chance to talk over goals of treatment with the nurse. However, as he improves, his role in the planning process assumes great importance.

One approach to teaching is to plan *for* the patient. In this approach,

> The nurse helps the patient through his crisis and attempts to relieve his anxiety so that learning can take place.

Discussion involves an
exchange of ideas
among persons.

the nurse transmits information and skills. It is assumed that the patient will be a generally passive but willing and grateful recipient of this information. Experience shows, however, that this is rarely the case. Few patients will change their behavior simply because someone has informed them as to why they should do something.

Determining priorities. Both patient and nurse have contributions to make to the planning process. Priorities should be set jointly, based upon the patient's felt needs and the nurse's professional judgment as to his most pressing learning problems. Further planning by the nurse should include a choice of content that is tailored to the patient's specific problems.

Lesson planning. There are many ways in which written lesson plans can be organized. They can be written in sentence or in outline form. The experienced nurse will usually need only a word outline to bring entire ideas to mind.

In preparing an outline, the nurse should make note of places where a specific teaching action should be taken. These actions include use of an audiovisual aid, a demonstration, or a particular question directed to the patient.

By writing the content and teaching actions side by side the nurse will be able to coordinate the two. She will clearly see where there are large blocks of verbal content that would be enhanced by visual aids. In some cases there may be too many aids for a small block of material. This also allows her to judge whether objectives can be met by the methods chosen. If the objective is that a patient learn how to breast-feed her newborn, it would hardly be appropriate for all the teaching actions to center upon discussion.

Choice of method. From their own experience, nursing students are familiar with various teaching methods. The best method of teaching a patient often combines individual and group instruction. At a Connecticut hospital, for example, classes as well as a planned program of individual instruction are conducted for diabetic patients and their families.[7] The nurse who organized the program assembled teaching materials that could be brought to the classroom or bedside in a basket. These included samples of urine-testing materials, recording charts, syringes and needles, insulin, medication vials and labels, alcohol sponges, dry cotton balls, etc. The basket may be used by any nurse instructing a diabetic patient or his family.

One-to-one instruction is of great value. For one thing, it allows the nurse to pace her teaching program according to the patient's progress.

[7]Lisa M. Trayser. 1973. A teaching program for diabetics. *American Journal of Nursing* 73:92.

However, it is often more convenient to teach in groups. This is usually the case when families are involved or if hospital staff is limited. If patients have specific questions, they should be encouraged to raise them during their next one-to-one contact with the nurse.

Group instruction, on the other hand, also offers many advantages. It provides thorough instruction for more patients, a definite time and place for learning, and a consistent presentation of instructions. In addition, it gives the patient support through contact with other patients who have similar problems.

An important part of both individual and group instruction is discussion. Discussion involves an exchange of ideas among persons. The best discussions are those in which all members of a group actively participate. Discussion also takes place in a one-to-one situation.

Group instruction allows patients to come in contact with and learn from others having similar problems. Here, a nurse conducts a discussion of the first trimester of pregnancy with parents at a Red Cross mother and baby care course. [Photo by Ted Carland, courtesy the American Red Cross]

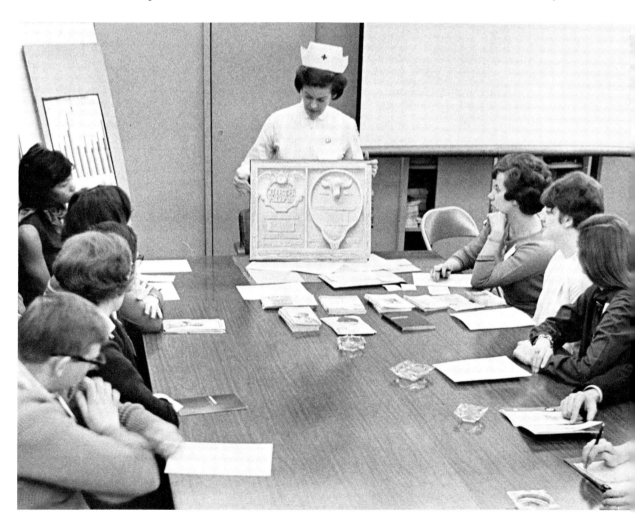

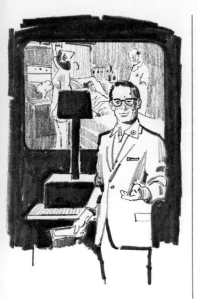

Most demonstrations will be helped by the use of various teaching materials.

During a discussion with a patient scheduled for a barium enema, for example, the nurse might show him the need for this procedure by asking him about his symptoms. She must show interest in what he wants to know about the entire experience. She should always take into account his feelings about undergoing such an uncomfortable procedure as well as his fears about the possible findings. This kind of give-and-take often provides strong motivation for the patient to learn about his condition. It also helps the nurse make sure that the patient understands what is happening to him.

Discussion may also involve demonstration. The demonstration-performance method of instruction is perhaps the simplest and most natural of all. It is particularly useful when manual skills or physical movements are to be taught.

A demonstration can be either formal or informal, planned or spontaneous. The informal method is used most frequently in one-to-one situations. The formal method requires more planning on the part of the teacher. It is most often used in group instruction.

When demonstrating a procedure, the nurse should go slowly through the entire process. She should explain each step thoroughly as she goes along. Uncommon terms should be avoided. If the patient appears lost, the nurse should stop the demonstration and go back over the material until it is clear in the patient's mind.

At the end of the presentation, the nurse should briefly summarize what she has said and done. This helps the patient to see the process as a unified whole rather than as a series of unrelated steps. In addition, it is important to make sure that the patient thoroughly understands a procedure before allowing him to try it himself. Most demonstrations will be helped by the use of various teaching materials.

Today, a wide variety of these materials is available in many hospitals. The nurse often has access to slides, tapes, filmstrips, and charts. These materials can be of great value in those illnesses where the patient must learn extensive self-care. However, these materials can never take the place of the nurse. She should consider them as aids to the development of an individualized teaching plan and be ready to follow up appropriately when necessary.

It is also important that the nurse supervise the patient's use of these aids. At Kaiser-Permanente Medical Center in Los Angeles, an Audiscan machine is used for some patient education programs.[8] Located at the patient's bedside, the small unit looks like a portable TV set and plays sound-and-slide programs. The nurse can stop the film whenever she wishes—if it proves upsetting or if questions arise. Filmstrips are available on a wide range of subjects, including emphysema, diabetes, and obstetric, coronary, and postsurgical care.

[8]Making the patient a part of patient care. 1973. *Modern Hospital* 121:108.

In using written materials, it is important to bear in mind the patient's reading ability. Experience has shown that people who have developed the habit of reading can be reached in many ways, including posters, newspapers, and other written materials. The person who does not read easily will often respond to radio and television.[9]

The use of complex medical terms can be confusing to many patients. If a patient does not understand the terms used by health professionals, he may turn instead to his roommate or his visitors for their "medical" opinions. This often leads to further misunderstanding and anxiety for the patient.

The nurse cannot always predict which terms will present problems to a particular patient. She should be aware, however, of the kinds of words that are often misunderstood. Certainly words such as "visualization," "contraindication," and "cathartic" should generally be eliminated from teaching materials.

The nurse should always make use of the talents of other members of the health care team. Nutritionists, physical therapists, and others all have valuable contributions to make to the development of any teaching plan. The nurse may call upon them to help her in developing her own knowledge and skill as well as to participate directly in patient teaching.

Timing. No matter which method of teaching the nurse selects, she must bear in mind that the patient is undergoing a difficult time in his life. She should try to avoid attempts to teach during times that may be stressful.

Teaching sessions should be kept short so that patient interest will be sustained. It is also important to have an unhurried manner. When the patient makes mistakes, he should be corrected gently and encouragingly with courtesy and tact.

Evaluation

As is the case with the other steps in the nursing process, evaluation requires a joint effort by patient and nurse. It also may involve the efforts of the patient's family and other members of the health care team.

Evaluation takes place in many ways. The following methods will be helpful:

1. The nurse should observe the patient to determine if he has mastered the tasks at hand. Can he now give himself his own insulin shots? Is he able to use his crutches properly?
2. The patient will often give verbal clues that indicate his level of understanding. These include questions—an obvious indication—and general comments, which may be more subtle.

[9]Redman, p. 78.

The nurse should always make use of the talents of other members of the health care team.

3. The nurse may question the patient directly. She should, however, avoid the impression that the patient is now being given a "final examination." Feelings of failure on the patient's part will only hinder the learning process.

4. The nurse should consider the observations of members of the patient's family and other health professionals who have come in contact with him.

There are several possible results of the evaluation of any teaching process. First, the patient may have responded as expected. The goals of the process may have been reached and the patient's problems resolved. No further teaching action may be needed. The nurse may, however, plan for a later follow-up to make sure that the problem has not recurred.

Second, it is possible that the immediate goals of the teaching process have been reached, but long-range problems remain to be solved. The nurse will then devise a new plan to deal with these long-term goals. The results of this new plan will then be evaluated.

Third, it may be found that the patient's problems remain unsolved. It is possible that certain patient problems were not foreseen. This situation calls for reassessment and a new plan.

Finally, it may be that new problems have arisen. Plans for dealing with these new problems must now be coordinated with efforts to solve the patient's original problems.

Modification

If evaluation reveals the need for changes in the teaching plan, the nurse will move into the modification phase of the nursing process. Modification involves a reassessment of the patient's needs and the drawing up of a new plan to meet these needs. Once the new plan has been decided upon and implemented, the nurse will once again enter the evaluation phase. If further modification is indicated, the whole cycle will repeat itself until the patient's learning problems are resolved.

SUMMARY

Teaching is an important part of the nurse's activities. It may include anything from giving general health information to providing specific facts about the patient's condition. Many hospitals hold formal group instruction sessions, particularly for certain types of patients such as pregnant women or emphysema patients. However, it is often during informal moments that the nurse finds her best opportunities for effective teaching.

The nurse collects data on the patient's learning needs throughout the course of her contact with him. She does this through observation, listening, and exploration. Once the necessary information is at hand, the nurse develops her specific teaching plan. At all stages she is sure to involve the patient in the planning, implementation, and evaluation of his own care. The success of her plan will depend to a large degree on this involvement.

Before putting her teaching plan into effect, the nurse evaluates the patient's readiness to learn. She must take note of his intelligence as well as his awareness of his condition. She must also bear in mind his psychological state. The fact of illness itself may create anxiety that will block the patient's ability to learn. In addition, patients pass through a series of psychological stages, each of which influences their readiness to learn.

A number of techniques are effective in teaching. Among these are discussion, demonstration, and performance. The use of written, graphic, and audiovisual materials is also helpful. The nurse must always consider the individual needs of the patient when choosing her teaching methods.

As the teaching plan is implemented, the nurse obtains constant feedback from the patient. She evaluates the success of her plan and, if necessary, modifies it to better meet his needs.

STUDY QUESTIONS

1. What is learning? Briefly define the two steps that make up the learning process.
2. Identify four of the conditions that must be met if teaching/learning is to take place.
3. How does the nurse establish teaching goals for herself? How does the nurse establish learning goals for the patient?
4. Name three methods of teaching a nurse may use. Suggest situations in which each might be appropriate, and explain why.
5. Draw up a teaching plan for a 55-year-old married male patient who has been placed on a low-sodium diet for hypertension.

SELECTED BIBLIOGRAPHY

Aiken, Linda Harman. 1970. Patient problems are problems in learning. *American Journal of Nursing* 70:1916–18.

Combs, Arthur W.; Avila, Donald L.; and Purkey, William W. 1971. *Helping relationships: Basic concepts for the helping professions.* Boston: Allyn and Bacon.

Haferkorn, Virginia. 1971. Assessing individual learning needs as a basis for patient teaching. *Nursing Clinics of North America* 6:199–209.

Pohl, Margaret L. 1973. *The teaching function of the nursing practitioner.* Dubuque, Iowa: Brown.

Staton, Thomas F. 1960. *How to instruct successfully: Modern teaching methods in adult education.* New York: McGraw-Hill.

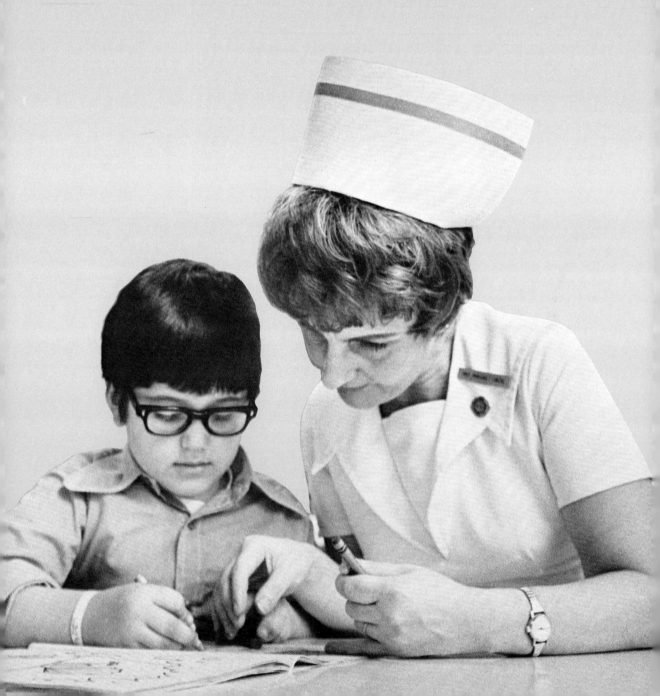

Part Four

The therapeutic environment

Charlotte had always considered herself a bargain-hunter on her many trips to Europe. But one souvenir she had never bargained for was a case of infectious hepatitis.

A few days after returning home from her latest trip, she began to develop chills, fever, abdominal cramps, and vomiting. The events of the next week all ran together in her mind. There was the visit to the doctor, after which her symptoms seemed to subside. But then they flared up again, worse than ever, and suddenly she developed jaundice. At that point, she was admitted to the isolation wing of the local hospital.

At first, isolation had almost seemed welcome. It was a chance to read, rest, and daydream. But after a week, Charlotte had had quite enough. Even reading and television were not enticing any more. Then the doctor suggested that she keep a diary to help pass the time.

Monday: Have been sleeping badly the last few nights. There's so much time during the day to do nothing except nap that I'm slept out by nightfall. I don't even dream anymore, except about escaping from this room. I might feel better if I weren't so bored, but I don't seem to have the energy to do anything to relieve the boredom. The fluorescent light in the room doesn't even change the sound of its buzz.

The night duty nurse came in and talked with me for a while last night. She says she understands how I feel, that night duty can be deadly boring too. It's so quiet, and the subdued night lights make everything look gray. But at least her shift ends at 7A.M. My "shift" seems to be going on forever.

Wednesday: Didn't feel like writing yesterday. I was dozing off in the afternoon and suddenly it seemed as though the ticking from the wall clock was a herd of wild animals charging into my room. I woke up screaming and it took the nurse a while to calm me down. She said I had been hallucinating and that it happens sometimes to people in isolation.

On top of that, I think I'm getting worse instead of better. They've taken my temperature 6 times instead of the usual 4. An extra stool culture was sent down to the lab, and everyone seems to be taking a lot more care

245

about washing their hands before and after treating me.

Thursday: Had to stop writing yesterday because my food tray came. The food seems to be getting worse and worse. I get to choose the menu, but since I'm on a low-fat diet, it's like asking a kid to choose between spinach and liver!

Sometimes these days I flare up at the silliest things, or at the wrong people. It's just so frustrating not to be able to decide my own actions. Maybe it wouldn't bother me so much if I weren't used to being so independent.

Saturday: I'm being moved to a semiprivate room today. Don't know who my roommate will be. I hope she doesn't have a lot of visitors coming in while I'm trying to sleep.

A few days after moving into the semiprivate room Charlotte was released from the hospital. The health care team explained to her the danger of bringing on a relapse by overextending herself. Charlotte didn't think that was likely. Most of her energy went into thinking about what she wanted to do. She just didn't seem to have enough energy left over to actually do it.

During the first few days at home, Charlotte almost missed the hospital. Its routine seemed so safe and secure. She had no worries there. Anita and some friends stopped by regularly to help out, and the visiting nurse came daily for a stool culture. But Charlotte found herself depressed by the effort it took to do even simple things. She wondered if she would ever get back to her normal life.

What safety precautions and infection control measures should be taken for a patient in isolation?

What are the patient's rights in this situation?

What precautions should be included in discharge planning?

---

12 Patients' rights in the health care system

History of interest in patients' rights

The concept of **patients' rights** is a rather recent phenomenon. To a large extent it is a by-product of two trends in twentieth-century America: legal redefinition of previously protected relationships, such as landlord-tenant or employer-employee, and the rise of the consumer movement.

Frequently, supporters of these trends have referred to principles of human or personal rights. For example, truth-in-lending laws are based on the idea that the customer has a right to know the true interest rate he will be charged. Many people are beginning to insist that the health care consumer also has certain rights, which have been largely disregarded in the past.

During the past few years in particular, the vague concept of patients' rights has been brought into sharper focus. For example, in 1973 "A Patient's Bill of Rights" was approved by the American Hospital Association (AHA), and public reaction was almost universally favorable. Also in 1973, the American Medical Association endorsed the institution of patient grievance mechanisms.

Hospitals have begun to respond to the patients' rights movement in many different ways. Some now distribute booklets to inform patients that they can expect to be treated with courtesy and efficiency. In New York, the first patients' rights workshop in the city's history was carried out with remarkable success. In Pennsylvania, a "Citizens' Bill of Hospital Rights" was released in 1973 by the state insurance commissioner. This was the first public statement of its type. And a national consumer group, Public Citizen, Inc., has turned its attention to the health care field. It has demanded more information about medical procedures and better quality care. Members of this group also insist that the hospital be made more accountable to the consumer.

At the national level, the Secretary's Commission on Medical Malpractice, Department of Health, Education and Welfare, released a report

Upon completing this chapter, the reader should be able to:

1. Place the current status of the patient's Bill of Rights in the historical context of the trend toward human rights.

2. Explain the ethical and legal considerations involved in patients' rights.

3. Discuss specific patients' rights and current mechanisms designed to protect them.

A
Patient's
Bill
of
Rights

Approved by the
House of Delegates
of the American
Hospital Association,
February 6, 1973

The American Hospital Association presents a Patient's Bill of Rights with the expectation that observance of these rights will contribute to more effective patient care and greater satisfaction for the patient, his physician, and the hospital organization. Further, the Association presents these rights in the expectation that they will be supported by the hospital on behalf of its patients, as an integral part of the healing process. It is recognized that a personal relationship between the physician and the patient is essential for the provision of proper medical care. The traditional physician-patient relationship takes on a new dimension when care is rendered within an organizational structure. Legal precedent has established that the institution itself also has a responsibility to the patient. It is in recognition of these factors that these rights are affirmed.

1 The patient has the right to considerate and respectful care.

2 The patient has the right to obtain from his physician complete current information concerning his diagnosis, treatment, and prognosis in terms the patient can be reasonably expected to understand. When it is not medically advisable to give such information to the patient, the information should be made available to an appropriate person in his behalf. He has the right to know, by name, the physician responsible for co-ordinating his care.

3 The patient has the right to receive from his physician information necessary to give informed consent prior to the start of any procedure and/or treatment. Except in emergencies, such information for informed consent should include but not necessarily be limited to the specific procedure and/or treatment, the medically significant risks involved, and the probable duration of incapacitation. Where medically significant alternatives for care or treatment exist, or when the patient requests information concerning medical alternatives, the patient has the right to such information. The patient also has the right to know the name of the person responsible for the procedures and/or treatment.

4 The patient has the right to refuse treatment to the extent permitted by law, and to be informed of the medical consequences of his action.

5 The patient has the right to every consideration of his privacy concerning his own medical care program. Case discussion, consultation, examination, and treatment are confidential and should be conducted discreetly. Those not directly involved in his care must have the permission of the patient to be present.

FIG. 12-1 *The bill of rights for a patient.*
[© 1972 by the American Hospital Association. Reprinted by permission.]

in 1973 recommending the adoption and distribution of a patient's bill of rights. It also advocated the development of institutional patient grievance mechanisms.

What is the basis for defining patients' rights?

The rationale for patients' rights includes both ethical and legal considerations. One legal provision is that the patient has the right to informed consent. In other words, he is entitled to an explanation of the treatment he is about to undergo and has the right to refuse it.

6 The patient has the right to expect that all communications and records pertaining to his care should be treated as confidential.

7 The patient has the right to expect that within its capacity a hospital must make reasonable response to the request of a patient for services. The hospital must provide evaluation, service, and/or referral as indicated by the urgency of the case. When medically permissible a patient may be transferred to another facility only after he has received complete information and explanation concerning the needs for and alternatives to such a transfer. The institution to which the patient is to be transferred must first have accepted the patient for transfer.

8 The patient has the right to obtain information as to any relationship of his hospital to other health care and educational institutions insofar as his care is concerned. The patient has the right to obtain information as to the existence of any professional relationships among individuals, by name, who are treating him.

9 The patient has the right to be advised if the hospital proposes to engage in or perform human experimentation affecting his care or treatment. The patient has the right to refuse to participate in such research projects.

10 The patient has the right to expect reasonable continuity of care. He has the right to know in advance what appointment times and physicians are available and where. The patient has the right to expect that the hospital will provide a mechanism whereby he is informed by his physician or a delegate of the physician of the patient's continuing health care requirements following discharge.

11 The patient has the right to examine and receive an explanation of his bill regardless of source of payment.

12 The patient has the right to know what hospital rules and regulations apply to his conduct as a patient.

No catalogue of rights can guarantee for the patient the kind of treatment he has a right to expect. A hospital has many functions to perform, including the prevention and treatment of disease, the education of both health professionals and patients, and the conduct of clinical research. All these activities must be conducted with an overriding concern for the patient, and, above all, the recognition of his dignity as a human being. Success in achieving this recognition assures success in the defense of the rights of the patient.

The nurse's understanding of patients' rights can be guided to some degree by an understanding of her own legal status. State laws that regulate nursing are called practice acts. Some of these acts define and specify limitations of the functions of the professional and practical nurse.

In New York, for example, the role of the professional nurse is defined as the performance of paid services to a patient, requiring the "application of nursing principles depending on biologic, physical, and social sciences."[1] The act holds that the nurse is responsible for supervision of patients. It

[1] Sidney Willig. 1971. Nursing and the law. In *Nursing: Concepts of practice,* ed. Dorothea E. Orem, p. 183. New York: McGraw-Hill.

also provides that she must be skilled in the observation of symptoms and reactions and able to describe and communicate them by accurately recording the facts. She is authorized to carry out treatments and give medications as prescribed by a licensed physician. She is also expected to apply "nursing procedures involving an understanding of cause and effect" in order to safeguard the life and health of the patient.

Although it is not a legal document, the AHA's widely acclaimed bill of rights is perhaps the most important reference point in a discussion of patient rights. According to one analyst, this bill "says what we in nursing have been saying for years, but it says it emphatically to all who would be patients and to those who are accountable for making those rights available—the hospital administrator and the physician who practices medicine in that hospital."[2]

Specific patients' rights

The right to adequate health care

According to the AHA bill of rights, a patient is entitled to "considerate and respectful care."

It may seem surprising that such a right needs definition at this time. Today, medical technology is advancing at a rapid pace, and people have a better chance than ever in history to recover from serious illness. Nonetheless, "quality of care" is a rather vague concept.

Once a physician or nurse undertakes the care of a patient, the courts maintain, it is his or her duty to render care that meets present-day standards. Under current law, doctors or nurses can be liable for any problems that may arise when they were aware of an abnormal physical finding and failed to inform the patient. However, there is no written law requiring that the patient be treated with consideration.

Physicians and hospital administrators often think of the patient's needs in purely clinical terms. How accurate is the diagnosis? Are advanced treatments available? The patient, on the other hand, is more likely to take a humanistic point of view when he evaluates quality of care. Of course he wants to be treated with the best of equipment and by the most qualified personnel. But he also wants health care to be delivered in a respectful and dignified manner, at a price he can afford.

When then Pennsylvania insurance commissioner Herbert S. Denenberg published his own bill of patients' rights in 1973, he called for "quality of care." He pointed out that the public has a right to top medical treatment delivered according to standards that are continuously monitored and reviewed. He also stressed that the public has the right to economical care,

---

[2] American Hospital Association. 1973. Patient rights, nursing responsibilities. *Hospitals* 47:102.

delivered efficiently and without unnecessary services. Commissioner Denenberg pledged to use the full regulatory authority of the state's insurance department to see that his bill of rights was implemented.[3]

As a result of these and other demands for health care, patients are no longer accepting without question whatever treatment is handed out to them. Many now refuse to sign blanket consent forms. Rather, they demand an explanation of what they are signing.

The new trend has also seen the emergence of a new specialist, the "patient representative," "ombudsman," or "patient advocate." This is a health professional whose primary responsibility is to act as the patient's representative in the health care system. The patient advocate serves two functions. He informs the patient of what to expect from the people treating him, and he attempts to change the system where injustices exist.

In some hospitals, grievance committees have been formed to provide a forum for patients' concerns and complaints. Hospital public relations departments have revised their follow-up questionnaires to include items that allow a former patient to voice his opinion on all phases of his hospitalization.

Of particular significance to the nurse is the fact that patient education is becoming an important and regular part of the patient's care plan in many hospitals. It is coming to be recognized that an informed patient is generally a more receptive patient who tends to respond better and more quickly to treatment.

An informed patient is generally a more receptive patient who tends to respond better and more quickly to treatment.

The right to privacy and confidentiality

Protection from exposure. The courts have emphasized that all members of the health team treating or caring for a patient must act with decency and respect. They must also arrange for the greatest possible degree of privacy. The patient has the right to be seen, observed, and examined only by those persons essential to his care or treatment. When he is moved through hospital corridors or into examination or treatment rooms, he should be covered and not exposed unnecessarily to other hospital personnel. This also holds true in wards and shared rooms.

When a patient dies, he has the right not to be observed, not to undergo any operation, such as autopsy, and not to be touched by unauthorized persons. His rights of privacy pass to the surviving relatives, who may sue if these rights have been violated.

Consent must be obtained from the patient to photograph him or to publish his photograph. A photographer should not be admitted to the room without the patient's consent.

A hospitalized patient can request that only his physician be present

---

[3]Nancy Quinn and Anne R. Somers. 1974. The patient's bill of rights: A significant aspect of the consumer revolution. *Nursing Outlook* 22:242.

for any examination. He can also ask that visitors be restricted. No one should be admitted to the patient's room unless the patient gives his approval.

It is the nurse's responsibility not only to protect the patient's privacy but also to help him deal with the loss of privacy that is inevitable in certain situations. Although the nurse cannot always prevent the occurrence of embarrassing situations, she can help the patient maintain his poise. For instance, one man who had suffered a heart attack said that the kindest thing a nurse had done for him was to busy herself with flowers during the few moments when he cried.[4]

People differ in the extent to which loss of privacy distresses them and in the type of exposure that is most threatening to them. Some people are more intimidated by the need to discuss personal affairs than by the need to expose their bodies. The more helpless the patient—whether physically, emotionally, or both—the greater the likelihood that problems will arise from this loss of privacy.

Sharing information appropriately. The rights of a patient in a hospital or a physician's office run parallel to the rights accorded an American citizen by the Constitution and the Bill of Rights. For example, the patient's records can be shown without his permission only in special legal circumstances. The patient can request that any discussions about medical care be held in private. He has control over any information that the hospital's public relations department wants to release about him. A signed statement must be obtained by anyone—a lawyer, insurance agent, social worker—who wishes to see the patient's records.

It is important for the nurse to explain how information is handled before the patient pours out a great deal of personal information to her. Usually, the patient is able to understand that it is necessary for the nurse to share information with other staff members. However, he has the right to object if he does not wish certain information to be shared.

Sometimes a nurse is obliged to discuss information the patient has volunteered even though he objects. A common example is the fact that he has decided not to take his medication. In most hospitals the nurse would be expected to communicate this fact to the physician—with an explanation to the patient about why she must do so.

Of course, it is not always possible or advisable to mention to the patient every detail of information that is shared about him. The degree of the patient's illness affects such a decision, as does the type of information involved.

Some information is by its very nature protected. If a physician asks an unmarried woman whether she has ever been pregnant, he must regard her answer as confidential. At other times the nurse must be sensitive to the fact that the patient considers certain information confidential even when it would appear not to be. A patient may wish, for example, that it not be commonly known that he wears a toupee, or has artificial dentures.

All efforts should be made to arrange for privacy when the patient wants to discuss a confidential matter. In a multiple-bed room, the nurse can move a chair close to the patient's bed or wheel him to a lounge or into a hall. Some patients find it easier to confide in one member of the staff than others. For example, an elderly woman may wish to talk to an older nurse's aide rather than to a young nurse. Instead of trying to change such a situation, a professional nurse works with it by carefully guiding the person whom the patient selects as confidant.

A final legal note. Whenever discussing a patient with colleagues, one should take care that doors are closed. Gossiping about a person or making unauthorized communications about him can be considered invasion of privacy; it can also be regarded as defamation of character.

The right to information and explanations in understandable terminology

Diagnosis. According to the American Hospital Association's bill of rights, the patient has the right to obtain from his physician complete information concerning his diagnosis, treatment, and prognosis. This information is to be provided in terms he can reasonably be expected to understand.

Sometimes it is not medically advisable to give such information directly to the patient. In that case, it must be given to an appropriate person, usually the next of kin.

Treatment, including procedures

Informed consent. Anyone who treats with medicine, gives advice, or performs an operation without the expressed or implied consent of the patient is liable to suit. An exception is when a medical emergency exists and there is no one available to give consent.

The patient can consent to treatment in four basic ways:[5]

1. *By expression, oral or written.* If the patient is a child, a parent may sign a consent form. With oral consent, a witness should be present.
2. *By implication, through action.* If a patient comes to a physician's office for help, his very presence implies that he will accept care by the physician.

[5]Paul S. Derian. 1973. Do patients have rights? *Southern Medicine*, December 1973, p. 12.

> The nurse must be sensitive to the fact that the patient considers certain information confidential even when it would appear not to be.

3. *By implication, in emergencies.* If a patient is unconscious after an accident, the physician is justified in assuming that he has the patient's consent for treatment.
4. *By consent of a parent or guardian.* A person under age 21 must obtain permission to receive any medical care other than emergency treatment.

The basic difference between consent and informed consent is that the latter refers to a precaution which a physician takes when he suspects the patient may sue him for **malpractice.** His suspicions could be grounded in the nature of a particular procedure or in the character of the patient.

According to the AHA, wherever possible a patient should be given an explanation of specific treatments or procedures. He should also be told what medically significant risks are involved and how long he can expect to be ill. In addition, he has the right to an explanation if alternatives for care or treatment exist. For example, women with breast cancer are today demanding a choice between the simple and the radical mastectomy, as no definitive proof has yet been offered that one is better than the other in terms of survival.

On the other hand, the patient also has the right not to know what medical care is being given in certain situations. For example, a person may not wish to know that he has a terminal cardiac condition. It is up to the physician to exercise discretion in deciding whether serious emotional harm may result from such a disclosure.

When medications are prescribed, the patient can and should question their need and effectiveness. He should also be given as direct an answer as possible about their purpose, side effects, dosage, and schedule.

Legally, it is the physician's responsibility to explain a treatment or procedure. Often, however, a patient will ask the nurse for additional information. For this reason it is essential that she be thoroughly familiar with procedures such as X-rays, electrocardiograms, and cardiac catheterization in order to describe them accurately to the patient.

Here are some suggestions that help protect the patient against harm, and the nurses, doctors, and hospital against lawsuits:[6]

1. Be sure there is a signed, dated, and witnessed consent on file within a reasonable time before the procedure is done.
2. Take action if there is reason to believe the patient signed the consent while under sedation or other medication that might affect his mental ability.
3. Raise a question if it appears that the patient has not been properly informed. Perhaps his knowledge of English is limited. If the nurse

[6]Michel Lipman. 1972. "Informed consent" and the nurse's role. *RN* 35:92.

suspects the patient does not understand the risks of surgery or a diagnostic procedure, she should call this to the attention of the physician.

Studies have shown that patients who bring suits usually have real or imagined grievances other than dissatisfaction with the procedure about which they are suing. Often, considerate nursing care and a willingness to listen to complaints can do much to improve the quality of patient care and help prevent the unpleasantness of a suit.

Human experimentation. The AHA bill of rights states that the patient is entitled to be advised if the hospital proposes to engage in human experimentation affecting his care or treatment.

Current ethical principles governing the use of human subjects in medical research were articulated in 1966 by the U.S. Department of Health, Education and Welfare. HEW issued a series of directives that covered the following areas:

1. Voluntary consent of the human subject
2. Qualifications and responsibilities of the investigator
3. The relationship between potential risk to the subject and potential value of the investigation

According to these guidelines, it is up to the investigator to supply the patient with the information needed to decide whether or not to participate. He must also give the patient as accurate an idea as possible of the amount of time and energy that will be involved.

The patient must also be warned if his participation may entail a loss of dignity or autonomy, mental or physical privation, pain or discomfort, or physical or emotional injury.

Today, the question of human experimentation is still surrounded by controversy. One question: Is it ethical to randomly divide patients into two groups—those treated with a particular drug and those who are not—when the drug is generally considered to be of value? Strict scientific procedure demands that studies be "double blind." That is, the investigator should not know which patients are receiving which treatment, and the patients are likewise ignorant. However, this method has raised a cry of protest from those who consider it unethical.

Continuity of care. Today, patients are demanding the right to reasonable continuity of care. They should know in advance what physicians and appointment times are available and where. They should be told while still in the hospital how to safeguard their health after release from the hospital.

As a result of pressure from patient interest groups, many hospitals have begun to reevaluate their discharge planning procedures. In an Illinois hospital, a committee developed a program based on three concepts:

1. The need for an interdisciplinary team approach to the problems of discharge planning
2. The conviction that continuity of care involves helping a patient with his nonmedical as well as his medical needs
3. The philosophy that programs implemented by an institution are most likely to succeed when they are developed from within that institution

Now, four social service staff members devote their entire time to discharge planning. When possible, head nurses schedule conferences with the social workers to discuss patients' problems in depth. These and other innovations have significantly affected patient satisfaction with continuity of care.[7]

Prognosis

The patient has the right to refuse any or all parts of the treatment proposed to him. If he decides not to undergo a particular procedure, the physician may ask him to sign a form releasing both hospital and physician from responsibility. The patient is not obliged to sign such a release, however. If he refuses treatment and also refuses to sign a release, the physician and the hospital may consider transferring him out of the hospital. Until that time, he must be given normal care.

The most common instance of a competent adult refusing treatment is the case of someone who, for religious or other reasons, refuses a blood transfusion. The courts have held that this is the right of the individual, unless the patient is pregnant, has minor children, or is not mentally able to make such a decision.

Names of personnel

According to the AHA bill of rights, the patient is entitled to know by name the physician responsible for coordinating his care. In addition, he should know the names of other personnel caring for him.

Institutional rules, regulations, and policies regarding patient's care

The patient also has the right to know what hospital rules and regulations apply to his conduct as a patient. He has the right to expect that,

[7]Helen Thomson. 1973. Assisting patients with posthospitalization plans. *Hospitals* 47:43–45, 98.

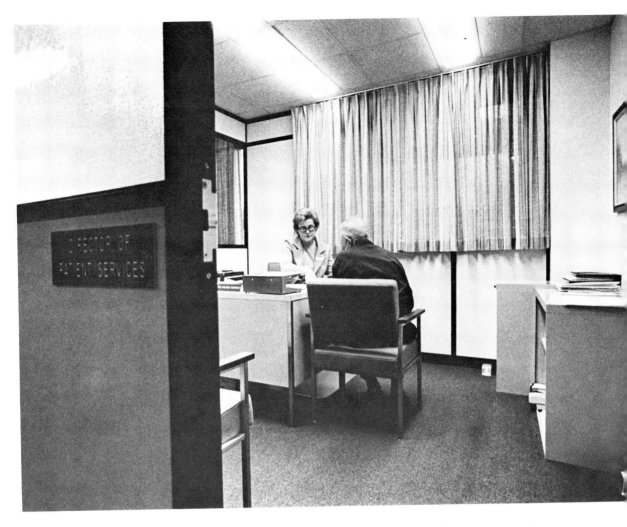

within its capacity, a hospital will respond to his requests for service. The hospital must provide evaluation, service, and/or referral as indicated by the urgency of the case.

When medically permissible, a patient may be transferred to another facility only after he has received complete information and an explanation of the need for such a transfer as well as alternatives. The institution to which the patient is to be transferred must first have accepted the patient for transfer.

Bills

The patient has the right to examine and receive an explanation of his bill regardless of source of payment. He is entitled to an explanation of the cost of treatment, the general length of hospitalization for his illness, whether any consultations are to be requested, and the reason for any laboratory studies.

A patient has the right to a complete explanation of his bill.

[Photo reproduced, with permission, from *Hospitals, Journal of the American Hospital Association*, April 1, 1974, p. 179]

Educational and health care agencies associated with patient's health care

The patient has the right to obtain information concerning any relationship between his hospital and other health care and educational institutions insofar as his care is concerned. He has the right to know of the existence of any professional relationships among individuals who are treating him.

SUMMARY

The concept of patients' rights is a relatively new arrival on the American health care scene. In the past, patients have more or less accepted the treatment offered, not daring to question its wisdom or to ponder alternatives. Today, in the wake of the consumer movement, patients are beginning to realize that they are customers and that they have the right to examine what they are paying for.

Much of the impetus for the patient movement stems from a list of demands approved by the prestigious American Hospital Association, which in 1973 enumerated "A Patient's Bill of Rights." The bill is not a legal document, but it carries great moral force. Already, hospitals have begun to respond noticeably.

An unquestioned right of patients, which the courts have upheld, is the right to privacy and confidentiality. A patient is entitled to protection from unnecessary exposure of his body or his emotions. His confidences to the nurse should be treated as such, except in unusual circumstances.

The patient is also entitled to a thorough explanation concerning his diagnosis, treatment, and prognosis, in terms that are understandable to him. He has the right to complete information when his participation in a medical study is requested and he can refuse to take part. The patient can also refuse medical treatment unless he is not mentally capable of doing so, or, in the case of a woman, if she is pregnant or has minor children.

The nurse plays an important role as guardian of patients' rights. She protects the patient's privacy, provides explanations, and investigates mechanisms for continuity of care. In many ways she serves the function of "ombudsman" or "patient representative," a new class of professional whose ranks have been swelling in recent months. It is the ombudsman's function to make sure the patient understands what kind of treatment he is entitled to, and to initiate change where his rights are not properly regarded.

STUDY QUESTIONS

1. What are the major provisions in the American Hospital Association's "A Patient's Bill of Rights"?
2. What is informed consent? In what ways can a patient give his consent to treatment?

3. What is a patient advocate?
4. Define "continuity of care." In what ways can the nurse ensure continuity of care for her patients?
5. According to the AHA, a patient has the right to information and explanations in terms he can understand. Explain in lay terms:
   a. The action of a diuretic
   b. The purpose and procedure of an electrocardiogram
   c. The importance of an adequate intake of carbohydrates

SELECTED BIBLIOGRAPHY

Annas, George J., and Healey, Joseph. 1974. The patient rights advocate. *Journal of Nursing Administration* 4:25–31.

Quinn, Nancy, and Somers, Anne R. 1974. The patient's bill of rights: A significant aspect of the consumer revolution. *Nursing Outlook* 22:240–44.

Regan, William A. 1965. The legal side of confidential information. *RN* (June 1965). Reprinted in *Nursing fundamentals,* ed. Mary E. Meyers, pp. 69–73. Dubuque, Iowa: Brown, 1967.

Willig, Sidney, 1971. Nursing and the law. In *Nursing: Concepts of practice,* pp. 175–220. New York: McGraw-Hill.

13 Maintaining a safe environment

What is man's environment?

The term "environment," when used in its widest sense, refers to the entire range of internal and external influences that act upon an individual. These include the air he breathes, the chair he sits on, the food he eats, the rate at which his heart pumps blood throughout his body.

Man has several regulatory systems within his body that enable him to adapt internally to the world in which he lives. These include the renocardiovascular system (the kidneys, heart, and blood vessels), the pulmonary mechanisms, and the adrenal mechanisms. (These systems will be discussed in chapter 15.) Man has also found ways in which to control artificially the temperature, light, and ventilation in his external environment. The following are some of the external environmental factors to which man's body must adapt.

Temperature

"Comfortable" external temperature is a relative term, varying from individual to individual and even from culture to culture. For example, Americans generally favor an office temperature of about 20°–25° C (68°–77° F). Englishmen, on the other hand, feel they function best at 17°–22° C (63°–72° F).[1] Extremes of heat and cold cause man to react in a number of predictable ways. He works inefficiently, loses his temper more readily, becomes ill more quickly.[2]

Ordinarily, man's own body temperature varies only about 2° from the standard of 98.6° F. However, such conditions as infection or sunstroke can disrupt the normal functioning of his heat-regulatory mechanisms (see chapter 25).

[1] Harold Hillman. 1973. The optimum human environment. *Nursing Times* 69:693.
[2] Ibid.

Humidity

Humidity is the amount of moisture in the air. Although high humidity causes a certain amount of discomfort, it is only dangerous when combined with extreme external temperatures. When temperatures are low, high humidity is considered a contributing factor in hypothermia, arthritis, and bronchitis. When combined with high temperatures, it encourages the spread of bacteria.

The use of air conditioning, which is now common in American homes and office buildings, reduces humidity. As a result, people who live or work in air-conditioned environments often complain of dry throats.

Light

The amount of available light is an important consideration in carrying out detailed work, such as surgical procedures. Poor lighting reduces the contrast of objects. Many headaches are caused by attempting to do fine work without sufficient light.

Noise

Like "comfortable" external temperature, "noise" is a relative term. A teen-ager's stereo can be his father's raging headache. However, sound levels above 120 decibels are painful and, indeed, damaging to everyone's ears.[3] Researchers have found that older people living in remote, quiet villages have considerably less hearing loss than those living in busy, noisy cities. This had led many to believe that the taken-for-granted hearing loss in elderly people is really due to the damage of everyday noise rather than solely to the aging process itself.[4]

Noise pollution forces people to shout in order to be heard. This constant effort to be heard becomes a stress in itself. It is especially hard on those who must wear hearing aids. Turning up the device increases the volume of background noise, causing confusion and discomfort.

Ecological concerns

Today, it is impossible not to be conscious of the problem of environmental pollution. This pollution is increasing because man now uses greater amounts of the energy that runs the biosphere. Also, man is filling the biosphere with more and more toxic substances that further reduce available energy.[5]

[3] Ibid., p. 694.
[4] Ibid.
[5] Carter L. Marshall. 1973. *Dynamics of health and disease*, p. 311. New York: Appleton-Century-Crofts.

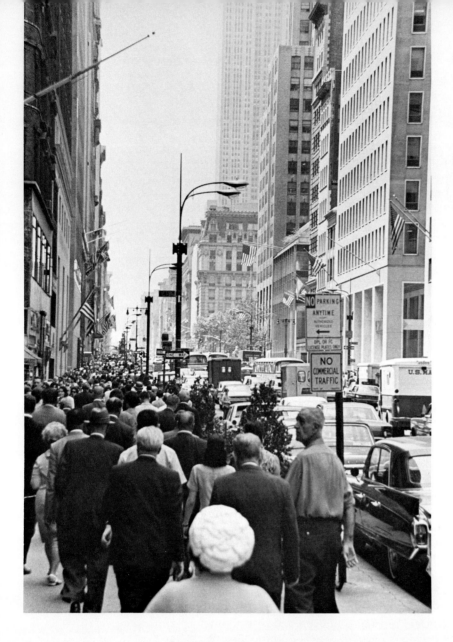

Overcrowding, of both people and vehicles, is a major problem faced by modern American society.
[Photo by Merrim from Monkmeyer Press Photo Service]

Dust and bacteria. Dust and bacteria pose a threat to health in certain situations. In mines and asbestos factories, dust causes irritation, which may lead to silicosis, asbestosis, and a host of other industrial diseases. Dust and water droplets are also dangerous in overcrowded housing. Under these conditions, meningitis, tuberculosis, colds, and influenza can be carried easily from one person to another.

Smoking. The dangers of smoking have been widely discussed and publicized. People who smoke have a higher death rate than nonsmokers, particularly from heart disease and lung cancer. Chronic bronchitis and pulmonary emphysema are also significantly affected by smoking. Even if the individual does not die from these diseases, the chances are he will be severely impaired by them.[6]

The dangers of smoking are not confined to smokers alone, however, The carbon dioxide level in a smoke-filled room has been shown to exceed the standard for safety set by the federal government.[7] Other products of cigarette smoke can be dangerous for nonsmokers who suffer from bronchial and heart conditions.

Smog. Smog is caused by dust-laden water droplets. This condition contributes to chest diseases of all kinds, particularly bronchitis and emphysema. In many locations, local and national legislation has forced factories and cars to absorb more of the hydrocarbons from fuel before discharging them into the atmosphere. These regulations consequently have brought about a considerable decrease in atmospheric dust levels.

The patient's immediate environment

The nurse must be aware of the many environmental factors that affect human health. In addition, she must be aware of the requirements for the specific environments in which she works, including patients' homes, hospitals, and other agencies.

The spread of infection from one patient to another and from nurse or family to patient can pose a major threat. (See chapter 14 for a discussion of infection control.) The most important of the nurse's defenses against the spread of infection is proper handwashing technique. In addition, the nurse must be familiar with proper techniques for the use of gloves, masks, and gowns.

Isolation is an important part of infection prevention. The patient with an infectious disease should be separated from the general population, along with all equipment used by him. The techniques for isolation also will be discussed in chapter 14. All of these procedures are intended to promote the concept of safety—for patient, nurse, and family alike.

What is safety?

Webster's dictionary defines safety as "the quality or condition of being safe; freedom from danger, injury or damage; security."[8] According to Maslow (see chapter 8), safety needs are second in importance only to basic

[6]U.S. Department of Health, Education and Welfare. 1971. *Facts: Smoking & health,* pp. 1-2.
[7]U.S. Department of Health, Education and Welfare. 1972. *Public exposure to air pollution from tobacco smoke,* p. 11.
[8]*Webster's new world dictionary of the American language,* 2d college ed. p. 1253. 1970. New York and Cleveland: World.

The most important of the nurse's defenses against the spread of infection is proper handwashing technique.

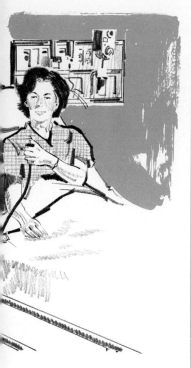

The patient whose call signal is not answered promptly will develop fears for his safety in an emergency.

physiological needs. "Safety as related to the patient has two aspects: (1) a real danger or threat to his welfare, and (2) his feeling that he is safe or in danger."[9]

The patient's safety may be jeopardized by threats from within or without. For example, an upset in his fluid and electrolyte balance (see chapter 22) may be life-endangering. His body may be unable to synthesize certain vital substances. Or he may have been exposed to an overdose of radiation.

The patient's feelings of safety or danger are directly related to past experience and to concern over unknown elements in his present situation. The patient with pains in his chest who fears he has had a heart attack is likely to be frightened while a diagnosis is being made. The hospitalized child needs reassurance that his mother will indeed return in the morning. The patient whose call signal is not answered promptly will develop fears for his safety in an emergency.

Characteristics of the patient that influence his safety

The safety of the patient is influenced by his own individual needs and problems. The following are some factors to be taken into consideration.

Age. Perhaps the most common threat to the older patient is the danger of falling. The increased frequency of falls among older people is caused in large part by the way in which they walk. Older persons generally use a gait characterized by a stooped trunk with the neck and head bent forward. This posture throws the center of gravity forward, thus upsetting the sense of balance.

In addition, the older person generally spends much of his time sitting, which leads to some degree of hip flexion contracture. This contributes even further to the forward-leaning posture. His ability to lose and regain his balance is quickly impaired. Many older persons drag their feet along the floor as a result. This problem of balance is also found in younger persons who have been bedridden for any length of time.

The nurse must always be on the lookout for situations in which falls are likely to result. Scatter rugs and slippery floors are especially hazardous. Items commonly used by the older patient should be placed within easy reach. The patient should also be taught to sit and stand up slowly. Sudden motion often causes a loss of balance.

Another important factor in falls is lack of adequate lighting. Since an older person's vision is often impaired, it is essential that proper lighting be provided. Bathrooms should be well lighted at night.

[9]Irene L. Beland. 1970. *Clinical nursing: Pathophysiological and psychological approaches,* 2d ed., p. 12. New York: Macmillan.

All of these precautions are especially vital for the patient who has had a previous fall or who is suffering from some form of brain damage. The elderly patient who has lost a limb or is deaf or has impaired vision is also particularly vulnerable. In addition, it is important to remember that the older patient generally has problems in adapting to changes in his routine and environment. This leads to a state of disorientation and confusion.

Children also require special attention. More children under 15 years of age die as a result of accidents than from disease.[10] Suffocation, falls, burns, scalds, poisoning, and drowning are typical accidents for this age group. Most accidents involving children are directly traceable to carelessness on the part of an adult.

The following general principles should be followed to ensure the safety of younger patients:

1. The child should always be put in the proper size crib or bed. A tall child should not be given a crib with sides so low that he can easily fall out. The sides on the crib should always be up whenever the child is left alone.
2. An infant should never be left alone in the bath or on a table from which he can fall. At home, he should never be left alone on a bed with no sides.
3. Dangerous objects, including scissors, safety pins, or breakable items, should never be left within the child's reach. Cleaning fluids, disinfectants, and other household poisons should be securely capped and stored out of the child's reach. They should not be poured into containers that previously held food, such as old soda bottles or juice containers.
4. Do not allow a child to place small objects in his mouth. Coins, beads, etc., all too often wind up stuck in small throats.
5. Do not leave the child alone when he is feeding himself.
6. Select toys with an eye for possible hazards. Loose button eyes, wheels that come off, and items made of easily breakable plastic should be avoided.
7. Children often resist attempts to give them injections or take their temperature rectally. Always have another person assist whenever resistance is encountered. When available, a member of the child's family is usually helpful at these times. Do not leave the child alone while a rectal thermometer is in place.
8. Check on the child frequently during the night and while he is resting during the day. Bedcovers should be securely fastened and unnecessary pillows removed to prevent suffocation.

[10] Alice L. Price. 1965. *The art, science, and spirit of nursing,* p. 103. Philadelphia: Saunders.

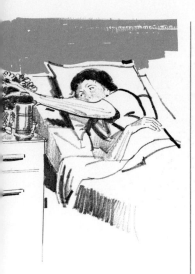

Sixty-five percent of all injuries to patients occur within 10 feet of their beds.

Degree of orientation and/or level of consciousness. The degree to which a patient is conscious of his surroundings and is able to respond to them is an important safety consideration. Those who are comatose or are suffering from neurological impairments generally have the following problems that increase the danger of accidents:

1. Many of these patients are totally or partially paralyzed. This paralysis leads to rigidity in movement and loss of sensation. The patient cannot tell, for example, that he is being burned because his heating pad is turned up too high.
2. The neurologically impaired patient often has episodes of confusion. Mental deterioration, temporary or permanent, may have occurred.
3. These patients commonly are unable to communicate quickly and clearly. They may also be unable to comprehend instructions readily.

A few basic guidelines should be employed to guarantee the safety of these patients. Hot water bottles and heating pads should generally not be used on the unconscious patient or on the patient who is suffering from a loss of sensation. Burns can also be caused by ice bags and ice caps. Since the patient often does not realize he is being burned, the nurse must be sure to observe carefully for irritation, skin breakdown, or other signs of burns.

The restless or confused patient should be protected by the use of padded bedrails. Physical restraints should be used only when absolutely necessary, as they often increase the patient's agitation. They are also upsetting to his family. Both patient and family should receive a complete explanation of the need for restraining devices. Proper application and care of these devices are important. They should be removed at least once a day so that the patient's skin may be cleansed and powdered. The skin should also be inspected for signs of irritation and breakdown.

The objective of all restraining devices and procedures is to protect the patient from harming himself. This can often be accomplished simply by the presence of a family member or a staff person. In some cases, it may be necessary for the patient to be given sedatives.

Safety hazards in the patient's environment

Sixty-five percent of all injuries to patients occur within 10 feet of their beds.[11] Indeed, 41 percent of all patient injuries are the result of falls from the bed itself.[12] Many of these accidents are caused by the patient reaching for a faraway object or stumbling over equipment.

[11]Gustave L. Scheffler. 1962. The nurse's role in hospital safety. *Nursing Outlook* 10. Reprinted in *Nursing fundamentals,* ed. Mary E. Meyers, p. 168. Dubuque, Iowa: Brown, 1967.
[12]Price, p. 101.

Physical hazards

Litter and clutter. Good housekeeping techniques can make a vital contribution to patient and staff safety. Spilled liquids should be wiped up immediately. Broken bottles should be properly disposed of to avoid cuts. In the patient's room, tables and wastebaskets should be placed near the bed, but not where the patient may stumble over them. The patient's telephone, call signal, and radio or television should be accessible without stretching or leaning.

Furniture and equipment. The safe use of furniture and equipment depends upon two factors: (1) regular maintenance and (2) a thorough understanding by the staff of how the equipment works. Wheelchairs, mechanical lifts, and other devices used for carrying patients should always be inspected for loose wheels, broken parts, and other defects. The nurse should not attempt these repairs herself, but should refer them to the proper maintenance department.

Knowing how to use a particular piece of equipment safely not only promotes efficiency but also reduces the danger of accidents and damage. Many electrical devices, for example, are grounded to prevent shocks. Use of an ordinary extension cord, or wrapping the wire around a piece of pipe, defeats this grounding and exposes both nurse and patient to the danger of electrical shock. (See also section below on electrical appliances.) The nurse should also be on the lookout for possible design defects that may be hazardous.

Floors and lighting. As was mentioned in the section on elderly patients (see p. 264), nonskid floor coverings and well-lighted rooms help prevent accidents. Personnel and visitors must be warned when floors are wet. Furniture and other movable objects should always be kept out of passageways.

Electrical appliances. Improper use of electrical appliances can lead to injuries from shocks and burns. Defective equipment, worn or frayed cords, and improper insulation present special hazards. Wires should never be run under rugs or along doorsills. In addition, all electrical appliances should be provided with signal lights to indicate that they have been turned on. Care should be taken to ensure that too many appliances are not plugged into the same outlet, thus running the risk of overloading the circuit.

Because water is a good conductor of electricity, people often get shocks if they touch an appliance with wet hands. Water should also be kept from direct contact with the appliance itself in order to prevent short circuits. Likewise, metal objects should be kept from contact with these appliances, as metal is also a good conductor of electricity.

Knowing how to use a particular piece of equipment safely not only promotes efficiency but also reduces the danger of accidents and damage.

The best weapon
against fire is education
in proper preventive
methods.

Thermal hazards

Boiling water. Improper use of hot water bottles is the most common cause of burns or scalds from boiling water. The temperature of the water should never exceed 125° F or 52° C. (Remember that water does not boil at less than 212° F or 100° C.) As was indicated (see p. 266), hot water bottles should not be used on unconscious or otherwise disoriented patients. Nor should they be used on the old or on the very young, as their skin is thinner and less resistant to heat.

In the home, pots of boiling water should be placed toward the back of the stove with the handles pointed inward, not protruding outward. This prevents the possibility of their being knocked over. Such precautions are especially necessary when small children are present.

Fire. The best weapon against fire is education in proper preventive methods. A study of United States hospitals has shown that faulty electrical wiring and appliances cause the most fires, but that more patients die as a result of fires caused by cigarette smoking.[13] Electrical fires start because of defective equipment, faulty wiring, improper insulation, and overloading of circuits.

Careless handling of cigarettes and matches—by patients, staff, and visitors alike—is extremely hazardous. "No smoking" signs should be posted in rooms where oxygen or other gases are stored or in use. Sand-filled containers for cigarette butts should be provided in areas where smoking is permitted, as well as sufficient ashtrays. Patients who are permitted to smoke in their rooms should have someone with them while doing so, especially those who are incapacitated.

Proper training in escape procedures is vital. Frequent fire drills, even if not mandated by law, should be held. All hospital employees should know how to sound the alarm, operate fire extinguishers, and assist in removing patients from the area. One of the most important staff functions is to maintain calm; panic may cause more harm than the fire itself.

The following are the general procedures the nurse should follow in case of fire. Each hospital will have its own specific plan of action, and circumstances may dictate a change in the order in which these procedures are carried out.

1. Notify the switchboard or sound an alarm.
2. Assign one person to remain at the telephone.
3. Be calm and reassure patients and staff.
4. Have workers and ambulatory patients close all windows and doors leading to the fire site.

[13]Ena M. Morris. 1968. In case of fire emergencies. *American Journal of Nursing* 68:1498.

5. Turn off all oxygen equipment and electrical appliances.
6. Clear all possible exits.
7. Place wet blankets under closed doors, if necessary, to keep patients' rooms free of smoke.
8. Remove all patients who are close to the fire.[14]

Similar fire hazards to those in a hospital are also in the home. Once again, smoking in bed or careless use of matches is the leading cause of fatalities. Parents and children should plan escape routes and procedures together, and then conduct their own fire drills. Fire extinguishers should also be available for home use.

Chemical hazards

Drugs. Errors in the prescription, dosage, and administration of drugs can be hazardous, and even fatal. If the prescribed drug or its dosage seems to differ from the usual course of treatment, the nurse should question the order and, if necessary, refuse to carry it out. (See chapter 24 for a discussion of the administration of therapeutic agents.)

Poisons. Poisonous drugs should always be stored separately under lock and key. Ordinary cleaning fluids, which may be fatal if swallowed, are commonly stored on open shelves in workrooms, however. Since the possibility of accidental poisoning or suicide attempts is always present, the use of such substances should be kept to a minimum. Pest control, including the use of aerosol sprays, should be undertaken with appropriate caution.

In the home, cleaning fluids should be stored out of the reach of children in clearly marked, securely capped containers. Medicine cabinets should be locked and periodically cleaned out to remove all out-of-date medicines. Child-proof caps are now common for prescription and other drugs. Adults and older children should be taught not to take someone else's prescription.

Microbial hazards

The subject of infection has already been briefly referred to on p. 263. A full discussion will be presented in chapter 14.

As was mentioned, the single most important weapon the nurse has against infection is proper handwashing technique. Other measures for the prevention of the spread of infection include the use of masks, gowns, and gloves, isolation, and scrupulous aseptic techniques.

14Price, p. 100.

Errors in the prescription, dosage, and administration of drugs can be hazardous, and even fatal.

Radiation hazards

The use of radiation and radioactive substances is always potentially hazardous. The danger from exposure to large dosages of these materials has been widely publicized, but continuous exposure to small dosages may also be damaging. Proper safety techniques can keep such danger to a minimum level. Three important factors for the nurse to always keep in mind when dealing with radiation in any form are time, distance, and shielding.[15]

Time. Since the potential for damage from radiation increases with the amount of time a person is exposed, it is especially important that the nurse carry out needed procedures quickly and efficiently. This means that all nursing actions must be carefully planned in advance. Accurate records should be kept of the time the nurse spends with patients who are undergoing radiation treatments utilizing internal radioactivity. Accepted safety limits should not be exceeded. This can often be accomplished by rotating schedules so that one person does not spend too much time in the radiation area.

Distance. Patients being treated with radioactive implants or other radioactive substances should be given single rooms with outside walls if at all possible. If they must share a room with other patients, these should not be persons in the childbearing years. Pregnant nurses should not work with patients receiving such treatments.

Shielding. The use of lead drapes, aprons, and gloves will provide adequate protection for nurses assisting with X-ray and fluoroscope procedures. Heavier lead shields are needed when working with patients who are being treated with radium or cobalt. In the event that a radioactive implant becomes dislodged, it should be picked up with lead forceps and disposed of in a lead container. Dressings also should not be handled directly.

If a patient being treated with a radioactive implant or other radioactive substance should vomit, or if a urine specimen is accidentally spilled, the following general clean-up procedures should be used:

1. Paper towels or other absorbent material should be placed over the spill to prevent spreading.
2. Contaminated shoes should be removed before leaving the area.
3. Contaminated hands should be washed before using the telephone to call for assistance.

[15]Elisabeth H. Boeker. 1965. Radiation safety. *American Journal of Nursing* 65. Reprinted in *Nursing fundamentals,* ed. Mary E. Meyers, p. 226. Dubuque, Iowa: Brown, 1967.

4. The spill should be cleaned up from the outside in, minimizing the spread of contamination. Only a small amount of water or cleaning fluid should be used.
5. All cloths or other cleaning equipment used should be disposed of as radioactive waste.[16]

SUMMARY

The term "environment" refers to the entire range of internal and external influences that act upon an individual. When the nurse understands these many influences, she will be able to interpret how they apply to the hospitalized patient. She will also understand the ways in which the patient's adaptation mechanisms are affected by his situation.

Normally, our body temperatures adjust rapidly to the temperature in the air. If humidity is high and air temperature is low, people become more susceptible to hypothermia, arthritis, and bronchitis. A combination of high temperature and high humidity encourages the spread of bacteria.

Although people vary in the amount and kind of noise they can tolerate, a great deal of noise becomes a source of stress to most. Sound intensities above 120 decibels are painful to the ears and may be permanently damaging.

Atmospheric dust has been identified as a cause of silicosis, asbestosis, and many other industrial diseases. In overcrowded situations, a combination of dust and water droplets can encourage the spread of meningitis, tuberculosis, colds, and influenza.

It is a major responsibility of the nurse to protect the patient as much as possible from threats to safety arising from the hospital or home environment. In so doing, she must consider not only the characteristics of the environment but also those of the patient. For instance, older people are physiologically incapable of regaining balance quickly when they slip. This means that scatter rugs and slippery floors must be carefully avoided. Because often older people's vision is impaired, rooms and bathrooms should be well lighted.

Neurologically impaired patients or those who are comatose are often partially or completely immobilized. They must be carefully guarded from accidents caused by heat-giving appliances, ice bags, stretchers, or wheelchairs. If physical restraining devices are needed, they must be applied properly and removed and cleaned often. The skin areas that come in contact with these devices must also be cleansed regularly.

Various pieces of hospital equipment, such as adjustable beds, tables, bedrails, wheelchairs, and mechanical lifts, must always be kept in good repair. Spills on floors must be wiped up immediately and corridors kept free of clutter.

[16]Ibid., p. 230.

Electrical shocks or burns can result from frayed cords, defective equipment or wiring, or wet hands touching electrical equipment. Both hot water bottles and ice bags can cause burns. Fire can result from a number of causes, and fire prevention is an important concern of the nurse. In addition to keeping a watch for defective equipment, the nurse must monitor the smoking habits of patients, particularly those who are incapacitated.

Potent drugs and chemicals can potentially lead to disaster, and must be kept carefully out of general reach. Radiation treatments also require special precautions.

While the nurse's concern is basically for the safety of the patient, she must not forget to protect herself as well.

STUDY QUESTIONS

1. Briefly define the term "environment."
2. What are two of the major external environmental factors to which man must adapt? What are the means by which he is equipped to do so?
3. How does a patient's age influence his safety? What are some of the factors a nurse must consider when caring for a young child? an elderly person?
4. What factors in the hospital environment contribute to the danger of accidents? How can this danger be minimized?
5. What is the proper procedure for a fire drill in the institution in which you are studying?
6. Consider the following situation: An elderly hospitalized patient is confused and restless. He is trying to pull out his IV and his Foley catheter. He is crying out fearfully and hitting personnel who come near his bedside.
   a. What are the potential and actual threats to this patient's safety?
   b. What measures should be taken to increase his safety?
   c. What would be his possible reactions to these measures?
   d. What are the legal implications of these measures?

SELECTED BIBLIOGRAPHY

Boeker, Elisabeth H. 1965. Radiation safety. *American Journal of Nursing* 65. Reprinted in *Nursing fundamentals,* ed. Mary E. Meyers, pp. 224–33. Dubuque, Iowa: Brown, 1967.

Hillman, Harold. 1973. The optimum human environment. *Nursing Times* 69:692–95.

Morris, Ena M. 1968. In case of fire emergencies. *American Journal of Nursing* 68:1496–99.

Scheffler, Gustave L. 1962. The nurse's role in hospital safety. *Nursing Outlook* 10. Reprinted in *Nursing fundamentals,* ed. Mary E. Meyers, pp. 166–73. Dubuque, Iowa: Brown. 1967.

14 Asepsis and infection control

What is a pathogen?

By far the large majority of microorganisms are harmless to man. Many, in fact, are actually useful to him. These microorganisms, known as **flora,** are found in the mouth, throat, trachea, and nasopharynx. Among other areas, they are also present in the lungs, stomach, genitourinary tract, and the intestinal tract. They help the body by preventing the overgrowth of **bacteria** that might be harmful.

A small number of microorganisms cause disease. These are called **pathogens.** Whenever these pathogens invade the body, multiply, and overcome the normal flora, they cause infectious diseases. Just as the healthy body has built-in defense mechanisms against disease, so these pathogens also have safeguards. One of the most common is the ability to produce poisonous, disease-causing matter called **toxins.** Studies in **microbiology** provide more detail about these substances.

Assessment

Agent-host relationships

From birth, the human body develops relationships with a variety of microorganisms. These relationships are classified as symbiotic, commensal, parasitic, and obligatory.[1]

In a **symbiotic** relationship, the microorganism (the agent) and the body (the host) both benefit. For example, the flora living in the alimentary canal feed on its contents. At the same time, they synthesize vitamin K, which the body is unable to do for itself.

The microorganisms that live in a **commensal** relationship with the body are dependent upon their host, but neither harm nor help it. The normal flora in the gastrointestinal tract are believed to be commensals. There is some evidence, however, that certain conditions may lead them to cause infection.

[1]Irene L. Beland. 1970. *Clinical nursing: Pathophysiological and psychosocial approaches,* 2d ed., pp. 114–15. New York: Macmillan.

Upon completing this chapter, the reader should be able to:

1. Describe the relationship between microorganisms normally found in the body and those that are disease-producing pathogens.

2. Identify the factors that increase the susceptibility of a host or individual to pathogens.

3. Explain the relationship between the three stages of the infection process.

4. Discuss the nurse's responsibility in preventing infection and promoting infection control by strengthening the defenses of the host.

5. Discuss the factors that contribute to hospital-acquired (nosocomial) infections and the ways in which such infections can be eliminated or controlled.

The development of infection depends upon the relationship between the host, the agent, and their environment.

In a **parasitic** relationship, the agent feeds off the host, but the host derives no benefit from the agent. The agent in this type of relationship is called a **parasite.** In some cases, parasites are able to live independently of the host, as well as with it. These are classified as **facultative parasites.** **Staphylococci** and **streptococci** are common examples of facultative parasites.

A microorganism in an **obligatory** relationship is one that depends completely upon the host for survival and propagation. These microorganisms are called obligatory parasites. One of the most common is **Treponema pallidum,** which causes syphilis.

The elements of infection

The development of infection depends upon the relationship between the **host,** the **agent,** and their environment. The many complicated interactions in these relationships are still not clearly understood. Why is it that a usually harmless microorganism will sometimes cause disease? Why is it that known disease-producing microorganisms sometimes will not be harmful to the human body?

Despite these questions, there are certain processes that always must take place in order to produce an infection. These processes involve a cyclic relationship between the following elements:

1. The etiological agent (the pathogen)
2. The reservoir
3. A mode of escape from the reservoir
4. A means of transmission
5. A mode of entry
6. A susceptible host[2]

The etiological agent (the pathogen). The word "etiological" means "assigning or seeking to assign a cause." Thus, the **etiological agent** is the cause of the infection, or the pathogen. Since the body has its own, usually effective, defense mechanisms, the pathogen must be able to invade the body, break down the body's resistance, and then multiply itself. The pathogen's ability to do so is dependent upon the following factors:[3]

1. Morphology, or form. Some microorganisms, such as those causing botulism, tetanus, and gas gangrene, form **spores.** These spores are small, often unicellular structures that protect the microorganism from outside elements, including heat, drying, and chemicals. They also permit it to reproduce.
2. Physiology, including food and temperature requirements.

[2]Dubay and Grubb, pp. 11–12.
[3]Beland, pp. 119–21.

3. Resistance to physical and chemical agents.
4. Toxin production (see p. 273).

The reservoir. The **reservoir** is the environment in which the etiological agent lives and multiplies. This environment may be human, animal, or inanimate. The reservoir is also known as the source of infection.

A human reservoir may be provided by a person who is himself ill. It may also be provided by a person who appears to be well but whose mucous membranes or secretions contain pathogens. Such a person is called a **carrier.** "Typhoid Mary" is perhaps the most famous of these human reservoirs.

Animals may also serve as sources of infection. They have been carriers of plagues, rabies, and malaria. Pathogens may also be present in soil, air, food, water, milk, and feces.

A mode of escape from the reservoir. In man, the most common mode of escape is through the respiratory tract. Breathing, coughing, sneezing, and talking all permit pathogens to escape on droplets of moisture. This moisture evaporates, but the pathogen itself may remain suspended in the air for a considerable length of time.

Another common mode of escape is through the gastrointestinal tract. Pathogens may be expelled through this tract along with feces. Thus, adequate sanitary facilities are an important factor in infection control.

Once the agent has escaped, the danger of its spreading is dependent upon its ability to survive outside the reservoir. Facultative parasites, such as those that cause staphylococcus infections, have a high survival rate. Obligatory parasites, such as those causing syphilis, do not survive very long outside the reservoir.

A means of transmission. The simplest means of transmitting pathogens among human beings involves physical contact, such as kissing or sexual intercourse. Perhaps the most common means of transmission is contaminated hands. Physical contact does not necessarily involve touching, however. As was explained above, pathogens may also be transmitted by coughing or sneezing.

Pathogens may also be transmitted by contact with contaminated water, milk, drinking glasses, silverware, and so on. They are also carried by various insects, including mosquitoes (yellow fever), ticks (Rocky Mountain spotted fever), and flies (typhoid fever).

A mode of entry. The same routes that permit the pathogen's escape also provide for its entry. These include the respiratory and genital tracts; the mouth, skin, and mucous membranes; and wounds.

A susceptible host. Various factors influence the body's ability to resist invasion by pathogens. These include:

1. *Age.* Antibodies from the mother protect infants against infection for the first two months of life. After that, the body develops its own defenses against disease. Beginning at about age 50, however, the body's ability to resist infection begins to decline.
2. *Nutrition.* People who are undernourished are prone to infection. The incidence of tuberculosis, for example, is greater among the poorly fed than among those who receive an adequate diet.
3. *Sex.* Some diseases, such as pneumonia and meningitis, are found more commonly in men than women. Scarlet and typhoid fevers, however, affect more women than men.
4. *Medical treatment.* Individuals already receiving certain medical treatments are more susceptible to infection. These treatments include large dosages of **steroids, cortisone,** and **antibiotics.** Radiation treatments, which break down body tissues and depress the body's natural immune response, also lower the individual's resistance.
5. *Chronic diseases.* Uremia, diabetes, cancer, and leukemia are among the diseases that predispose an individual to infection.
6. *Shock.* Individuals in shock have a lowered resistance as a result of the breakdown of important body functions.

Signs and symptoms of the three stages of infection

Infectious diseases generally develop in three stages—incubation, illness, and convalescence.[4]

Incubation. Incubation may be defined in two ways: (1) It is the period between the pathogen's invasion of the body and the first visible signs of disease. (2) It is also the time in which the pathogen adapts itself to the host and begins to multiply. The length of the incubation period varies from disease to disease, but it is always roughly the same for a particular disease.

Illness. The period of illness, like the period of incubation, varies from one disease to another, but it is the same for a particular disease. This period begins with what is known as the **prodromal** stage. At this time, the individual experiences feelings of discomfort and impending illness, but does not manifest any specific symptoms of a particular disease. He may feel unduly tired, have muscular aches, or even a mild sore throat, for example. This may indicate that he has a simple cold or it may be the first sign of measles. It is also at this stage of the illness that he is most likely to spread his infection.

As the illness progresses to the **acute** phase, most individuals run a **fever.** This fever may be **constant, intermittent,** or **remittent** (varying but

[4]Ibid., p. 125.

not returning to normal). Accurate measurement and recording of fever are important factors in determining the phase of an illness.

Just as the length of the illness period varies from disease to disease, so the severity of symptoms varies from individual to individual. Some people experience only a mild attack. Indeed, in some cases, the individual may not even be aware that he is sick. This is the case, for example, for many individuals suffering from gonorrhea, which can be detected only through laboratory tests. Others become ill rapidly and perhaps die. A disease in which the symptoms are unusually severe and which leads rapidly to death is called **fulminating.**

Convalescence. The length of this period will depend upon how long the individual was ill and how his general condition was maintained during his illness. Some illnesses incapacitate the patient for only a short time, but may lead to a general weakening of his condition, thereby lengthening the period of convalescence.

Planning, implementation, and evaluation

Strengthening and supporting the defenses of the host

A person in good health has a vast arsenal of defenses that can be marshaled against invasion by disease-producing microorganisms. If the nurse is familiar with these defenses, she will better understand how they can be strengthened against infection, broken down by illness, and built up again.

Skin. Very few microorganisms are able to pass through healthy, unbroken skin. In addition, there are skin secretions that actually kill certain types of bacteria. If care of the patient's skin is neglected, an area of injury may become acutely inflamed and infected. (See chapter 16 for a discussion of the care of the skin.)

Eyes. Microorganisms are flushed out of the **conjunctiva** (the lining of the eyelids) by the constant washing of tears and the blinking motion of the lids.

Lungs. The lungs are protected by the mazelike structure of the nasal passages combined with moist membranes and **cilia** (short, hairlike growths). The act of sneezing causes dust and bacteria to be driven out along with membrane secretions (see p. 275). Coughing causes material from the lower respiratory tract to be expelled.

Gastrointestinal tract. Gastric juices and bile secretions contain chemicals that destroy invading pathogens in the gastrointestinal tract.

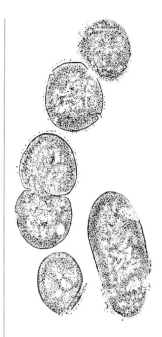

A person in good health has a vast arsenal of defenses that can be marshaled against invasion by disease-producing microorganisms.

Genitourinary tract.   The naturally acidic nature of the genitourinary tract is an important factor in overcoming infections in this area. Additional protection is provided by mucous secretions.

Leukocytes and tissue cells.   A vital body defense mechanism is provided by certain leukocytes and tissue cells. Some of these act as "scavengers" of foreign particles, such as bacteria or dead tissue cells. Certain substances in the blood, such as **properdin,** also provide the body with chemical protection against disease. When viruses are present in tissue cells, the cells are stimulated to produce a virus-killing protein called **interferon.**

Inflammation.   Inflammation is a defensive response of living tissue to any irritating or injuring agents. Inflammation is easily recognized by four signs: redness, swelling, heat, and pain. In the inflammatory process, exudate and cells seep from the dilated vessels into the surrounding tissue. This mass of cells releases enzymes that liquefy the cells and cause **pus** to form. As other blood substances are released and **fibrin** is formed, a wall is created that protects the body from the inflamed site. However, if the pus is not incised and drained, an **abscess** may form. Infectious material can then travel through the body via the bloodstream and infect more areas.

Immunity.   Immunity, the body's resistance to infection or disease, usually refers to protection of the individual against invasion by organisms. There are two kinds of immunity: passive immunity and active immunity. Babies are immune to certain diseases for the first 2 months because they have been supplied with antibodies from the mother's bloodstream. This is known as **passive immunity.**

Active immunity may be acquired naturally—through recovery from a communicable disease—or artificially—through immunization. The immunization process works as follows: Foreign protein substances (antigens in the form of vaccines) are introduced into the bloodstream. This stimulates the body to produce a protective antibody. The reaction of the antigen-antibodies provides a person with defense against specific infections and diseases. After vaccination, immunity lasts according to the antigen used, the dosage, and the age and health of the individual.

Immunization, like the processes of pasteurization, sterilization, sanitation, and isolation, provides another means of interrupting the sequence of infection and thus of controlling or preventing disease.

Preventing hospital-acquired (nosocomial) infections

For many years, the problem of hospital infections was so severe that hospitals were considered last resorts for medical treatment. By the late nineteenth century, the introduction of **antisepsis** and **asepsis** had brought about some measure of control.

Today, there is still concern because of the rising incidence of hospital infection. It is higher now than before the introduction of **antimicrobial** drugs. In a study of 491 infections, 16.3 percent were hospital-acquired. More than twice as many occurred on the surgical unit than on any other unit. The common sites of infection were respiratory tract, wound and skin, and urinary tract, in that order.[5]

The four chief methods of infection surveillance for hospitals and health facilities are physician reporting, nurse reporting, nurse-epidemiologist reporting, and prevalence studies.[6]

Basically, physician reporting and nurse reporting follow the same procedures. A form is filled out when an infection is diagnosed and placed in the patient's chart. These forms are reviewed periodically by an infection committee.

Another form of surveillance is to employ a single nurse-epidemiologist, who may spend from a third to all of her time in the surveillance and control of hospital infections. She collects surveillance data from a variety of sources and makes daily ward visits to review with the head nurse the current status of patients.

Prevalence studies, a fourth form of surveillance, are conducted every 3 to 6 months by an infection committee. This committee might also comment critically on the value of antibiotics. It should supervise training of hospital employees in infection control.

In an outbreak situation, two or more patients are affected by the same bacterium or virus. Sometimes an outbreak is dramatic, spreading rapidly to involve a large number of people, for example, with acute infantile gastroenteritis. Other outbreaks may be far less obvious, causing only a few lesions in a few patients. Staphylococcal wound infections are an example.

Obviously, affected patients must be treated at once. Unaffected patients in the area should also be given prophylactic antibiotics and perhaps transferred to another unit. They may even be discharged until the outbreak is over.

Some people become offended when told that they are harboring dangerous bacteria. Others may unjustifiably blame the staff of a patient unit undergoing an outbreak of infection. Therefore, the nurse must call upon reserves of tact, diplomacy, and firmness in dealing with affected patients in such outbreak situations.

[5]M. J. McNamara et al. 1967. A study of the bacteriologic patterns of hospital infections. *Annals of Internal Medicine* 66:481. In Irene L. Beland, *Clinical nursing: Pathophysiological and psychosocial approaches*, 2d ed., p. 137. New York: Macmillan, 1970.
[6]Theodore C. Eickhoff. 1967. Hospital infection control begins with good surveillance. *Hospitals* 41:118.

The following are some specific methods for controlling hospital-acquired infections:

1. All hospital personnel who have active staphylococcal lesions should be excused from work.
2. Antimicrobial agents should be used sparingly. Only well-defined reasons should justify the use of corticosteroids, immunosuppressive agents, and antineoplastic drugs.
3. Local procedures that greatly increase the host's susceptibility to infection should be performed only when absolutely necessary. These procedures include tracheotomies and venous cutdowns. Nasopharyngeal or tracheal suction should also be reserved for extreme cases.
4. Patients with active infection should be isolated. Hospital personnel and visitors coming into contact with infected patients should wear gowns, gloves, and masks. Protective isolation procedures should also be used for patients with exfoliating skin diseases, widespread burns, or agranulocytosis.[7]

Handwashing

General techniques. In normal clinical care, the following procedure for handwashing is generally observed:

1. Standing well away from the sink, turn on the water and adjust it to the desired temperature.
2. Wet hands and wrists thoroughly, holding them downward over the sink to allow the water to run toward the fingertips.
3. Take a generous portion of soap from the dispenser. If bar soap is used, it must be rinsed before being returned to the dish.
4. Scrub each hand with the other, creating as much friction as possible by interlacing the fingers and moving the hands back and forth. Continue the scrubbing action for 1 or 2 minutes, until areas between the fingers, the backs of hands, the palms, and areas around the fingernails are clean. Clean nails by working them against the palms or with an orangewood stick.
5. Rinse hands thoroughly by holding them under the running water with elbows higher than the hands so that the water flows downward to the fingertips. All soap should be carefully removed so as not to dry the skin.
6. Dry wrists and hands with paper towels, working from the area of the wrists to the fingertips. Discard each towel after one motion from wrist to fingertips.
7. Because the faucet handle is considered contaminated, turn off the water by using a dry paper towel to cover the faucet handle.[8]

[7] Beland, p. 142.
[8] Ibid., pp. 29–30.

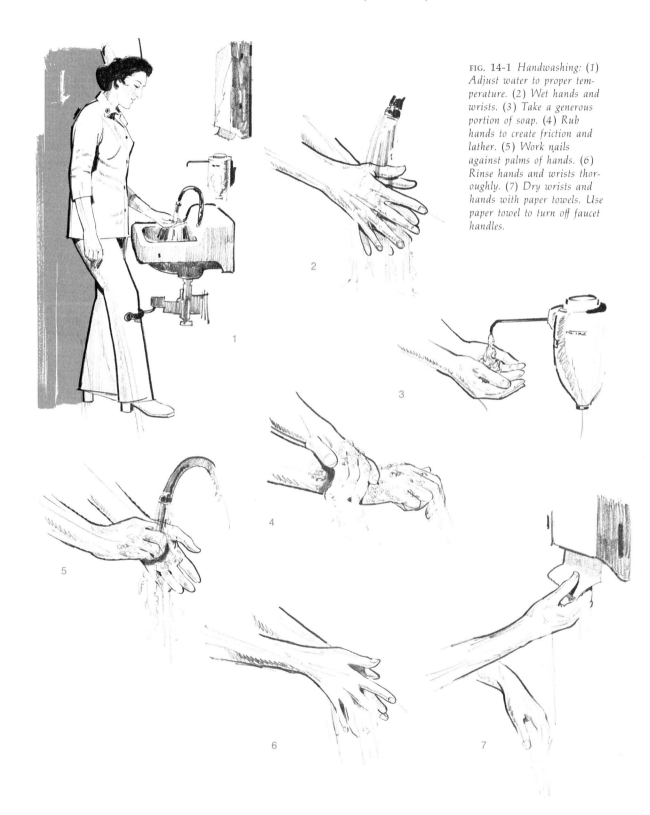

FIG. 14-1 *Handwashing:* (1) *Adjust water to proper temperature.* (2) *Wet hands and wrists.* (3) *Take a generous portion of soap.* (4) *Rub hands to create friction and lather.* (5) *Work nails against palms of hands.* (6) *Rinse hands and wrists thoroughly.* (7) *Dry wrists and hands with paper towels. Use paper towel to turn off faucet handles.*

Other sterile techniques

Gloves, masks, and gowns. The nurse puts on clean but unsterile gloves in order to protect herself from contamination. Gloves are used when inserting vaginal or rectal suppositories or rectal tubes and before handling extremely soiled dressings.

Sterile gloves prevent contamination of the patient during procedures requiring surgical asepsis or in the postoperative care of surgical wounds. Usually, gloves are packaged in a billfold-type muslin or paper wrapper, and are folded to form a cuff around the top. Hands must be washed and dried before sterile gloves are put on. An assistant should open and hold the wrapper so that the nurse touches only the wrapper and the gloves.

Gowns are worn in the operating room or in the presence of a patient with a communicable disease. The gown should cover clothes entirely and should open in the back.

Masks, which act as filters, are worn to minimize the danger of transmitting airborne disease-producing organisms. In the operating room, masks protect the patient from infection via droplets. On the medical units, they protect the nurse from a patient with an infectious disease. The mask should fit the face closely to prevent the escape of air around the sides. It should be worn only once, and then just for a short period.

Isolation

The extent to which a patient with a transmissible disease is isolated depends upon the nature of his illness, as well as on the physical facilities of the hospital. The following are some suggestions that can be applied in almost any isolation situation:[9]

1. The patient is segregated from others, and all equipment needed for his care is kept in the unit. Unnecessary equipment and furniture should be removed.
2. All food is transferred from the clean dishes and tray to dishes kept on a tray in the patient's unit. Dishes, basins, and similar articles should be disinfected before storage or use by others. If the patient has no sink in his room, a basin with a disinfectant solution should be kept in the unit and the solution changed several times daily.
3. Linen used by the isolated patient is kept separate. Feces and other body excretions can usually be poured directly into the hopper. Solid waste materials, such as food, soiled tissues, or old newspapers, should be collected in paper bags and burned. Articles too large for sterilization should be washed with a detergent and aired for 12 hours.
4. Items such as a nurse's watch will stay free from contamination if placed in a plastic bag.

[9] Audrey L. Sutton. 1969. *Bedside nursing techniques in medicine and surgery,* 2d ed., p. 108. Philadelphia: Saunders.

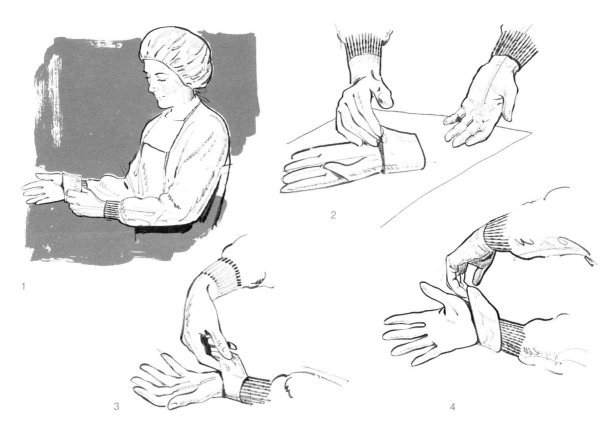

Reverse isolation. This is a technique used for patients who are extremely susceptible to infection. These include persons with extensive burns, for example, or those receiving massive chemotherapy, which causes bone-marrow depletion. For these patients, it is vital to provide an environment as free as possible from disease-producing organisms.

One type of reverse isolation unit includes the use of a plastic tent, which is placed over the patient's bed. A ventilating unit provides him with filtered air. An advantage of the unit is that it eliminates the need for gowns, masks, and other impediments. Visitors need not be restricted. Of course, the patient's physical activity is limited by the boundaries of the tent. Many patients in reverse isolation are extremely ill, however, and not able to move much in any event.[10]

Disinfection and sterilization

Basically, there are four different sterilizing procedures: chemical, pressure steam, dry heat, and ethylene oxide. The process of sterilization

FIG. 14-2 *Putting on sterile gloves by the open method: (1) After washing and drying her hands, the nurse slips her right hand inside the right glove. She must take care to prevent contamination of the exterior part of the glove. (2) She places her gloved hand beneath the cuff of the left glove to put it on. (3) She places the gloved right hand beneath the cuff of the left glove to unfold it and pull it over the cuff of the gown. (4) Similarly, she pulls the cuff of the right glove over the cuff of the gown.*

[10]Miriam K. Ginsberg and Maria L. LaConte. 1964. Reverse isolation. *American Journal of Nursing* 64:88–90.

is usually carried out in a central service area. However, the nurse should be aware of which type will be used so that she can bag equipment properly.

Steam sterilization is generally used for glass, metal, or stainless steel equipment, including all nonmetal bedside utensils, bedpans, wash basins, and emesis basins. Gas sterilization is used for delicate instruments, oxygen or suction gauges, blood pressure apparatus, stethoscopes, and plastic items. Caps should be removed from all glass bottles before sterilization.

SUMMARY

Infections are caused by disease-producing organisms called pathogens. Normally, the body harbors many organisms that are not harmful and are often beneficial. However, when the ecological balance between organism, host, and environment is upset, the organism can become a menace.

The process of infection follows a predictable sequence of events. If there is a break in the chain, infection may not occur. First, the pathogen must be invasive enough to break down the host's resistance. Then it must find a hospitable reservoir in which to flourish, a mode of escape from this reservoir, a means of transport, and a way of entering the host.

Even after this sequence of events has taken place, disease will not necessarily result unless the host is susceptible. Certain people whose resistance is lowered are more likely to contract disease than others. These include the very old and young, those who are malnourished, those with certain diseases, and those who are taking medications. Factors such as the sex and age of the host can also influence susceptibility.

The infectious process evolves in three stages: incubation, illness, and convalescence. The duration of incubation and illness varies from one disease to the next but is the same for a particular disease. Thus, it is possible to predict that measles will incubate over a period of 10 to 14 days and that the victim will be ill for about a week.

Prevention and control of infection are major responsibilities of the nurse and involve a wide variety of tasks and much specific knowledge. The nurse should understand the many natural defenses with which the body is equipped, the most important of which is the skin. When skin is properly cared for, the chance of bacterial invasion is greatly reduced. In addition to natural defenses, the body can be artificially supplied with immunity in the form of injections of vaccines. Vaccination, like pasteurization, sterilization, sanitation, and isolation, provides an important means of interrupting the infectious process.

Hospital-acquired infection is a major source of concern in every American hospital. Of course, in an environment where almost everybody is ill, it is extremely difficult to control the spread of infection from one patient to another or from patient to staff. The nurse's role in this regard is crucial. Not only is she charged with containment and prevention functions, she also is expected to provide information to staff and patients and to carry out various reporting duties.

The mainstay of infection control is proper handwashing. Whether she is working on the wards or in the operating theater, the nurse should be scrupulous in carrying out the recommended procedures for keeping her hands free of contamination. In addition, she must know how to put on and remove gloves, masks, and gowns.

When a patient has a communicable disease, he should be isolated from other patients. Specific procedures protect both the nurse and other patients from contamination. For example, all equipment used in the infected patient's room is either sterilized before being taken away or is carefully double-bagged before being sent to central service. Linen used in the isolation wards is kept separate, and solid waste materials are collected in paper bags and burned.

In implementing the techniques of asepsis, the nurse must bear in mind that a completely contamination-free environment is not possible, and that bacteria will invade no matter how strenuous her efforts. Nevertheless, these efforts are vital if the hospital is to remain a generally safe environment. All of these procedures can be modified for patients in their home environment.

STUDY QUESTIONS

1. What is a pathogen?
2. List and briefly define the four major types of agent-host relationships discussed in this chapter.
3. List the steps involved in good handwashing technique.
4. What are the stages of an infectious disease?
5. What is reverse isolation? How does this technique differ from standard isolation procedures?
6. Devise and describe in detail (including rationale) an effective, practical isolation plan for a member of your family with a salmonella infection. Take into consideration the characteristics of your actual residence and family members when drawing up the plan.

SELECTED BIBLIOGRAPHY

Beland, Irene L. 1970. *Clinical nursing: Pathophysiological and psychosocial approaches,* 2d ed., pp. 110–48. New York: Macmillan.

Dubay, Elaine C., and Grubb, Reba D. 1973. *Infection: Prevention and control.* St. Louis: Mosby.

Eickhoff, Theodore C. 1967. Hospital infection control begins with good surveillance. *Hospitals* 41:118–20.

Sutton, Audrey L. 1969. *Bedside nursing techniques in medicine and surgery,* 2d ed., pp. 101–11. Philadelphia: Saunders.

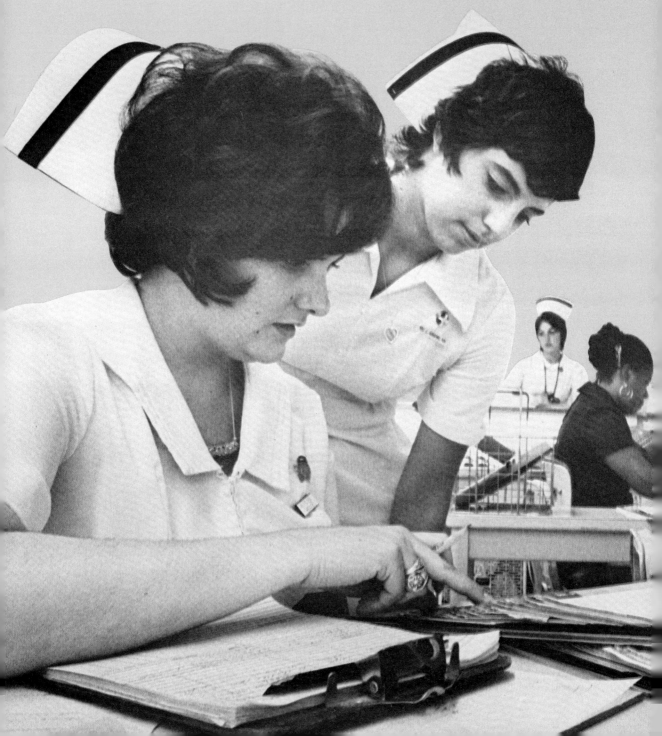

Part Five

Health maintenance in the health care system

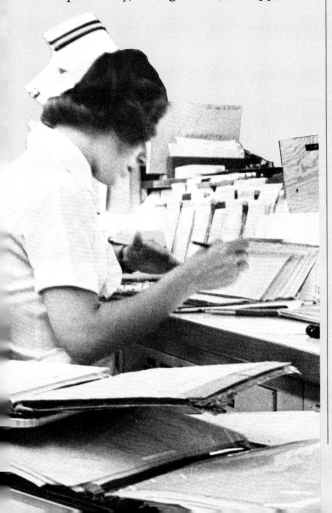

Estelle Tanner had been meaning to get rid of the old scatter rug in her front hall for years. Now she had slipped and fallen on it, fracturing her hip. Luckily, a neighbor had dropped by the same afternoon and found her lying helpless on the floor. An ambulance was called and Estelle was taken to the hospital. A few days later she was operated on.

During the first week after her operation, new discomforts appeared every day. For a while, it was necessary to feed her intravenously. Since she was unable to move herself, the nurses changed her position regularly and guided her in passive exercises. Estelle felt very helpless, even hopeless, at times. But the nurses explained that she would gradually improve, especially once she was able to move around and practice walking. In time, Estelle came to accept the enemas, the unfamiliar food, and the pain in her hip as part of a typical hospital stay.

What really worried her, however, was the thought of being dependent on a wheelchair or a walker for the rest of her life. She had trouble dressing herself, bathing, or even going to the bathroom alone. The thought of having to cope with such domestic tasks as grocery shopping and cooking was simply overwhelming.

After an extended period of twice-a-day

physical therapy, Estelle got around well enough with her walker to be able to leave the hospital. Because she felt she couldn't manage alone, and hiring a full-time companion was financially impossible, it was decided that she should come and stay with Anita and Richard for a while. She would have the bedroom on the first floor, and Steve and Paul would share a room temporarily.

Anita and Richard tried to make Estelle feel comfortable, but their way of doing things just wasn't the same as hers. Estelle had always regretted living so far away from her family, but now they seemed too close. The children's stereo bothered her, along with their late hours on the weekend. And she certainly didn't approve of those filthy old jeans that Paul ran around in all the time. Above all, Estelle sometimes felt like she was another child in the family, with everyone telling her what was best for her.

With the help of the family and a visiting nurse, Estelle continued with her daily physical therapy routine. Soon she was able to walk with the aid of only a cane, although stairs were still a problem. Much as Estelle appreciated the attentions of her family, she looked forward to the day when she would be back in her own home. It was decided to hire a part-time housekeeper to help with the cooking, cleaning, and other household chores. The visiting nurse promised to make the necessary arrangements through a social service agency in Estelle's town.

What are Estelle's health care needs while she is in the hospital? after she is discharged?

What nursing actions can be taken to meet these needs?

How is stress handled by each person and by the family as a whole?

What are the factors favoring physical and emotional homeostasis in this situation? What are the factors opposing homeostasis?

---

15 Homeostasis, stress, and adaptation

What is homeostasis?

Homeostasis is the process of continually changing to maintain internal stability and to adapt to external conditions. In the healthy organism, the drive to maintain a stable state is a very powerful force. In man, any imbalance is corrected quickly and subtly by the body's own regulating mechanisms. These regulating mechanisms are extremely sensitive to any change in the external or internal environment.[1]

Hippocrates, the father of medicine, believed that such regulating mechanisms existed. He asserted that the body was cured by "natural powers." The modern concept of homeostasis dates back only a hundred years, however. The term "homeostasis" (from the Greek *homoios*, like, similar; plus *stasis*, position, standing) was first used by an American physiologist, Walter B. Cannon. He wrote of the "wisdom of the body" in regulating itself. Somewhat earlier, a French scientist, Claude Bernard, emphasized the role of the inner environment in establishing and maintaining steady states in the body.[2]

In principle, homeostasis is not limited to living organisms. It has been applied also to the fields of sociology, economics, and ecology. Also, it does not imply only physiological balance. In psychology, it refers to the condition of psychological integration. However, the psychological regulatory mechanisms are less well understood than those of physiological regulation.

Physiological homeostasis

Physiological homeostasis involves the response of the body to a variety of stimuli. The study of physiological homeostasis is concerned with how the body maintains steady states of blood pressure, body tem-

[1] Audrey Burgess. 1970. *The nurse's guide to fluid and electrolyte balance,* p. 42. New York: McGraw-Hill.
[2] L. L. Langley. 1965. *Homeostasis,* p. 2. New York: Van Nostrand Reinhold.

Upon completing this chapter, the reader should be able to:

1. Explain and give examples of physiological and psychological homeostatic mechanisms.

2. Discuss the six features common to all homeostatic mechanisms.

3. Give five examples of variables that influence an individual's capacity for adaptation.

4. Define the three stages of Selye's general adaptation syndrome.

5. Relate nursing intervention to the nursing process in the case of a patient with problems of homeostatic imbalance.

6. Discuss the relationship between stress, adaptation, and homeostasis.

perature, body weight, respiration, body fluids, and hormones. It is concerned with the checks, balances, and feedback mechanisms that resist change and regulate interchange.

There are five major physiological homeostatic mechanisms. These are

1. The pituitary, or the "master gland" of the endocrine system
2. The parathyroid gland
3. The renocardiovascular system (the kidneys, heart, and blood vessels)
4. The pulmonary mechanisms
5. The adrenal mechanisms

The lungs regulate oxygen and carbon dioxide. Since carbon dioxide comes from the carbonic acid in the blood, the lungs thereby help maintain the important balance between acids and bases in the extracellular fluids. The kidneys give off chemical wastes and remove a large number of foreign substances from the extracellular fluid. The adrenal glands, located above the kidneys, secrete hormones essential to the excretion and retention of water and electrolytes, such as sodium, chloride, and potassium (see chapter 22). The pituitary gland directly affects the body's conservation of water through secretion of antidiuretic hormones (ADH). The parathyroid gland regulates the level of calcium in the extracellular fluid.[3]

Because of these regulating systems, changes occur automatically when imbalance arises. For example, when the body temperature begins to fall, **autonomic** (involuntary) nerves carry impulses that cause blood vessels in the skin to constrict, thereby conserving heat. If the carbon dioxide level in the blood rises, breathing automatically deepens, bringing more oxygen into the lungs.[4]

Another type of response takes place when the body senses a local burning sensation. The nerve receptors in the finger pick up the message of heat when the finger touches a hot object. This message is carried via the nervous system to the spinal cord, which sends back directions to the muscles. The muscles of the hand and arm pull the finger away from the source of stimulation, thus discontinuing the nerve impulses.[5]

Psychological homeostasis

The concept of homeostasis also applies to states of psychological balance. (This is called emotional or psychological homeostasis.) This balance is maintained by a variety of psychological processes and mecha-

[3]N. M. Matheny and W. D. Snively, Jr. 1974. *Nurse's handbook of fluid balance*, p. 10. Philadelphia: Lippincott.

[4]Theodore Lidz. 1968. *The person: His development throughout the life cycle*, p. 533. New York: Basic Books.

[5]Valentina G. Fischer and Arlene F. Connolly. 1970. *Promotion of physical comfort and safety*, p. 45. Dubuque, Iowa: Brown.

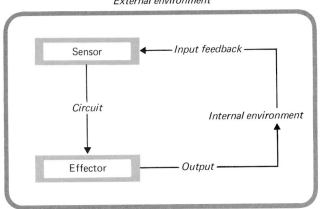

FIG. 15-1 *Basic elements of homeostasis.*

[From L. L. Langley, *Homeostasis,* p. 15. New York: Van Nostrand Reinhold, 1965. Copyright © 1965 by Litton Educational Publishing, Inc. Reprinted by permission of the publisher.]

nisms that regulate and restore psychological stability in a changing environment.

There are certain nonmaterial needs that must be met in order to maintain psychological stability. These include needs for self-esteem, love and belongingness, and safety and protection. (These were discussed in chapter 8.) When the fulfillment of these needs is threatened, psychological agents work to counter the threat.

How does a homeostatic mechanism work?

There are several features common to all homeostatic mechanisms.[6] The first is a sensing device that detects disturbances in the internal and external environments. This device is called a **receptor.** The stimulus that affects the receptor is called **input.** (Man's receptors are specialized tissues that respond to certain types of input. The skin responds to changes in temperature, pressure, etc.) There must also be a **circuit** to communicate these responses to an **effector mechanism.** (Man's main circuit is his nervous system.) The effector mechanism then acts to correct the disturbance. The action taken by the effector mechanism is called **output.** Figure 15-1 shows a typical homeostatic mechanism.

L. L. Langley has compared the homeostatic mechanisms in the body with the thermostat that controls a home furnace and air-conditioning system (see Fig. 15-2).[7] In the case of the thermostat, cold air (the input) outside the house causes the temperature to drop below that to which the thermostat has been set. This change in temperature is detected by the thermostat (the receptor), which is wired (the circuit) to a furnace. The thermostat then turns on the furnace (the effector mechanism), which produces heat (output). This causes the temperature to rise. When the desired temperature is reached, the thermostat automatically shuts off the

[6]Langley, p. 15.
[7]Ibid., pp. 12–15.

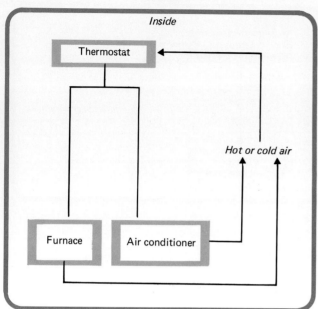

Inside

Thermostat

Hot or cold air

Furnace

Air conditioner

FIG. 15-2 *Control of house temperature.*

[From L. L. Langley, *Homeostasis*, p. 13. New York: Van Nostrand Reinhold, 1965. Copyright © 1965 by Litton Educational Publishing, Inc. Reprinted by permission of the publisher.]

furnace until more heat is needed. In warm weather, the thermostat triggers an air-conditioning system, which produces cold air.

Also important in homeostasis is **feedback.** There are two types of feedback: negative and positive. Most homeostatic mechanisms are regulated by **negative feedback.** In negative feedback, change in one direction triggers change in the opposite direction. The result is a state of balance between the opposing extremes. A mechanism that regulates itself through negative feedback is called a "self-correcting" mechanism. For example, the eating of glucose (sugar) causes the level of glucose in the blood to rise. This acts as a stimulus to a blood-glucose-lowering mechanism, which causes the level to fall. In this way, the level of glucose in the blood is returned to normal. Almost all of the body's homeostatic mechanisms are controlled by negative feedback.

In a **positive feedback** system, one change causes more of the same. This is known as a "self-perpetuating" system, or a "vicious cycle." It often leads to instability and death. For example, if a person loses a great deal of blood, he will not have enough left for his heart to pump effectively. The resulting fall in blood pressure causes even less blood to flow through the vessels to the heart. This, in turn, weakens the heart, which then pumps still less blood, and so on.

Influences on homeostasis

Homeostasis can be maintained only if certain physiological requirements are met. An adequate supply of substances such as water, oxygen, and nutrients must be available to the cells. Certain operating conditions, such as an appropriate glucose level, body temperature, and hydrogen ion concentration, must be present. Finally, conditions in the external environment must be within the limits to which man can adapt.

Physiological homeostasis also can be influenced by other than physical factors. Sociocultural conditions can lead to malnutrition, drug addiction, and air pollution. All of these can alter the body's chemical balance. Certain emotional states, such as fear, anxiety, aggression, or hostility, especially when they occur over a period of time, can damage the smooth operation of the homeostatic mechanisms. Extremes of these conditions may lead to permanent changes. These can result in the development of peptic ulcers, hyperthyroidism, or bronchial asthma.[8] Other disturbances in psychological homeostasis, such as depression, migraine headaches, and conversion reactions, can disturb physiological homeostasis. Mild habit disorders, such as nail-biting or thumb-sucking, can also have an effect on physiological homeostasis.

What is stress?

As it is commonly used, the term **stress** refers to "a burden or load under which a person survives or cracks."[9] It has also been defined as any internal or external influence that interferes with satisfaction of basic needs or that disturbs or threatens to disturb homeostasis.[10] Still another explanation defines stress as any disturbance in the body homeostasis general or severe enough to produce a coordinated body response.[11] This response includes renal, respiratory, metabolic, sympathetic, and circulatory reactions. These reactions can be brought about by physical or mental disturbances, including cold, hunger, and physical exertion. They can also result from infection, chemical or mechanical injury, or mental stresses, such as excitement. Both a crucial interview and an emotion-laden movie could be called stress-producing.

Even Hans Selye, pioneer of the stress concept, had difficulty defining stress. Stress, he finally concluded, "is essentially the *wear and tear* in the body caused by life at any one time."[12] Stress is a universal phenomenon; it cannot and should not be avoided. A painful blow or a kiss can be equally

[8]Irene L. Beland. 1970. *Clinical nursing: Pathophysiological and psychosocial approaches,* 2d ed., p. 45. New York: Macmillan.

[9]Lydia Rapoport. 1962. The state of crisis: Some theoretical considerations. *The Social Service Review* 36. Reprinted in Howard J. Parad, ed., *Crisis intervention,* p. 23. New York: Family Service Association of America, 1965.

[10]Harry W. Martin and Arthur J. Prange, Jr. 1962. Human adaptation—a conceptual approach to understanding patients. *The Canadian Nurse* 58. Reprinted in Margaret E. Auld and Linda H. Birum, eds., *The challenge of nursing: A book of readings,* p. 50. St. Louis: Mosby, 1973.

[11]Burgess, p. 43.

[12]Hans Selye. 1956. *The stress of life,* p. 254. New York: McGraw-Hill.

Stress is a universal phenomenon; it cannot and should not be avoided.

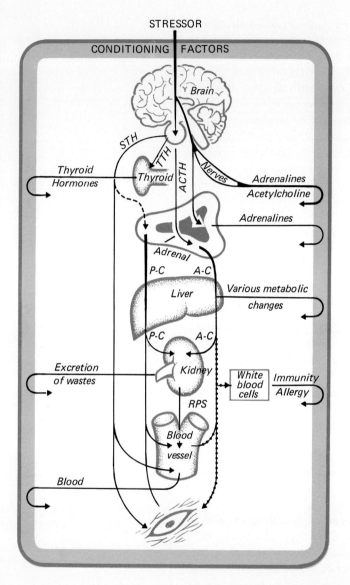

STRESSOR

CONDITIONING FACTORS

Brain

STH

TTH

ACTH

Nerves

*Thyroid
Hormones*

Thyroid

*Adrenalines
Acetylcholine*

Adrenalines

Adrenal

P-C   A-C

Liver

*Various metabolic
changes*

P-C   A-C

Kidney

White
blood
cells

*Immunity
Allergy*

*Excretion
of wastes*

RPS

*Blood
vessel*

Blood

FIG. 15-3 *Selye's concept of
the stress syndrome.*

[From Hans Selye, *The stress of life,*
p. 113. New York: McGraw-Hill,
1956. Copyright 1956 by Hans
Selye. Reprinted by permission of
the publisher.]

stressful. "Crossing a busy intersection, exposure to a draft, or even sheer
joy are enough to activate the body's stress mechanism to some extent."[13]

According to Selye, the body responds to stress of any kind with a
unified defense mechanism. This mechanism is characterized by specific
structural and chemical changes. The agents of stress that bring about this
reaction are called **stressors.** (See Fig. 15-3.) The entire stress syndrome—

[13]Ibid., p. vii.

the threat and the body's reaction to it—Selye called the **general adaptation syndrome** (see p. 297).

"Fight or flight"

An important part of the body's reaction to stress is the concept of "fight or flight," which was discussed in chapter 8. In this reaction, the adrenal medulla produces an instantaneous physiological response. Adrenal catecholamines (epinephrine and norepinephrine) prepare the body for action by directing blood toward the brain and muscles. The organism becomes alert and sensitive to stimuli.[14]

When stress is mental in origin, as it is so often in today's highly complex society, it may seem inappropriate that the response is still largely physical, involving muscles, heart, and intestines. But mental changes also occur in response to a threat. These include clearer thinking, resistance to mental fatigue, and resistance to the disruptive effects of conflicting emotional forces.[15]

Reaction to stress can occur primarily on a psychological or physiological level, although it is difficult to make a clear-cut distinction between the two. A threat to psychological homeostasis occurs whenever a person experiences a failure in adaptation in the face of some challenge. This might be a failure in marriage or a failure at work. Unless psychological repair efforts are successful, emotional aftereffects of the failure will interfere with future adaptive efforts in the same area.[16] Homeostasis can be maintained by avoidance of the situation or by the use of such defense mechanisms as projection or denial (see chapter 8). In psychosis, homeostasis is maintained at the expense of the individual's perception of reality.

What is adaptation?

Adaptation is the process by which an organism responds to its environment. It includes all conscious and unconscious forms of adjustment. It is the means by which an organism defends its individuality. All concepts of adaptation include the ideas of change, response, and the environment.

Adaptation has been defined as "the process of change whereby the individual retains his integrity—his wholeness—within the realities of his environment. A truly integrating system within the organism must be one that responds to environmental change, yet in the process defends the

[14]Lidz, p. 527.

[15]S. V. Boyden, ed. 1970. *Impact of civilisation on the biology of man*, p. 179. Toronto: University of Toronto.

[16]Bernard C. Holland and Richard S. Ward. 1966. Homeostasis and psychosomatic medicine. In Silvano Arieti, ed., *American handbook of psychiatry*, vol. 3, p. 345. New York: Basic Books.

Adaptation is the process by which an organism responds to its environment.

wholeness of the individual. The purpose of integration is to establish order and organization within the organism in harmony with its external environment."[17]

There are numerous examples of man's successful adaptation to a variety of conditions. The short, stocky frame of the Eskimo and the layer of fat under his skin serve to protect him from heat loss. The heavy muscles of the manual laborer or the professional wrestler illustrate an adaptation to activities requiring muscular effort. Enlargement of the myocardium in hypertension is another illustration of biological adaptation to increased work.[18]

Although man has a wider range of adaptive powers than other species, the extent of possible adaptive modes is limited. Physical adaptation is limited by **morphology** (form and structure) and **physiochemistry.** Man's ability to adapt to extremes of temperature, high altitude, and physical trauma is limited. Sociocultural adaptation is often restricted by traditions that retard the development of new solutions to social problems. Psychological adaptation is limited by psychological heredity and previous experiences with important figures in the individual's past.

The measure of man's ability to adapt has been called "adaptation energy."[19] This capacity is influenced by many factors.

Heredity determines the organism's potential for growth and development. Through the effect of cellular biochemical activities, genes affect adaptive ability. For example, genetic factors are involved in the transmission of sickle-cell disease and diabetes mellitus.

Another important factor is the extent to which the individual's *psychological* needs have been met in the past, especially in early life. "A child who is seriously deprived of love is susceptible to failure to develop emotionally."[20]

Achievement of adaptive potential depends also on the individual's level of *learning*—how well he has learned to satisfy his needs when confronted with the environment.[21] Flexibility promotes easier adaptation, and positive learning contributes to the development of flexibility.

Anatomical integrity is another factor affecting adaptability. An individual who is born with a brain injury may be less able to cope with emotional and physical demands than a healthier person.

Age is also a factor. In most cases, adaptability is greater in youth and early middle life than it is at the extremes of life. In young children and in the elderly, adaptive capacity is lessened. In the former, it is immature; in the latter, "adaptive energy" declines.

[17]Myra E. Levine. 1969. The pursuit of wholeness. *American Journal of Nursing* 69:95.
[18]Beland, p. 47.
[19]Selye, pp. 65–66.
[20]Beland, p. 48.
[21]Ibid.

Adaptation processes

There are several features common to all adaptation processes. First, adaptation, for the most part, involves the entire organism. Response to imbalance within the body calls up a generalized reaction in defense. Second, the body is able to adapt to greater demands if these are gradually introduced. When called upon to react suddenly, adaptive responses are not as efficient. As mentioned previously, the more flexible the organism is in its capacity to adapt, the greater is its ability to survive. In adaptation, the organism generally uses the mechanism most economical of energy. Finally, the adaptive response may be adequate, excessive, or inappropriate.[22]

The principal areas of human adaptation occur on social, psychological, and cellular levels. At the cellular level, complex biochemical processes regulate the activities necessary for biological survival. These include ingestion, assimilation, excretion, and procreation. In the psychological sphere, adaptation requires the integration of learning and idea formation, perception, and conscious and unconscious processes. The social, or, more accurately, the sociocultural, level of adaptation involves the development of modes of human behavior in groups. It centers around interpersonal interaction, values, beliefs, norms, and symbols.[23]

All of these levels of adaptation are dependent upon one another. The following example illustrates this interdependence. An individual attacked by a paralytic poliovirus may suffer permanent damage that restricts his mobility and disfigures his body. In one respect, all this is simply cellular. However, much more is involved if one is concerned with the total individual. He must be cared for by others. The residual effects of his disease will limit, according to the amount of damage, his participation in society for the remainder of his life. Psychologically, the individual has to adjust to these changes and deficits by acquiring a different concept of himself.[24]

What are the stages of the general adaptation syndrome?

Selye has divided the general adaptation syndrome (GAS) into three stages:

1. The "alarm reaction," in which the defensive forces are mobilized
2. The "stage of resistance," which reflects full adaptation to the stressor
3. The "stage of exhaustion," which follows if the stressor is severe enough and applied for a sufficient length of time[25]

The principal areas of human adaptation occur on social, psychological, and cellular levels.

---

[22]Ibid., p. 49.
[23]Martin and Prange, p. 49.
[24]Ibid., p. 50.
[25]Selye, p. 31.

The alarm reaction. When an individual senses a possible threat, whether a bodily injury or an emotional trauma, the body prepares defensively. In this first phase of the GAS, signals are sent out from the **hypothalamus.** They travel to the **adrenal medulla,** the primary organs (heart, brain, liver, etc.), and the **pituitary gland.** The heart beats faster, the muscles enlarge, and the level of glucose in the blood rises. The level of **corticoid** production also rises dramatically. (Corticoids are the hormones secreted by the **adrenal cortex.**) This results in the "fight or flight" response, which was described on p. 295.

No living organism can maintain a constant state of alarm. "If the body is confronted with an agent so damaging that continuous exposure to it is incompatible with life, then death ensues during the alarm reaction or within the first few hours or days."[26]

The stage of resistance. During the stage of resistance, the organism achieves full adaptation to the stressor. According to Selye, adaptation is characterized by *"the delimitation of stress to the smallest area capable of meeting the requirements of a situation."*[27] In other words, once the body has identified the nature of a stressor, it concentrates all its efforts in that one area, eliminating unnecessary actions. Selye maintains that this is true of any effort man makes. Once he learns how to do something, in the future he does it much more efficiently and with much less effort.

During the stage of resistance, the corticoid level falls as dramatically as it rose during the stage of alarm. This activity is now maintained only at the level absolutely needed to combat the particular stressor that is at work.

The stage of exhaustion. If the stressor continues to act upon the organism for any great length of time, the particular defensive mechanisms used during the stage of adaptation begin to wear down. The body's "adaptation energy" becomes exhausted at the point where the stressor is active. Once again, the generalized alarm reaction sets in, as the body attempts to make up for the damage to a particular area. Corticoid levels rise once more. If this stress continues, even these mechanisms will falter and fail. With all defense mechanisms exhausted, the organism must inevitably die.

The general adaptation syndrome can also be applied to stages of psychological or sociocultural adaptation. Built-in psychological defense and repair mechanisms protect the individual against psychological threats. These include denial, shock, and fainting. (See chapter 8 for a discussion of psychological defense mechanisms.) On a sociocultural level, interpersonal and group resources serve as defenses.[28]

[26] Ibid.

[27] Ibid., p. 120. Italics in original.

[28] James C. Coleman. 1973. Life stress and maladaptive behavior. *American Journal of Occupational Therapy* 27:171.

Helping the patient with problems of homeostatic imbalance

Assessing homeostatic problems

One of the nurse's primary functions is assessing the status of the patient's homeostatic mechanisms. In order to do so, the nurse must have a thorough knowledge of normal body functions so that she can recognize the abnormal. Proper assessment of homeostatic needs ensures that:

1. Signs and symptoms are correctly interpreted
2. Nursing problems are clearly defined
3. Nursing actions are based on an intelligent analysis of problems
4. Various therapies are carried out safely[29]

The correct interpretation of signs and symptoms is crucial in determining the actual physiological processes that are at work. These are sometimes reflected in misleading ways. For example, because of the stress reaction resulting in catecholamine secretion (epinephrine and norepinephrine), a seriously ill patient may appear deceptively stable and alert. It is important that the nurse recognize this, for often she is the first health care professional to evaluate a patient.

Intelligent analysis of the patient's problem demands that the nurse be familiar with the patient, his history, and his disorder. She must observe the patient's behavior and note the results of chemical examinations of his blood and other fluids. Intelligent analysis depends on her knowing what to observe, when to observe, and how to use her observations.

In supporting the patient's natural attempts to achieve balance, the nurse automatically increases the safety of her patient. For example, an increased temperature, possibly a sign of fluid imbalance in the body, would not be allowed to become elevated to a point of danger. Fluids would be replaced (intravenously or by mouth), and fluid depletion and possible cellular damage would be avoided. (See chapter 22.)

In addition, if the nurse carries out procedures in a safe, effective manner, psychological equilibrium of the patient is promoted. Patients feel reassured and secure when cared for by nurses with the ability to assess the situation quickly and to initiate prompt action. Such nurses appear to know what to do and take over when the patient is overwhelmed. They know how to do the "right thing."[30]

Restoring psychological homeostasis

The nurse can help the patient who has an emotional imbalance, and his family, through an understanding of normal reactions to stress. She

One of the nurse's primary functions is assessing the status of the patient's homeostatic mechanisms.

[29]Fischer and Connolly, p. 42.
[30]Beland, p. 235.

The nurse can help the patient restore psychological homeostasis by removing or decreasing the stressors that are acting upon him.

should also understand the psychological mechanisms by which man normally copes with stressful situations (see chapter 8). Often she can serve as a sympathetic listener. In so doing, she can arrest and partially reverse the chain of events that often leads from thwarted grief to guilt, depression, and illness.[31] One nurse writes of assisting the mother of a dying child by helping her to understand the natural psychological cycle of denial, hope, and acceptance.[32]

The nurse can help the patient restore psychological homeostasis by removing or decreasing the stressors that are acting upon him. For example, the threat of the unknown creates fear, anxiety, and emotional instability in the patient. This is especially true for patients who are scheduled for surgery. Patients who are thoroughly informed and counseled prior to surgery suffer far fewer postoperative complications and recover more rapidly than those who are not prepared. In some institutions, preadmission orientation programs are held for prospective patients and their families.

SUMMARY

Homeostasis is the process of continually changing to maintain internal stability and to adapt to external conditions. Man, along with other living organisms, has several internal mechanisms that enable him to maintain homeostasis. All of these mechanisms have certain essential features in common:

1. A receptor, or sensing device
2. A circuit, or means of communicating messages
3. An effector, which acts on the message and corrects the imbalance
4. A shut-off device, which terminates the activity when homeostasis has been restored

These mechanisms are controlled by either a negative feedback system (which is the most common) or a positive feedback system. In the negative feedback system, a change in one direction is opposed by a change in the opposite direction. In this way, a balance between extremes is maintained. In the positive feedback system, a change in one direction stimulates further change in that same direction. This is known as a self-perpetuating system, or a vicious cycle.

Maintenance of physiological homeostasis depends on a number of factors. These include a sociocultural and psychological environment conducive to homeostasis, as well as an adequate supply of necessary chemical ingredients, such as water, oxygen, and nutrients.

[31] Martin and Prange, p. 56.
[32] Linda Goldfogel. 1970. Working with the parent of a dying child. *American Journal of Nursing* 70:1675.

The technique used to maintain a state of homeostasis is called adaptation. This is the process of change and adjustment through which the organism is able to survive in a particular environment. Adaptation occurs on three interdependent levels—social, psychological, and cellular. One example of a physical adaptation is the Eskimo's conservation of heat by development of a layer of fat under the skin, and the evolution of a short, stocky frame. Although adaptation requires organismic change, one essential feature is the maintenance of the integrity—the wholeness—of the individual organism.

Unlimited adaptation by man, however, is not possible. He is limited by his innate biological adaptability, heredity, psychological factors, degree of learning and flexibility, anatomical integrity, and age.

Before adaptation can proceed, some stimulus must reach the sensing device. This is called a stressor, and it calls up a generalized bodily response to cope with the stimulus. This coordinated response of the renal, respiratory, metabolic, sympathetic, and circulatory systems was called the general adaptation syndrome by Hans Selye, pioneer of the stress theory. The general adaptation syndrome (GAS) occurs in three stages: the alarm reaction, the stage of resistance, and, if the stressor is severe enough and applied for a sufficient length of time, the stage of exhaustion. At this time, disintegration and death occur, since "adaptation energy," the ability to adapt to a variety of stressors, is finite.

In adapting to stress, two main processes occur through the hypothalamus in the brain. The adrenal medulla is stimulated by autonomic nerves to produce epinephrine and norepinephrine, preparing the organism for "fight or flight." At the same time, neurohormonal messages from the hypothalamus stimulate the adrenal cortex to produce corticoids. The combination of processes regulates water and electrolyte balance, catabolism, and vasopressor action. They protect the body from damaging insult within limits.

Stressors can also be psychological or sociocultural in origin. Built-in defenses, learned coping patterns, and group resources protect the individual on these levels.

The nurse's role in homeostatic problems is to assess the status of the patient's homeostatic mechanisms, stressors, and available coping mechanisms. In helping to achieve homeostatic balance, she decreases or removes stressors, supports adaptive processes, or demonstrates more effective ones.

STUDY QUESTIONS

1. What are the five major homeostatic mechanisms of the human body? What are the functions of each?
2. What are the basic components of all homeostatic mechanisms?
3. What is a negative feedback system? Contrast this type of system with a positive feedback system. Give examples of each type of system within the human body.

4. Name and define four major factors that influence man's adaptation capabilities.
5. What are the stages of the general adaptation syndrome?
6. Referring to chapter 8 (Psychosocial and Emotional Needs of the Patient) and
   chapter 11 (Teaching-Learning Aspects of Nursing), draw up a plan to help
   restore the psychological homeostasis of an anxious, 15-year-old female
   patient who is about to undergo surgery for the removal of an ovarian cyst.

SELECTED BIBLIOGRAPHY

Holland, Bernard C., and Ward, Richard S. 1966. Homeostasis and psychosomatic
    medicine. In Silvano Arieti, ed., *American handbook of psychiatry*, vol. 3, pp.
    344–61. New York: Basic Books.
Langley, L. L. 1965. *Homeostasis*. New York: Van Nostrand Reinhold.
Levine, Myra E. 1969. The pursuit of wholeness. *American Journal of Nursing*
    69:93–98.
Rapoport, Lydia. 1962. The state of crisis: Some theoretical considerations. *The
    Social Service Review* 36. Reprinted in Howard J. Parad, ed., *Crisis intervention*,
    pp. 23–31. New York: Family Service Association of America, 1965.
Selye, Hans. 1956. *The stress of life*. New York: McGraw-Hill.

16 Meeting cleanliness and comfort needs

Cleanliness may not necessarily be next to godliness, but it is an important element in promoting health and well-being. We have already seen how proper handwashing techniques are a vital defense against the spread of infection. Keeping the patient clean not only makes him more comfortable, it often speeds his rate of recovery and prevents complications.

Assessment of the skin, nails, and hair

Skin

Examination of the skin requires good light. Daylight is preferable, but a stand light with a bulb of at least 60 watts will do. (Fluorescent light can make even healthy people look cyanotic.) The examination of the skin should take the following factors into account:

1. Color
2. Turgor
3. Texture
4. Integrity[1]

Color. Changes or abnormalities in color should be noted. Among the more common abnormalities are cyanosis, jaundice, and pallor. Cyanosis is generally symptomatic of pulmonary disease, heart disease, or hypoglycemia. Jaundice may be caused by liver disease, drugs, or carotenemia (eating too many carrots or other yellow vegetables). Pallor is usually associated with anemia. It may also be caused by internal hemorrhaging.

It is also important to check for variations in skin color, including variations in pigmented areas. In adults, the use of makeup may conceal color variations as well as lesions (see below).

[1]Marie S. Brown and Mary M. Alexander. 1973. Physical examination, part 3: Examining the skin. *Nursing '73* 3:40.

Upon completing this chapter, the reader should be able to:

1. Relate the assessment of skin, hair, and nails to the assessment of the individual's total health status.

2. Relate the bath and other cleanliness procedures to the opportunity for further evaluation of the patient's physical and mental status.

3. Identify measures designed to meet the patient's physical comfort needs.

4. Discuss the relationship between physical comfort measures and emotional well-being.

5. Describe the four types of decubitus ulcers in terms of their appearance, cause, treatment, and techniques for prevention.

Turgor. The **turgor** of the skin can be estimated by pinching the lower abdomen or the inner forearm. Normal skin will quickly fall back into place when it is released. Skin that is dehydrated will stay pinched for 30 seconds or longer. Edema, which may be due to heart failure, kidney disorders, or malnutrition, can be detected by pressing a finger firmly against the skin, particularly in the ankle region. If the impression remains after the finger has been removed, edema is most likely present.

Texture. Normal skin is smooth, soft, and flexible. Dry, scaly skin may indicate eczema, ringworm, vitamin A deficiency, or hypothyroidism.

Integrity. Skin **lesions** may be concealed by cosmetics, clothing, or jewelry. Occasionally, a patient will associate the development of a lesion with an action for which he feels guilty. It is therefore important that the nurse maintain a nonjudgmental attitude toward such patients. Individuals with disfiguring lesions may also be reassured by the nurse's willingness to touch these areas.

Besides touch, the nurse should also use her sense of smell to identify lesions. Distinctive odors are associated with streptococcal infections, for example. Certain behavioral characteristics, such as scratching, rubbing, and picking, are also clues to skin lesions or other disorders.[2]

Nails and hair

The condition of the nails and hair is an indicator of a person's state of health. Normally, the nail beds should be pink. Cyanosis is indicated when the nail beds are bluish in color. The darkening of a nail may result from hemorrhaging due to trauma. Nails should normally be convex. The normal angle between the fingernail and nail bed is 160 degrees.

Healthy hair is clean, shiny, and generally all the same color, although growth patterns and exposure to sun will cause a slight variation in shade and color. Dark hair tipped with a reddish-rust color may indicate a recent severe protein deficiency. Coarse, brittle, dry hair often suggests hypothyroidism or nutritional deficiency. Unusual hairiness over the arms, legs, and other parts of the body may be an inherited trait. It may also be indicative of excess vitamin A intake, hypothyroidism, or Cushing's syndrome.

Changes during the life cycle

Aging causes a number of changes in the skin, nails, and hair. The extent of these changes varies from individual to individual and seems

[2]Lora B. Roach. 1974. Assessing skin changes: The subtle and the obvious. *Nursing '74* 4:64.

to depend primarily upon a person's genetic makeup. Other changes in the skin take place in those areas that are continuously exposed to the sun.

The aging process causes a decrease in the resiliency of the skin. This is demonstrated by the fact that if an older person pinches his skin, the fold will remain for a minute or two. The skin also loses some of its ability to stretch and to absorb moisture. In addition, the time necessary for a wound to repair itself and for new skin to grow almost doubles between the ages of 20 and 40.

A slowdown in the growth rate is also found in the nails and hair. The nails of a 20-year-old grow at the rate of 1 mm per week. By the time he is 80, his nails will grow at only half that rate. Changes take place in the appearance of the nails as well. The older person's nails tend to be ridged and grooved. Brittleness may also be a problem. In addition to growing more slowly, the hair tends to become thinner and lose color.

Individual habits

An important part of the assessment process for the nurse is to familiarize herself with the patient's particular hygiene habits. Frequency of bathing and shampooing, general grooming, and use of makeup are all closely linked to socioeconomic and cultural background. Religion may be a factor, too, as in the case of Orthodox Jewish women, who are required to take a ritual bath following the menstrual period.

The nurse should also remember that in addition to her own cultural and economic background, she has probably adopted the hygiene habits of the health profession as her own. These are not necessarily those of the general public. Even a simple concept such as washing one's hands may have an entirely different meaning for a nurse than it has for an adolescent or a manual laborer.

Planning, intervention, and evaluation

Bathing

Bathing a patient can serve many purposes in addition to the maintenance of good hygiene. A patient will often look upon the person who gives him physical care, who touches him, as the one who cares about him the most. He will usually be more responsive to such a person than to someone who spends less time with him.

If a nurse with strong interpersonal skills cares for him—assists him in a way he can experience—she can use his openness to his own advantage. The giving of a bath can be such an experience. Through it, the nurse can establish

Bathing a patient can serve many purposes in addition to the maintenance of good hygiene.

While giving a patient a bath, a nurse has an excellent opportunity to observe him.

rapport and, as a result, be in a position to more easily observe physiologic and psychologic phenomena. Needed nursing intervention can then follow.[3]

Assisting a patient with bathing gives the nurse an excellent opportunity to observe him. She can take note of the characteristics of his skin, hair, and nails. She can assess his motor skills, the factors that may be inhibiting them, and whether or not movement is painful. She can also measure the rate and depth of his respiration.

At this time, the nurse can begin to build a picture of the patient's emotional state. She can judge his response to touch, and assess both his ability to cope with his condition and his readiness for rehabilitation. She can also observe his orientation to time and place.

Bathtime is also a particularly good time for teaching (see chapter 11). For example, the nurse may use the opportunity to show a diabetic patient how to take care of his feet. The patient's confidence that his listener is totally involved with his needs may prompt him to ask questions he had previously withheld.

Lotion baths. Normally, patients are bathed with a mild soap and water. But some patients, particularly older patients, may show signs of irritation due to dry skin. In these cases, it helps to use a preparation such as baby lotion. Baby lotion cleanses the skin thoroughly, is nongreasy, and has a pleasant fragrance. In addition, there is no need for an accompanying pan of water. The moisturizing and massage that accompany the use of this lotion are also helpful in the prevention of decubitus ulcers (see p. 316).

The following technique has been developed for giving a bath with baby lotion:[4]

1. Place a large towel under the part of the body that is being bathed. (A few tissues should be kept at hand for wiping off smaller areas.)
2. When washing the patient's arms, apply extra lotion and massage well into the elbows.
3. When washing the feet, give special consideration to the heels.
4. After the bath, sprinkle the patient well with baby powder to leave his skin smooth and fresh. The use of powder also cuts down on any friction, rubbing, or sticking of the skin against sheets and bedclothes. It is especially important to powder in crease areas, under breasts, between the buttocks, and in the folds of skin on the abdomen.

Patients who have poor circulation will benefit from periodic **lotion baths.** This technique is also useful for those in casts, splints, or braces, or for those who are paralyzed. Emaciated or obese patients, or those with edema, will also find it helpful.

[3]Ellen D. Davis. 1970. Give a bath? *American Journal of Nursing* 70:2367.
[4]Jean Hardy. 1974. Bathing patients without soap and water. *Nursing Care* 7:25–27.

Perineal care. Sexual taboos are still a strong force in modern American society. As a result, care of the perineal area has been a frequently neglected subject. Yet poor perineal care has been found responsible for the high incidence of bladder infection among patients with indwelling catheters. Even if no infection develops, the resulting odor, discharge, and skin breakdown will prove embarrassing and discomforting to the patient. Proper care of the perineal area helps prevent skin irritation and breakdown due to residues of perspiration, urine, or feces on the skin.

In caring for female patients, the following routine should be observed:[5]

1.   Place a bath towel lengthwise under the patient's hips. One end can be used for drying the perineal area and the other for drying the anal region.
2.   Ask the patient to flex her legs, and then cover them with a bath blanket.
3.   Cleansing should be accomplished with cotton balls dipped in warm soapy water. Additional balls should be dipped in clear warm water for rinsing.
4.   Wipe from the pubic area toward the rectal area, using one cotton ball for each stroke.
5.   The outer perineum and the area between the thighs and the labia should be washed first. They should then be dried and powdered.
6.   Now separate and wash the labia minora on each side. Then cleanse the urinary meatus and the vaginal orifice. Always use a new cotton ball for each stroke and always wipe from front to back. These areas should then be rinsed and dried.
7.   Next, place the patient on her side, separating the buttocks, and wash the posterior region. Pay special attention to the anal region. This area should also be powdered when dry.

Some nursing texts state that male nursing personnel are responsible for finishing the bath for male patients unable to care for themselves. Given the still small percentage of male nurses in the United States, this statement will probably not apply in the majority of situations. Even where male personnel exist, they may not always be available. Consequently, the following technique should be used when giving perineal care to male patients who are unable to provide their own perineal care:[6]

1.   A bath towel and blanket should be used and arranged as described for female patients above. Cotton balls should be used, as described earlier.

[5]Gertrude E. Gibbs. 1969. Perineal care of the incapacitated patient. *American Journal of Nursing* 69:124–25.
[6]Ibid., p. 125.

2. Wash the penis first. If the patient is uncircumcised, the foreskin should be pulled back and the glans and prepuce washed and dried. The foreskin should then be pulled back to cover the end of the penis once again.
3. The outside of the foreskin and penis, including the posterior side, should be washed next. Separate the patient's legs and lift the scrotum gently upward and forward. The thighs should be cleansed at the same time. All areas should be rinsed well, dried, and then powdered lightly.
4. The patient should now be turned on his side, separating the buttocks. Now wash the area from scrotum to anus. This area should also be dried and powdered.

Oral hygiene

Although there are no societal stigmas attached to care of the gums and teeth, this is another area that is frequently neglected in a hospital situation. Even when they are only mildly ill, as with a cold, for example, many people neglect their usual oral hygiene routines. If this neglect continues for any period of time, the result may be gum disease. This leads to bad breath, bleeding gums, and the inability to chew food properly. Eventually, this neglect may result in the loss of several teeth or even all of them.

Poor dental care is particularly hazardous for older patients. Such patients usually experience a decrease in the output of their salivary, mucous, and other glands. Normally, these secretions provide a vital protective and cleansing action. Their decrease leaves the patient more vulnerable to cavities, gum disease, and even upper respiratory infection. Those who are crippled, have unsteady hands, or are stroke victims also have special oral hygiene problems. They may find it difficult to manipulate a toothbrush. They may not be aware that food has collected in the paralyzed side of the mouth. Even if physically capable, confused or disoriented patients may neglect mouth care.

For all of these reasons, oral hygiene should always be a part of any nursing care plan. If the patient is unable to brush his teeth, the nurse should do it for him, as follows:[7]

1. If there is any food debris in the patient's mouth, he should rinse his mouth before brushing. A bulb syringe may be used if the patient is unable to rinse his mouth himself.
2. The patient's lips should be retracted with one hand.
3. A soft-bristle nylon brush should be placed at a 45-degree angle to the gums and vibrated back and forth horizontally about 10 times. A sweeping motion should then be made away from the gums. Brush

[7] Marie Reitz and Wilma Pope. 1973. Mouth care. *American Journal of Nursing* 73:1728–30.

the front and back surfaces of the teeth in the same manner. The top surfaces should be brushed with a horizontal stroke.
4. Dental floss should be used after brushing. This ensures adequate cleaning of the areas between the teeth, a common site of cavities and gum disease.

In addition to cavities and gum disease, hospitalized or homebound patients are particularly prone to dehydration. Many of these patients are not being fed by mouth or may be anorexic. As a result, the stimulation needed for salivation is largely absent. Breathing through the mouth, which causes the moisture on the tongue to evaporate, contributes still further to this condition. After a while, the lips, tongue, and teeth become coated with thickened mucus. Bacteria may develop, leading to an infection of the parotid (salivary) glands.

Dehydration and resulting bad breath can be prevented by the following means:[8]

1. Mucus should be removed with a sodium bicarbonate solution. This solution should be swabbed over the tongue, lips, gums, and inner surfaces of the cheeks. A wooden spatula should be used for retracting the cheeks and lips, thus making sure that all surfaces are reached.
2. A pleasant-tasting antiseptic should be used to moisten the mouth.
3. Cracking of the lips may be prevented by the application of petroleum jelly or liquid paraffin.

Certain types of patients require special care in this area. Among them are those with bleeding gums or those whose jaws are wired together. Irrigation with a syringe or a dental squirt is usually indicated in the latter case. Patients with uremia have brown, dry tongues, and the taste and smell of urine will be present in the mouth.

Dentures. If the patient has removable bridges, these must be taken out and brushed thoroughly with cold water and dentifrice or soap before being replaced. Dentures, too, should be scrubbed with soap and water or with a dentifrice, using a denture brush. At night dentures may be soaked in a denture-cleaning solution, but during the day plates or bridges made of plastic should be kept in a dry container. This container should be clearly labeled to avoid embarrassing mix-ups. Some older patients may still have dentures made of vulcanite, which is porous and absorbs food debris, giving the dentures a sour odor. Soaking these dentures in a 1 percent ammonium hydroxide solution once a week will help to eliminate odor. When not worn, they should be kept in a container of water to which a few drops of essence of peppermint have been added.

[8]Winifred Hector. 1970. Care of the teeth: The nurse's view. *Nursing Times* 66:1611.

The patient's dentist should be consulted if the dentures begin to fit loosely. Also, older patients should be encouraged to wear their dentures every day to prevent changes in facial contour. Dentures should always be removed before surgery.

Shampoo and daily hair care

The nurse must learn to take care of all kinds of hair—to comb it and keep it clean. Care of the hair supports the patient's feeling of well-being and builds his morale.

Many white nurses are not accustomed to caring for the hair of black patients. The following are the basic principles of hair care they need to know:[9]

1. After shampooing, comb the hair thoroughly before drying, to prevent tangling.
2. Since the hair is usually of a thick texture, it should be combed with a large-toothed comb and brushed with a firm-bristled brush.
3. The hair is usually dry and needs oiling. If the patient does not have his or her own hair oil or conditioner, small amounts of white petroleum jelly or mineral oil may be applied.
4. For styling, hair may simply be rolled on regular curlers or strips of brown paper. However, if the patient will be hospitalized for a long period, the hair is usually braided to prevent matting and tangling.

Patients of any race who have mild dandruff probably require no treatment other than regular shampoos. More severe cases should be treated with a medicated shampoo containing tar. Shampoos containing selenium sulfide are very effective but must be rinsed out very carefully, as there is a slight risk of damage if they are left on too long or used too frequently.

Pediculosis capitis (also head lice and **scabies**), often a problem among schoolchildren, is characterized by a maddening itch. Look for patches of lusterless, dry hair in pruritic areas of the posterior scalp. Secondary bacterial infections with cervical lymph node swelling may also be present, especially in girls.

Gamma benzene hexachloride USP (Kwell shampoo) is nearly 100 percent effective for scabies. Wet the patient's hair thoroughly and shampoo vigorously, using about two tablespoons and working in the lather. Rinse the hair thoroughly to rid it of organisms loosened by the shampoo. This regimen should be repeated at four-day intervals if the first application is not effective.

[9]Sarah F. Giles. 1972. Hair: The nursing process and the black patient. *Nursing Forum* 11:86–87.

Meeting comfort needs

Characteristics of bed and mattress

Rest is often part of the patient's treatment, sometimes the most important part. (See chapter 17 for a discussion of the effects of bed rest.) To assure maximum rest, the bed must be constructed to allow for comfort and good posture. It should also be durable, lightweight, easy to move, and easy to clean.

To meet the requirements for comfort, most authorities suggest, the bed should measure 6 feet 6 inches long, 3 feet wide, and 26 inches from the floor to the springs. Hospital beds today are usually of the **Gatch** type, equipped with a spring frame and a crank so that they can be raised, lowered, and adjusted to different positions. Button-operated electric beds function the same way.[10]

A hospital bed may have at the head a towel rack or other equipment for holding solutions during treatment. Rubber-tired wheels make the bed easy to move, and brakes keep it from sliding.

The mattress may be of cotton, wool, curled hair, kapok, or sponge rubber. Today, those made with inner springs or the sponge-rubber type are preferred, because they are comfortable, firm, and wear well. The mattress is covered with sturdy ticking, preferably waterproof. A quilted pad is used for most home beds, and some hospitals now provide them. The pad makes the bed more comfortable for the patient and also protects the mattress. Mattress covers should not cover the side carrying handles, which may be needed in an emergency.

Special beds. A number of beds are available for patients with special problems; some of them can be duplicated at home. The **Stryker frame** is an apparatus consisting of two frames with a pivot device at each end, which permits turning the patient. It is used for patients with vertebral fractures, spinal injuries, burns, or bedsores, or for those who must be turned frequently.

The **CircOlectric** bed is an electric bed on a circular frame, which operates on much the same principle as the Stryker frame. This bed permits lateral turning of the patient and can be operated by the patient when his condition allows it. The bed is used to place a paralyzed patient in a standing position.

In recent years, many hospitals have begun to use **water beds** for patients with decubitus ulcers, for those who are chronically bedridden, or for burn, stroke, or paraplegic patients. The patient literally floats on water contained in a nylon bag. The principle of alternating pressure is used for the **air bed,** which also provides uniform support of the body.

Rest is often part of the patient's treatment, sometimes the most important part.

[10]Claire P. Hoffman et al. 1968. *Simplified nursing,* 8th ed., p. 169. Philadelphia: Lippincott.

Making the bed

Making an unoccupied bed. Hospitalized patients often spend a great part of their time in bed. Many of their activities take place there, including eating, bathing, elimination, and medical treatment. Obviously, it is vital that the patient be as comfortable as possible in the place where he is spending so much time. If the bed is bumpy and wrinkly, with top covers improperly placed, he may feel uncomfortable and develop physical and emotional complications.

In a skillfully made hospital bed, wrinkles are minimal. The patient can get in easily despite physical disabilities, and it is easy for hospital personnel to put a helpless patient into it.

The basic hospital bed is made the same way as a hotel bed. However, patients have individual needs that may require modification of the standard approach. If the patient's back is painful, he may need a bed board placed under the mattress to provide support for his back. If he is confused and disoriented, crib sides will keep him from falling out of bed. If he has difficulty moving and turning, he may need an alternating pressure mattress to prevent the development of sores.

A patient who is paralyzed on one side of his body will have trouble getting in and out of bed, so his bed is lower than normal. A patient whose legs are in pain may need a cradle (frame) placed over his feet to keep the weight of the bedclothes off his legs.

The following is one method of preparing the basic hospital bed:[11]

1. Place a mattress pad on the bed.
2. Put a sheet on the bed, even with the foot of the bed. Fold the excess under the head of the mattress and miter (tuck under at right angles) the corner on one side to hold it in place.
3. Put another sheet on the bed, even with the head of the bed. Fold the excess under the foot of the mattress and miter the corner to hold it in place.
4. Place a blanket over the sheet (about 6 inches from the head of the bed). Fold the excess under the mattress at the foot of the bed, and miter the corner to hold it in place.
5. Finish making the side of the bed as follows. First, put on a spread even with the head of the bed. Then, fold in the excess under the mattress at the foot of the bed. Finally, miter the corner to hold it in place.
6. Go to the opposite side of the bed and repeat steps 2 to 5.
7. Fold the spread in and over the blanket at the head of the bed. Fold the sheet back over this fold to make a 4- to 6-inch fold at the head of the bed. Then fold the top covers halfway down to the foot.

[11]Gertrude D. Cherescavich. 1968. *A textbook for nursing assistants,* 2d ed., pp. 25–29. St. Louis: Mosby.

8. Put pillowcases on a firm pillow and a soft pillow and place the pillows at the head of the bed.

Most important is that the bed be smooth—free of wrinkles and uneven surfaces—so that the patient does not develop pressure areas and decubitus ulcers. This means that bedclothes under the patient must be pulled tight and anchored well under the mattress.

In making a bed, avoid shaking, waving, and pulling linen about. Such activity permits any bacteria on the linen to be thrown into the air. Also, remember that the hospital floor is not clean or free from bacteria. If sheets or pillowcases fall on the floor, discard them in the linen hamper.

Making an occupied bed. Since patients often spend much of their time in bed, it is often necessary to change some of the linen while the patient is still there. In that case, the following procedure is suggested:[12]

1. Remove used linen from the bed, as follows. Lower the siderail, then place a bath blanket over the patient and the top covers. Loosen the top covers at the foot and remove the spread, blanket, and top sheet.
2. Move the mattress to the top of the bed, as follows. If the patient is able, ask him to grasp the head of the bed with his hands and pull when you give the word. Grasp the side edge of the mattress with both hands and move it toward the head of the bed.
3. Move the patient to the far side of the bed, then make the foundation of the bed on one side. Move the patient to the clean side. Then go to the other side of the bed and finish making the other side.

Giving a back rub

A back rub has two main purposes: to stimulate circulation in tissues that are under pressure and in muscles that are at rest, and to relax the patient.

The bedridden patient uses his back in much the same way a normal person uses his feet, that is, almost all the time. The skin on the back cannot sustain the pressure of body weight indefinitely and therefore requires added nourishment from increased circulation. This is one excellent reason for rubbing a patient's back. A second reason is to help him to rest or sleep. A good back rub relieves tension and may also relieve headaches due to tension in the neck and shoulders.

In addition to its physical benefits, a back rub can have a soothing psychological effect and can often aid in the development of an interpersonal relationship. The sensation of touch helps build rapport between patient and nurse much more quickly than word exchange alone can do.

A back rub can have a soothing psychological effect and can often aid in the development of an interpersonal relationship.

[12]Lucille A. Woods, ed. 1972. *Nursing skills for allied health services,* vol. 1, pp. 153–56. Philadelphia: Saunders.

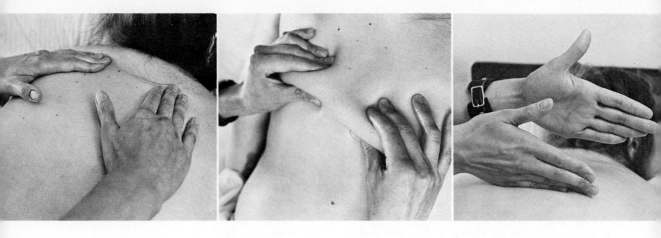

The three major strokes used in the back rub: (1) effleurage, (2) pétrissage, (3) tapotement.

[Photos by Dan Bernstein]

A back rub can remove anxiety not only from the patient, but from the nurse. There will be times when a nurse cannot immediately think of an appropriate response to a patient's questions. The silence that occurs while she is thinking is not so distressing when she is performing a physical action. Many nurses feel more comfortable working physically with a patient in addition to talking to him. Back rubs can also serve as the occasion for adding to a nursing history.

There is no one technique for administering a back rub that must be followed. Three basic strokes are used, alone or in combination:

1. **Effleurage.** This is a smooth, long stroke that is used in moving the hands up the spine and then lightly down the sides.
2. **Pétrissage.** In this stroke, large pinches of about 3 inches of skin and muscle are taken. The fingers move up the sides of the vertebral column and then over the entire back.
3. **Tapotement.** The edge of the hand is used in a hacking motion over the surface of the back.

Whether a back rub is sedative or stimulating depends on which of these three motions predominates, the amount of pressure the hands exert, and the speed of the strokes. The back rub will stimulate if it consists of rapid, firm strokes, primarily pétrissage and tapotement. It will relax if more long, stroking motions are used. If the back rub is intended to improve circulation, the strokes should follow the muscle in the direction of the return flow of circulation.

Each of these methods of massage should be used at least five times in order for the procedure to be called a back rub. Simply applying lotion to the patient's back and massaging lightly is an application of lotion, not a back rub. Many patients have refused back rubs simply because they are both disappointed and uncomfortable with nothing more than cold, wet lotion on their backs.

The time spent giving a back rub can be relaxing for the nurse as well as the patient. If the nurse positions the patient well and assumes a relaxed posture, using good body mechanics, her physical exertion is not great.

(See chapter 18 for a discussion of body mechanics.) Also, during this time she is separated from the busy activities of the unit, and is not likely to be interrupted.

Positioning

Proper positioning of the patient is not a cut-and-dried matter. The nurse must make sure that the patient is not only comfortable, but also free of the threat of decubitus ulcers, contractures, muscular debilitation, infection, or circulatory or respiratory problems. Each time the nurse arranges him in a bed, chair, or wheelchair, she must know exactly where to place every part of his body.

The principles of body alignment will be discussed more fully in chapter 18, but the following is a brief summary of each of the four major positions:

Supine. There are four main concerns in positioning the patient comfortably on his back:[13]

1. Toes should be pointed upward so that he does not suffer footdrop.
2. Heels should not rest heavily on the bed—this could cause decubitus ulcers.
3. Legs should be extended and aligned to prevent hip and knee contractures.
4. The head should be kept in line with the spine to prevent neck contractures.

Most patients find the supine position comfortable. Those who find it uncomfortable include patients with incisions, tumors, or injuries or deformities on their backs.

Prone. Although uncomfortable for patients with certain problems, the prone position offers the advantage of placing no tension on the head, neck, and shoulders. It also maintains the limbs in a relaxed, normal position.

Care should be taken that the patient does not suffer **torsion** of the neck. Watch for aspiration of blood, mucus, or vomitus. The patient's shoulders and abdomen should be supported so that he can breathe easily. His toes should be suspended over the edge of the mattress to prevent **plantar flexion.**

The patient's head should be positioned laterally, in good alignment with the trunk. A pillow should not be placed under the head, since this may interfere with respiration. To prevent permanent torsion of the neck,

Each time the nurse arranges the patient in a bed, chair, or wheelchair, she must know exactly where to place every part of his body.

[13]How to negotiate the ups and downs, ins and outs, of body alignment. *Nursing '74* 4:46.

the patient's head should be turned from side to side about every two hours.[14]

Side-lying. There are three major concerns when the patient is in the side-lying position:[15]

1. Proper head and body alignment so that he does not experience discomfort and contractures
2. Resting the upper arm on a pillow so that its weight on his chest does not interfere with breathing
3. The slight flexion of all extremities for greatest comfort and least risk of contractures

Twisting of the spine is a potential danger when using this position. This can be prevented by supporting the front of the patient with pillows, making sure to position him with the top arm and leg slightly flexed. His head should be in good alignment with his trunk, with the neck neither flexed nor extended.

Patients who have been lying supine or prone for a long time welcome a change to the side-lying position. The change brings new muscles into play and relieves skin pressure.

Sitting. Sitting up can improve the patient's general strength, activate his joints, and improve his circulation. It also stimulates bladder and intestinal functioning, relieves pressure, and improves respiration. In positioning, the nurse's concerns for the seated patient include:[16]

1. Avoiding plantar flexion
2. Positioning hands, feet, and limbs to avoid contractures and poor circulation
3. Ensuring good alignment to prevent contractures

If the patient is to sit in a wheelchair, it must be wide enough, with footrests that are even and are adjusted to the proper height. Wristdrop and contractures of the hands can be prevented by placing a pillow in the patient's lap. Padding the footrests with towels or having the patient wear slippers or shoes will avoid scrapes and bruises on the feet.

Decubitus ulcers

Decubitus ulcers are caused by capillary damage or blocked capillary circulation. Normal circulation depends on the force with which the blood

[14] Ibid., p. 48.
[15] Ibid., p. 49.
[16] Ibid., p. 51.

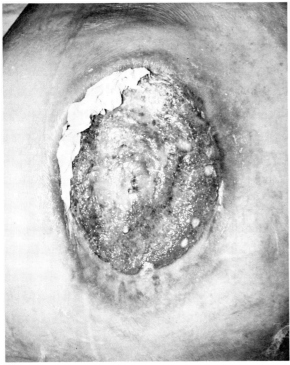
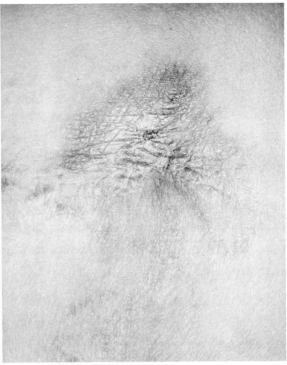

is pumped, the viscosity of the blood, and capillary resistance to flow. Nursing care should be planned to maintain normal function in these three areas.

There are four general types of decubitus ulcer. Progressing in severity, they are classified as **superficial, subcutaneous, anoxic,** and **pregangrenous.** A superficial ulcer is a break that occurs in the skin if it becomes too dry or if adjacent skin surfaces are not kept separated. If a superficial ulcer becomes infected, it soon goes deeper into the skin and becomes a subcutaneous ulcer.

Anoxic ulcers form soon after spinal cord injuries, as a result of damage during or immediately after the injury. Pregangrenous ulcers are a particular threat to patients with peripheral vascular disease or diabetes. These ulcers take the form of a thickened, dark scab, usually on a heel, metatarsal joint, or even toes.

Prevention. Although some patients are very susceptible and will develop decubitus ulcers despite the best of care, decubitus ulcers are usually the outcome of nursing neglect. In most instances they can be avoided.

Specialists have devised many techniques and devices for the prevention of decubitus ulcers, each with certain advantages and limitations. Among them are bed cradles and pillows, special mattress pads, heel pads, water beds, turning beds, air beds, **hyperbaric oxygen treatment,** and **Gelfoam pillows.** *Whatever specific techniques are used, however, the importance of turning the patient regularly cannot be overestimated.*

Decubitus ulcer before and after treatment.

317

Treatment. Superficial ulcers often heal in less than a week if the patient's position is changed frequently. The ulcer is cleansed with hydrogen peroxide and exposed to rapidly circulating warm air supplied by a hair dryer placed on an overbed table. A mild ointment or powder is applied, and a light dressing is fastened with nonallergenic tape.

The treatment for a subcutaneous ulcer is irrigation. Infection clears from this type of ulcer within a week or two, but healing is slow unless a local application of a nutrient is introduced with a packing. Additional ascorbic acid may also aid healing, and a balanced diet is important.

Anoxic ulcers can be treated with compresses of half-strength Eusol solution kept on for one hour and applied three times daily. A dressing with an ointment containing enzymes—Elase or Varidase—should be applied generously between compress treatments. As soon as it is possible to lift even a corner of the scab, the ulcer can be irrigated and packed, or Cicatrin powder can be blown under it. The same general treatment is used for patients with pregangrenous ulcers, who in addition must be maintained in a prone position.

SUMMARY

Keeping the patient clean and comfortable not only promotes his health and well-being, it often speeds the rate of his recovery. Because many of the procedures involve intimacy between nurse and patient, it is important that the nurse be scrupulous in her performance and sensitive in her attitude.

For example, giving a bath can provide the opportunity for an intimate sharing of concerns and feelings. This is a time when the patient feels the nurse is interested in his comfort and not afraid of caring for his personal needs. The nurse often has an excellent chance to observe specifics of the patient's physical and emotional state.

Hospitalized patients are susceptible to dry skin, which is uncomfortable and contributes to the formation of decubitus ulcers. The nurse must therefore consider alternatives to the traditional soap-and-water baths. Lotion baths are often highly successful for patients with dry skin. They are also therapeutic for those with poor circulation. The nurse, whatever bathing technique she uses, must take particular care to provide proper cleansing of the perineal area, for both male and female patients. This will prevent infection, skin irritation, embarrassment, and discomfort.

Daily attention to the patient's hair is also important in maintaining his sense of well-being. Daily care of the mouth and teeth is vitally important as well. If the patient is unable to brush his teeth or take care of his dentures, the nurse must do it for him. She must also take measures to keep the patient's mouth from becoming dehydrated, thus cutting off the flow of cleansing salivary juices.

A major element in maintaining the patient's physical comfort is the use of the appropriate type of bed, properly made up. Today, many different types of beds are available to meet the demands of particular disease states. Whatever type is used, the bed linens and covers must be properly arranged to ensure maximum comfort. Most important in making any bed is that it be kept free of wrinkles or uneven surfaces that might lead to skin irritation.

Back rubs can be given either to stimulate the patient's circulation or to relax his muscles. Back rubs provide both physical and psychological benefits. The close contact and the experience of touching and being touched help build rapport between patient and nurse.

Proper positioning of the patient keeps him both comfortable and free of the threat of decubitus ulcers, muscular debilitation, and other problems. Careful consideration should be made of the demands of his illness before placing the patient in a particular position.

Decubitus ulcers are a constant threat, most often the result of in-attentive nursing care. Superficial ulcers may heal in less than a week when properly treated. More severe cases, however, require many months of treatment and are painful and exhausting to the patient. Most important in both prevention and treatment of decubitus ulcers are frequent turning and proper positioning of the patient.

STUDY QUESTIONS

1. What information can the nurse obtain by observing the color, turgor, texture, and integrity of the patient's skin?
2. What are the steps in giving a patient a lotion bath? What is the purpose of using this technique?
3. What are the steps in making an occupied bed? an unoccupied bed?
4. Briefly outline the procedure for giving a back rub, including definitions of the three major strokes.
5. What functions are served by proper positioning of the patient? What are the consequences of improper positioning?
6. What are the common causes of decubitus ulcers? How can the nurse help prevent them from forming? What steps should she take if these ulcers develop?

SELECTED BIBLIOGRAPHY

Brown, Marie S., and Alexander, Mary M. 1973. Physical examination, part 3: Examining the skin. *Nursing '73* 3:39–43.

How to negotiate the ups and downs, ins and outs, of body alignment. *Nursing '74* 4:46–51.

Reitz, Marie, and Pope, Wilma. 1973. Mouth care. *American Journal of Nursing* 73:1728–30.

Roach, Lora B. 1974. Assessing skin changes: The subtle and the obvious. *Nursing '74* 4:64–67.

17 Meeting rest, sleep, and sensory needs

Upon completing this chapter, the reader should be able to:

1. Identify the conditions that must be met before an individual can rest.

2. Identify and discuss the stages of sleep.

3. Describe the behaviors that may result from sleep alteration or sleep deprivation.

4. Define the four levels of consciousness.

5. Compare and contrast sensory deprivation, sensory overload, and sensory distortion.

6. Discuss the role of the nurse in meeting the patient's sensory needs.

What is rest?

Bed rest commonly is prescribed as part of the treatment for many illnesses. Simply restricting a patient's activity, however, does not automatically ensure that he is actually "at rest." In fact, providing an environment in which the patient can truly rest is probably one of the most difficult nursing problems. Being at rest implies tranquillity, calmness, and freedom from anxiety. It does not necessarily imply inactivity, which is the cessation or avoidance of physical exertion. Another term for rest is repose, or relaxation without emotional stress.[1]

Assessment

How can the nurse tell if the patient is truly at rest? There are six characteristics of rest that apply to nearly every patient situation, although, of course, every patient has his own specific requirements for rest. These six characteristics summarize the meaning of rest.

1. A person can rest when he feels that things are under control, both in his personal life and in his hospital (or other health care facility) environment. He is relaxed if he feels that the people caring for him are competent.

2. A person can rest when he feels accepted. He must feel he is important to the staff and that they are concerned with the personal problems that interfere with his rest.

3. A person can rest if he understands what is happening to him. This means that he must be kept informed of what is going on at all times.

4. A person can rest if he is free from irritation and discomfort. This means that he is free from wrinkled sheets, lack of privacy, and alternating periods of rushing and waiting.

5. A person can rest if he has a satisfying amount of purposeful activity.

[1] Amasa B. Ford. 1965. The meaning of rest. *Cardiovascular Nursing* 1:11.

6.   A person can rest if he knows he will receive help when it is needed. This help must be freely given and easy to accept.[2]

What is sleep?

Assessment

Sleep is a natural, periodically recurring physiological state of rest. It is characterized by relatively little physical and nervous activity, various levels of consciousness, and lessened responsiveness to external stimuli. It is not a suspension from life, however, but a progression of rhythmic cycles representing different phases of neural function.[3]

Sleep is a universal phenomenon, present in all living organisms and revolving around biological rhythms. This rhythm in man is called **circadian** (from the Latin *circa dies,* meaning "about a day"). The rhythm starts from about the third month of life, and is perhaps inherited from the mother's cycle. Because of this rhythm, human beings, regardless of culture or location, sleep between 5 and 8 hours at a time, usually at night.

Although human beings differ in their sleep habits, normal people show roughly the same overall pattern. Age, fatigue, illness, emotional upset, alcohol, and drugs can alter that pattern. Any marked deviation may indicate a serious disorder.

The function of sleep, although not entirely clear, appears to be one of restoration and integration. Physiologically, hormone release, cellular replenishment, and other metabolic changes that occur during sleep prepare the body for another day. Psychologically, sleep may assist the person in problem solving, coping, and reenergizing his powers of concentration and interest in daily tasks. The function of sleep can be observed by noting the effects of sleep deprivation. People who have been deprived of sleep generally are irritable, depressed, highly sensitive to pain, apathetic, disoriented, and confused.

While the individual's body sleeps, researchers have found that his mind does not "sleep." Actually, it is quite active in some stages of sleep. This brain activity during sleep is measured by **electroencephalograph (EEG)** tracings. Electrodes placed at various sites on the skull transmit activity through changes in the electrical potential of large numbers of cells in the cortex of the brain. (The action of individual cells is not measured.) The electroencephalograph amplifies shifts in this potential to magnetic tape or to a row of ink pens. Each pen moves up when the electrical charge is negative and down when the electrical charge is positive. These up and down movements, called **brain waves,** are recorded on tracing paper. The

[2]Barbara W. Narrow. 1967. Rest is . . . . *American Journal of Nursing* 67:1645.
[3]U.S. Department of Health, Education and Welfare. 1965. *Current research on sleep and dreams,* p. 9. Washington, D.C.: U.S. Public Health Service.

waves will show whether the potentials are shifting in a regular, harmonious manner, or whether, on the other hand, the changes are fast and disorganized.

The stages of sleep. When the normal person falls asleep, there are predictable **stages of sleep** that can be detected by these EEG tracings. At first, the individual becomes drowsy. He feels relaxed, serene, and pleasant, but is easily aroused. A regular rhythm, known as **alpha rhythm,** appears on the EEG paper. Quickly he goes into what is called the first stage of sleep. The brain waves become smaller and change rapidly. The individual feels he is "drifting." Physiologically, his bodily processes are slowing down. The heart rate decreases, the pulse becomes even, and his respirations are regular. In stages two and three, the pattern changes, the muscles are very relaxed, and the body continues to slow down. Large, slow **delta waves** appear in stage four, which occurs approximately 20 minutes after falling asleep. The individual is very relaxed and rarely moves. The dream state, or the state of **rapid eye movements (REM),** is the last stage. The individual moves in and out of the non-REM (or vegetative) stages and the REM stage throughout the period of sleep.

The flow of stages of a typical night's sleep may be from stage one $\longrightarrow$ three $\longrightarrow$ four, retracing back to stage two $\longrightarrow$ REM, back to stage four $\longrightarrow$ REM, and back again to an earlier stage. There is a swing from light to deep sleep and back again about five times in a normal 7- to 8-hour period of sleep. The swings usually occur in 90-minute cycles—the time span of many other biological cycles.

The REM stage of sleep is perhaps the most incongruous of sleep stages, since the body is hardly at rest. This is called the "activated sleep state." It is a time of autonomic excitement, metabolic acceleration, and dreams. The EEG tracing resembles that of a person who is awake but who is in deep concentration. The eyes move (as measured by an electrode placed near the eye), respiratory and pulse rates increase and are irregular, and blood pressure fluctuates. The body temperature rises. The fine muscles of the face and extremities contract frequently. The brain metabolism, especially oxygen consumption, is increased over that occurring in other stages. The brain temperature also rises. Hormone levels and serum constituents change. Hormone release during this stage is an important determinant of vitality and fatigue, metabolism, and the ability to resist infection. It also influences the transmission of nerve impulses.[4]

If awakened during the REM stage, the individual reports a vivid dream. If awakened in other periods, he reports no mental activity or less dreamlike activity. REM is the stage in which patients report angina pain and in which episodes of peptic ulcer attacks occur.

[4]Donna A. Grant and Cynthia Klell. 1974. For goodness sake—let your patients sleep. *Nursing '74* 4:56.

The probable function of the REM-dream stage is one of organizing—programming memory traces recently acquired or retrenching old memories.[5] Early in life, a large percentage of sleep is in the REM stage, but this percentage declines rapidly with age.

Some of the physiological changes that occur during the various stages of sleep have been noted previously. In addition, secretions of the nose, mouth, and throat diminish. In the urinary tract, the volume of urine secretion decreases. Perspiration increases somewhat. The digestive system seems to be little affected by sleep, and hunger contractions are just as strong and frequent as in wakefulness. Body movements may occur at times of strong stomach contractions. The sigmoid colon is relatively quiet, but intestinal movement continues as it does in the daytime.[6]

Respirations during sleep are noisier than those in the awake state. This may be related to the altered muscular tone in the upper respiratory passages.

Reflexes seem to weaken, and reflex time is lengthened. The cough reflex remains, but tendon reflexes disappear or diminish.

The **basal metabolic rate (BMR)** is lowered 10 percent during sleep. Heat production decreases with muscular relaxation, and the heart rate parallels the temperature curve. (It is estimated that a change of 1°F in body temperature causes a change of 10 to 20 heartbeats per minute.)

The pupils of the eyes are constricted in sleep, and the eyes themselves roll. They do not hold a fixed position throughout the night.[7]

During stage four, there is an increase in secretion of growth hormone. In addition to regulating growth, **somatotropic hormone** influences fracture healing, lowers the blood cholesterol, and stimulates tissue healing.

Results of sleep deprivation. Lack of certain parts of sleep, then, can be as important as total lack of sleep. If sleep is disrupted in a hormone-release stage, hormones may enter the system, but not at the right biological time. If this happens to a hospitalized patient, he may awaken to greet the new day only with malaise. When deprived of REM sleep, the patient may be continually fatigued and be unable to concentrate. He may be disoriented and confused. In epilepsy, REM sleep deprivation lowers the seizure threshold, and it can sometimes precipitate psychosis. When deprived of stage four sleep, the individual becomes apathetic and depressed.

Individual needs for sleep

Although the mean number of hours per night for a normal adult is $7\frac{1}{2}$ hours, some people sleep only 3 hours a night. Others complain of

[5]Rudolf Kaelbling. 1972. The mysterious world of sleep and dreams. *Medical Insight* 4:48.

[6]Roche Laboratories. 1966. *The anatomy of sleep,* p. 43. Nutley, N.J.

[7]Ibid., p. 47.

When sleep disorders arise, they appear to originate from a variety of sources involving a person's behavior, training, environment, body chemistry, and brain activity.

insomnia even after sleeping 8 hours, and a small percentage of people habitually sleep more than 10 hours at a time. An infant may sleep 16 hours out of 24, while a 3-year-old sleeps only 10 hours. It is believed that the need for sleep decreases with increasing age. Thus, the amount of sleep, per se, does not determine whether a sleep disorder exists.

There are also variations in what individuals consider as the optimal periods of wakefulness and sleep. Some people consider themselves "night owls," working or just staying up most of the night. Others, "early birds" or "larks," retire early and do their best work in the early hours of the morning.

When sleep disorders do arise, they appear to originate from a variety of sources involving a person's behavior, training, environment, body chemistry, and brain activity.

Deviations from normal sleep

Insomnia. According to an old Egyptian proverb, one of the world's greatest stresses is to be in bed and not be able to sleep.[8] **Insomnia** is not the total lack of sleep. It usually means poor sleep, or unrefreshing sleep. It affects people in all countries, in primitive as well as in industrial societies. Insomnia victimizes the poor as well as the rich, the intelligent as well as the less intelligent. In one study, a third of the adults in the United States claimed to worry about being able to sleep, and a quarter of the people said they felt too exhausted to get up in the morning.[9]

It is thought that insomniacs have a more "aroused" sleep than the typical sleeper. Measures of autonomic functions, such as the blood pressure, heart rate, and so on, are higher than in good sleepers.

There are two types of insomniacs: those who cannot fall asleep and those who cannot remain asleep. In investigating the origin of sleep disorders, several possibilities should be considered. These include drug dependence, **restless leg syndrome** (tingling and pain in the legs causing restlessness at night), and **nocturnal myoclonus** (jerking of leg muscles). Also to be considered are **sleep apnea** (periods of cessation of breathing) or **idiopathic insomnia** (sleeplessness without apparent reason).

The use of drugs is estimated to cause some 40 percent of insomnia problems. Insomnia occurs in people who are heavy drinkers or who habitually take drugs, such as barbiturates, for sleep. A tolerance develops quickly, and more and more of the drug is required to facilitate sleep. If the person tries to fall asleep without the drug, a problem arises. Alcohol and many sleeping pills depress the normal REM stage of sleep. Once free of the drug's influence, the brain tries to make up for all the lost REM sleep. This is a highly agitated bodily state, and the patient experiences

---

[8]Julius Segal. 1973. Insomnia. *Medical Insight* 5:17.
[9]Ibid.

increased dreaming and terrible nightmares. Sometimes convulsions occur with total drug withdrawal.

There are some drugs that, if given in specific dosages, do not significantly suppress REM sleep. They are chloral hydrate 500 mg and 1,000 mg; flurazepam hydrochloride (Dalmane) 30 mg; chlordiazepoxide hydrochloride (Librium) 50 mg; and diazepam (Valium) 10 mg.[10]

Nocturnal enuresis (bed-wetting). This is primarily a disorder of childhood. It occurs in some 5 to 15 percent of preadolescent children, mostly male.[11] The etiology is not known, but it has been associated with limited bladder capacity, increased nitrogen content of the urine, unusually deep sleep levels, and genetic makeup. Some drugs, social and psychological support, treatment of underlying organic diseases, bladder training, and enuresis alarms (that awaken the child for midnight voiding) have been found helpful in treating **enuresis.**

Somnambulism. **Somnambulism,** commonly known as sleepwalking, is also primarily a disorder of childhood. Most patients eventually outgrow the problem. The actual walking is thought to take place in non-REM sleep, and the person is not aware of walking in his sleep. The immediate concern is to protect the individual from hurting himself when the episodes occur.

More uncommon deviations from normal sleep patterns include teeth grinding, childhood night terrors, and **narcolepsy,** which is the tendency to fall asleep quickly and at inappropriate times.

Sleep deprivation

Sleeplessness alone can cause deterioration in behavior, and it can aggravate the symptoms of already existing psychiatric illness. It is accompanied by biochemical changes in the body.

Subjects who have been deprived of sleep exhibit certain common behaviors. Their speech is slurred and rambling, and they fail to recognize or correct mispronunciation. Sleeplessness is similar to drunkenness. Subjects bump into objects with their eyes open or stumble on nonexistent steps. Their speech is listless, lacks normal inflection, and is inappropriate to the situation.[12] The person is ill-tempered and may perform assigned tasks inaccurately or inefficiently. The EEG demonstrates that light periods of sleep occur in the sleep-deprived person even when he is seemingly awake.

Physiological measurements taken of sleep-deprived subjects have yielded mixed results. In general, the central nervous system appears to

[10]Anthony Kales and Joyce Kales. 1970. Evaluation, diagnosis, and treatment of clinical conditions related to sleep. *Journal of the American Medical Association* 213:2233.

[11]*Current research on sleep and dreams,* p. 31.

[12]Roche Laboratories, p. 24.

Sleeplessness alone can cause deterioration in behavior.

deactivate. The blood pressure and temperature decline. In one study, after 120 hours without sleep, some of the measurements began to rise, illustrating a possible mechanism to cope with sleeplessness. Other studies of respiration, muscle tension, and skin conductance show either no change or mixed responses.

Promoting rest and sleep

Planning, implementation, and evaluation

Today, the trend in medical care is away from the indiscriminate use of "complete bed rest." It has been realized that there are many ill effects of restricted activity. Often, allowance of limited activity is less stressful and requires less energy than that required for restricted bed rest. For example, in heart disease, the use of a bedside commode requires less energy than the use of a bedpan.

Nevertheless, adequate rest and sleep are important factors in promoting convalescence and recovery. Because of the new environment of the hospital, the numerous interruptions necessary for nursing care, and the concomitants of the individual's illness, sleep problems are common in hospitalized patients.

Sleep difficulties in the hospital, whether they originate from emotional, physical, or environmental causes, can be managed by nursing attention to the factors that disturb sleep. Each shift of nursing personnel can help the patient in the following ways.

Day staff:
1. Encourage naps in the morning rather than in the afternoon. Afternoon naps consist mostly of deep sleep—stage four sleep—and short periods of this sleep generally leave the patient feeling groggy. Morning naps, however, are mostly a continuation of REM sleep. Because it is light sleep, the patient usually awakes feeling refreshed.
2. Keep the patient as busy during the day as his condition permits. This way he will be tired by evening.

Evening staff:
1. Find out what the patient's sleep routine was at home and, whenever possible, try to follow it. Certain "rituals" can promote sleep.
2. Offer backrubs.
3. Straighten or change linen when necessary, and offer an extra blanket. The additional blanket is not only for warmth but also gives many patients a feeling of security.
4. Offer a sleeping medication.
5. With patients' permission, unplug telephones.

Meeting rest, sleep, and sensory needs   **327**

6. Close the patient's curtain enough to block out light from the unit.
7. Close the door if possible.
8. If a patient requires medication for pain, try to give it early enough so that it takes effect before he gets the sleeping medication. That way he will be relieved of pain and relaxed so that the sleeping medication will be more effective.

Night staff:
1. Find out who is not sleeping and why.
2. Be sure unit lights are dim and unnecessary ones are out.
3. When checking on patients, make as little noise as possible. Be well organized so that disturbances will be minimal.
4. When a sleeping pattern has been established that works for each patient, write it down so that every nurse will know to do the same.[13]

Alterations in consciousness

Assessment

Consciousness is a graded continuum of awareness that ranges from alertness to coma. Each point on the continuum has a characteristic clinical appearance, as determined by the functioning of various cerebral cortical (cortex) and subcortical structures.

The **alert** person is in full possession of his senses. **Drowsiness** resembles a state of continued sleep. The person can be aroused, but when left alone he tends to return to sleep. This is also called lethargy.

Stupor is a state of seemingly total loss of consciousness. It is possible to arouse the stuporous patient, but it requires vigorous, usually painful, stimuli. When aroused, he may resist stimulation. Awareness is limited, memory is inadequate, and thinking is confused. The patient's orientation is disturbed, his comprehension impaired, his attention span short, and his perception distorted.[14]

The **comatose** patient cannot be aroused, no matter how vigorous the stimulus. Basic autonomic systems function, but no voluntary movements occur. Reflex muscular contractions, withdrawal movements, or changes in breathing rate and depth may be the only responses to painful stimuli. Corneal reflexes may be present. Pupil reactivity may be absent or minimal. Cough reflexes are absent and swallowing is impaired.[15]

A sleeping person differs from one in coma. Although asleep, a person may still respond to stimuli, and he is capable of the mental activity of

[13]Grant and Klell, p. 57.
[14]Robert R. Gifford and Martin R. Palut. 1973. On describing altered states of consciousness. *Journal of Neurosurgical Nursing* 5:18.
[15]Ibid., pp. 19–20.

It is important that close observation and accurate descriptions of the patient's responsiveness and behavior be made.

dreaming. The comatose person is probably unaware of external stimulation, with the exception of severe pain. The sleeping person can be recalled to consciousness when stimulated. The comatose person cannot.

The levels of consciousness as described above are not so clear-cut when observing an actual patient. In addition, a diagnosis may be difficult for the physician when the patient is unconscious. Because of these factors, it is important that close observation and accurate descriptions of the patient's responsiveness and behavior be made.

First, close *observation* by the nurse will enable her to recognize early changes in brain function. This can lead to prevention of irreversible changes through early medical intervention. Second, precise nursing *description* provides an exact record of the pattern of consciousness. Any change, of course, should be reported immediately.

The following observations should be noted and charted in detail:

1. Any change in the level of consciousness as manifested by the patient's spontaneous behavior, resistance to care, or response to noxious stimulation
2. Voluntary motion of the extremities and any change in muscular tone or position of the body or head
3. Equality of pupils, their size, and reaction to light
4. Changes in the color of the face, lips, extremities, and trunk
5. Changes in texture, temperature, and moisture of the skin; early evidence of pressure sores
6. Quality and rate of pulse and respiration
7. Rectal temperature every 2 to 4 hours, depending on the need of the individual patient
8. Blood pressure (taken as ordered every 30 to 60 minutes according to the condition of the patient)
9. An accurate measure and record of fluid intake and output
10. Accurate and complete description of focal or generalized convulsions
11. Early signs of edema of the face or around the eyes, especially after head injury or cranial surgery
12. Signs of meningeal irritation, stiffness of neck, and so on
13. After intracranial operations, dressings checked frequently for bloody drainage or leakage of cerebrospinal fluid.[16]

Planning, implementation, and evaluation

When caring for unconscious patients, the nurse assumes the responsibility of performing totally the care that the patient would ordinarily assume himself.

[16]Esta Carini and Guy Owens. 1974. *Neurological and neurosurgical nursing,* p. 141. St. Louis: Mosby.

Safety and protection. The nurse is concerned with the prevention of further injury to the patient from accidents (see chapter 14). Side rails should be up at all times. Sometimes they are padded to prevent injury from unexpected movement or from convulsive activity.

If the patient is not comatose, he can be assisted out of bed to a chair. A chest harness or other type of restraint should be placed around the torso to prevent him from falling. A proper sitting position should be maintained, with his head and arms supported.

Eye secretions diminish and the corneal reflex may be lost during the period of unconsciousness. The cornea can become scratched unless it is protected. The eyes should be examined frequently for signs of irritation, cleansed with suitable solutions, and lubricated with mineral oil at frequent intervals.[17] An eye patch may be necessary.

The room temperature should be maintained at 70° to 75° F. Many unconscious patients are over 60 years of age and thus are more sensitive to atmospheric changes. They are also more susceptible to respiratory complications than younger patients. A warm environment is a comfortable environment for the patient whose consciousness level varies.

If the patient is restless and becomes a danger to himself, a light restraint or sedation may be necessary. It is recommended that the fingernails be kept short to prevent self-injury.

Hygiene. The skin and the mucous membranes of the unconscious patient demand special care (see chapter 16). It is essential to cleanse the skin of infectious agents that may be present from bowel, bladder, or respiratory tract contamination.[18] Bathing also stimulates the circulation. A sheepskin or alternating pressure mattress can be used to prevent skin breakdown. If the skin is dry, lanolin or cold cream should be applied daily.

Since the unconscious patient often breathes through his mouth, the membranes become dry and cracked. Mouth care, including lubrication, should be given every 2 to 4 hours. The patient's own teeth should be brushed, and dentures should be removed.

Ventilation. To make breathing easier, the nose should be kept free of mucus. Gentle cleansing and lubrication will keep the passages open. After a head injury, if bleeding is present, nasal cleansing should be done only with a physician's order. Suctioning may be necessary to keep the airway open. In prolonged unconsciousness, a tracheotomy may be indicated. The side position is preferable to the supine position to prevent the tongue from falling back and blocking the air passages.

Moving and positioning. A "turning sheet" should be used to move and position an unconscious patient every 2 to 4 hours. After positioning the

A warm environment is a comfortable environment for the patient whose consciousness level varies.

---

[17] Carini and Owens, p. 143.
[18] Ibid., p. 142.

During the time that the patient is comatose, it is to be remembered that hearing is one of the last sensations to diminish.

patient on his side, the nurse should check to make sure that the neck is not bent and that the lower leg is straight. The uppermost leg should be flexed with the knee at a right angle to the hip. A footboard is used to prevent foot drop, and support of the wrist will prevent wrist drop. Pillows are used to support the extremities. If the patient does not move at all, his extremities should be put through the complete range of motion exercises at least twice a day (see chapter 18). A cradle (or footboard) is placed over the foot of the bed to prevent pressure of the bedclothes on the extremities.

Nutrition. The comatose patient is not given nourishment by mouth. Nutritional needs are met through intravenous liquids, or **gastric tube** feedings (see chapter 19). Vitamins, antibiotics, and electrolytes are added to intravenous infusions. If giving feedings through a gastric tube, the nurse should instill 100 to 300 cc every 2 to 3 hours. Overfeeding is to be avoided, as the gastric contents can be regurgitated and aspirated. If not contra-indicated, a high-vitamin, high-protein feeding with 2,500 to 3,000 calories in about 2,500 to 3,000 cc of fluid every 24 hours is recommended for an adult.[19] Each feeding should be followed by a small amount of water to clear the tube. The tube should be lubricated at the orifice and changed every 5 days.

Elimination. The unconscious patient is usually incontinent of feces and urine. This increases the susceptibility to decubitus ulcers. A Foley catheter or external drainage apparatus is used to control urinary incontinence. To prevent constipation and impactions, a mild cathartic is given every second or third night, followed by a colon lavage the following morning. Prune juice may be given through the gastric tube.

As the patient begins to regain consciousness, a regimen for bowel training should be initiated. Adequate fluid and food intake, regular toilet-ing, and suppositories are effective in achieving regular bowel movements. See chapter 21 for a further discussion of elimination needs.

Emotional needs. During the time that the patient is comatose, it is to be remembered that hearing is one of the last sensations to diminish. Always assume that the person is conscious. Talk to him, but not about him, at the bedside. Family members also may have to be reminded of this. If possible, involve members of the patient's family in his care. This will help them feel less helpless and will give them something practical to do. They should be encouraged to express their feelings about the patient, and be allowed to question freely. Explanations of treatments should be given to family members. During this period of stress, the family will be reassured by the nurse's concerned, interested attitude.

[19]Ibid., p. 144.

If the patient begins to regain consciousness and becomes increasingly alert, the nurse must help him in progressively becoming more independent. It is important for him to become involved in activities of daily living and to reestablish his identity as an adult. During the period of convalescence, when he is partially independent but still limited in his activities, it is important to provide the patient with emotional support. The nurse can show the patient that she is interested in his well-being, and she can help the patient by reassuring him and stimulating his desire to get well.

Sensory alteration

Assessment

Sensory alteration is a state of changed perception in an individual. It occurs when the individual is exposed to an environment that is significantly different from the environment that he is accustomed to. The three major types of sensory alteration—**sensory deprivation, sensory overload,** and **sensory distortion**—are similar in that in all three the amount of *meaningful* stimuli is decreased. In addition, the behavioral changes that result from all three forms of sensory alteration are similar.

Sensory deprivation occurs when there is a decrease in the amount or intensity of the stimuli available to the individual's sensory organs. It may result from inadequate or monotonous stimuli (sensory underload), and it can occur in perfectly healthy people as well as in sick individuals.

Sensory distortion occurs when the stimulus is presented out of its usual time or spatial sequence. Sensory overload occurs when the sense organs are presented with multiple stimuli at higher than normal levels of intensity. In acute care units of many hospitals, the potential for sensory overload is especially high. It has been found that the stimulation from respirators, cardiac monitors, suction machines, and oxygen outlets constantly assaults the patient. The sound level produced by these machines exceeds the level of sound found in normal conversation and approaches levels of a noisy office or a radio playing at full volume.[20]

Reactions to sensory alteration. In the hospital, certain patients are prone to develop symptoms of sensory alteration. Isolated patients, laryngectomy or tracheotomy patients, patients on complete bed rest, or patients who are aged or terminally ill should be particularly observed for signs of sensory deprivation, distortion, and overload.

Typical reactions include hallucinations, delusions, illusions, increased sleeping, thought disorganization, anxiety, and panic. Examples of relatively simple effects include seeing dots, colors, and geometric shapes; hearing

[20]Ibid., p. 149.

Sensory alteration occurs when the individual is exposed to an environment that is significantly different from the environment that he is accustomed to.

Sensory stimulation
and its perception are
essential to well-being.

the sounds of wind and water; and feeling warmer and colder. More complex effects may include seeing meaningful objects, people, animals, and landscapes. Taste and smell experiences have been reported, including tasting or smelling something when it is not present.[21]

Sensory systems. A **sensory system** consists of the ability to receive mental impressions through the sense organs and the ability to organize the stimuli received (perception).

The biological aspect of the sensory systems is not limited to the standard senses of vision, taste, smell, touch, and hearing. It also involves general sensations of location in space, balance, degree of body mobility, and the feel of the extremities. The receptors for this sense **(kinesthesis)** are located in muscles, in joints, and in the inner ear.

Sensory nerves carry impulses from the receptor (for example, the eye) to the brain, where psychological selection and organization—perception—occur. This judgment is based on past experiences, knowledge, and attitudes. The initial impulse is then perceived (by the brain) as shape, color, space, movement, pain, heat, or cold.

Sensory stimulation and its perception are essential to well-being. The following is a description of the basic perceptual systems. Without fully functioning systems to sense and perceive, distortion of sensory input occurs.

1. The **basic orienting system.** The apparatus of the inner ear picks up forces of acceleration. These specify the direction of gravity and the movements of the body. This system cooperates with the other systems since it provides a basic framework.
2. The **auditory system.** This system responds to vibrations of the air. The input specifies the nature of vibratory occurrences, and allows the individual to locate the origin of the vibrations.
3. The **haptic system.** This apparatus consists of a complex of subsystems. It has no sense organs per se, since the receptors are located throughout the body. It is the sense of touching, and is essential for exploration.
4. The **taste-smell system.** The receptors of the nose and mouth work together in the activity of eating. Eating also includes feeling the food—a contribution of the haptic system.
5. The **visual system.** This apparatus combines with all the others and overlaps all of them in registering information. It functions in accommodation, pupillary adjustment, fixation, convergence, and exploration.[22]

[21]C. Wesley Jackson and Rosemary Ellis. 1971. Sensory deprivation as a field of study. *Nursing Research* 20:49.

[22]James J. Gibson. 1966. *The senses considered as perceptual systems*, pp. 51–52. Boston: Houghton Mifflin.

Planning, implementation, and evaluation

Since there are minimum and maximum levels of sensory stimulation necessary to well-being, the nurse must actively manipulate the environment to decrease or increase the stimuli available to patients. Orienting the patient to his environment, making stimuli meaningful to him, and keeping him in touch with himself and others are three general goals that are helpful.[23]

To orient the patient to the environment, the nurse can provide concrete reminders of time and place—a clock, calendar, radio, television, and magazines. If the patient is visually impaired, the nurse should announce her presence and describe all treatments performed. She can describe the environment to him as well—his food tray, his room, or what the weather is like. References can be made to the date and time. The family and other staff members can be encouraged to continue this orientation program.

Stimuli can be made meaningful by surrounding the patient with familiar objects brought from home—personal belongings, foods, or hobby equipment. Occupational therapy may be helpful. It is important that the nurse continue to communicate with the patient. This reassures him that he is in touch with himself and with those around him. It is also helpful for the patient to discuss his feelings of loneliness and fear.

SUMMARY

Rest and sleep, although essential to recovery and convalescence, are elusive and often difficult to provide for patients. Each person has his own unique requirements for relaxation, and often the hospital (or other health care facility) routine itself significantly interferes with a patient's established sleep patterns. Some of the characteristics necessary for rest are freedom from worry, discomfort, and irritation; adequate activity; and a feeling of being accepted and understood.

Sleep is a universal phenomenon, characterized in the normal person by predictable stages of drowsiness, light sleep, deep sleep, and dreaming. The body slows down in the first stages of sleep, and then activates in the dreaming (or rapid eye movement) stage. The functions of sleep are thought to be integrative and restorative, preparing the individual, psychologically and physiologically, for another day. Although there is a range of needs for sleep, the overall sleep patterns of most people are similar. Marked deviations from this pattern result in insomnia, nocturnal enuresis, somnambulism, and other sleep disorders. Sleep deprivation results in bizarre psychological changes in behavior and biochemical changes in the body.

The nurse must actively manipulate the environment to decrease or increase the stimuli available to patients.

[23]Cynthia F. Cameron et al. 1972. When sensory deprivation occurs . . . . *Canadian Nurse* 68:33.

Consciousness is the degree of awareness in an individual that can range from alertness to coma. Other states along the spectrum include drowsiness (lethargy) and stupor. In caring for the comatose patient, who is completely unresponsive, the nurse must attend to every body system. Skin care, hygiene, elimination, nourishment, circulation, and prevention of complications and accidents are all part of the care, in addition to observing and reporting any changes in condition. The principles of caring for the comatose patient are the same, regardless of the etiology of the condition.

In sensory alteration, the usual and customary environment of an individual is significantly changed. Changes in his perception of this environment also occur. This state can be a result of sensory deprivation (underload), distortion, or sensory overload, but they are all due to a decrease in the amount of meaningful stimuli available to the individual. The behavior that occurs—hallucinations, delusions, thought disorganization—is similar in all three types of sensory alteration.

The nurse can manipulate the environment to provide sufficient and varied amounts of sensory stimulation. Radios, newspapers, clocks, personal belongings, and recreational therapy can help the individual reorient himself. The goals of the nurse who cares for patients with sensory alteration are to orient the patient to his environment, make stimuli meaningful, and keep the patient in touch with himself and others.

STUDY QUESTIONS

1. What conditions must be met before a person can rest?
2. What are the stages of sleep? Describe each stage.
3. Define insomnia, nocturnal enuresis, and somnambulism. What are some methods the nurse may use in helping a patient overcome these problems?
4. Describe the four basic levels of consciousness. What methods are used to determine a patient's level of consciousness?
5. Compare and contrast sensory deprivation, sensory overload, and sensory distortion.
6. Using your own clinical experience, and referring to chapter 11 ("Teaching-Learning Aspects of Nursing"), draw up a plan for orienting a 50-year-old female patient, blind since birth, who has been admitted to the hospital for treatment of varicose veins.

SELECTED BIBLIOGRAPHY

Chodil, Judith, and Williams, Barbara. 1970. The concept of sensory deprivation. *Nursing Clinics of North America* 5:453–65.

Downs, Florence S. 1974. Bed rest and sensory disturbance. *American Journal of Nursing* 74:434–38.

Ford, Amasa B. 1965. The meaning of rest. *Cardiovascular nursing* 1:11–14.

Long, Barbara. 1969. Sleep. *American Journal of Nursing* 69:1896–99.

Narrow, Barbara W. 1967. Rest is . . . . *American Journal of Nursing* 67:1646–49.

18 Meeting motor needs

Assessment of activity and functioning

Activity, the state or condition of moving, is a basic, universal drive. It is thought to be related to almost every other physiological and psychological striving. It assists the individual immeasurably throughout all stages of life—infancy, childhood, adolescence, adulthood, and old age.

Optimal activity and functioning can be interrupted in many ways. These include disease, therapy, and factors within the patient and his environment. **Immobilization** implies any prescribed or unavoidable restriction of movement in any area of a person's life. The source of immobilization may be physical, emotional, intellectual, or social.

The entire body may be immobilized, as in a body cast. Or a single limb of the body may be immobilized, as with an arm cast or through paralysis of a leg and arm on one side as a result of a stroke. Immobilization results from the application of **traction** and **splints.**

Pain may also lead to immobilization when the individual splints, by reflex or by voluntarily curtailing muscle activity, a part of the body to prevent further discomfort. Weakness, fatigue, electrolyte imbalance, and general debility may result in low energy levels, another cause of immobilization.

Bed rest, part of the medical regimen for coronary infarction, rheumatic heart disease, and other conditions may lead to immobilization of healthy parts of the body when only some parts need the actual rest.

Confinement to a particular space is a form of physical restriction. The resultant restraint on normal patterns of social interation is called **social immobilization.**

Emotional immobilization can occur when stress exceeds the individual's coping ability. Until an adjustment is made, the person is unable to act. **Intellectual immobilization** results when there is a lack of knowledge-acquisition ability, such as occurs in mental retardation.

Effects of restricted activity

Prolonged inactivity predisposes the individual to specific complications and is accompanied by a progressive loss of function in normal

1. Identify and give examples of each of the four types of immobilization.

2. Discuss the effects of inactivity on each of the seven body systems.

3. Promote the patient's optimal motor function through regular active and/or passive exercises.

4. Use proper body alignment principles when positioning a patient.

5. Discuss the methods used to help a patient to walk with or without mechanical devices.

Prolonged inactivity predisposes the individual to specific complications and is accompanied by a progressive loss of function in normal organs.

organs.[1] Potentially, every organ system may be subject to dysfunction. The result may be permanent disability or delayed recovery. The following is a brief summary of the effects of inactivity.

Musculoskeletal function. With muscular inactivity, there is a profound effect on the musculoskeletal system, which, in turn, affects other systems.

If muscles are totally inactive, 3 percent of muscular strength is lost per day. **Atrophy** (wasting) of the muscles begins within 48 hours of inactivity. The muscle mass is decreased, **muscle strength** (the maximal tension that muscles can exert) and endurance declines, and a cycle of "deconditioning" begins. Inactivity leads to muscle degeneration, which leads to less activity, which means even further impairment.

In the bones, another degenerative process takes place with inactivity. Muscular inactivity depresses the normal buildup of **bone matrix** (the formative portion), while the removal of osseous tissue continues unabated. A process of decalcification **(osteoporosis)** begins, with the loss of calcium, nitrogen, and phosphorus from the bones. Even after activity is resumed, it may take months or years to restore osteoporotic bone.

Contractures result from prolonged immobilization of a joint in one position. With immobilization, the muscle fibers in a joint shorten in response to decreased activity. Instead of the loose connective tissue formed in normally active joints, dense tissue now fills the area. Trauma and edema of the joint hasten this process. Atrophy and limited movement follow the formation of dense tissue. When the process has just begun, measures can be taken to overcome its effects. If unchecked, however, tendons, ligaments, and the joint capsule eventually will become affected. At this point, the effects are irreversible.

Metabolic processes. The metabolic rate decreases in response to the decreased energy requirements of the cells during inactivity. Body buildup **(anabolism)** declines, but the breakdown processes **(catabolism)** accelerate. As protein is broken down, nitrogen (one of the protein end products) increases in the body. A negative nitrogen balance, or a state in which more nitrogen is being excreted than is being consumed, now exists.

Cardiovascular effects. Immobilization has dramatic effects on the cardiovascular system. This system is also affected by changes in other systems. For example, the calcium that is released from the bones may increase cardiac irritability.

The work load of the heart is increased because of a greater venous return. This produces an enlargement of the heart and an increased **stroke volume** (amount of blood ejected per heartbeat).

[1]Emily B. Campbell. 1970. Nursing problems associated with prolonged recovery following trauma. *Nursing Clinics of North America* 5:551.

Inactivity promotes **thrombus** formation because of stasis of the venous blood, injury to the innermost layer of the veins, and changes in the composition of the blood that predispose to blood coagulation.

After a period of inactivity, the ability of the autonomic nervous system to equalize blood supply when the individual resumes an erect posture declines. This is called **orthostatic hypotension,** and it is evidenced by a sudden drop in blood pressure on standing. In one study, a group of healthy men were kept on strict bed rest for 21 days. It took 5 weeks of resumed activity before the ability to equalize blood supply returned completely.[2]

As the basal metabolic rate decreases with decreased activity, less oxygen and carbon dioxide are produced. Respirations then lessen in number and depth. In all areas of the body, this causes tissue hypoxia.

In addition, the effort needed to breathe in the supine position is double that in the erect position. The patient therefore uses more energy to get less air. This means he takes even fewer deep breaths, which accentuates the already decreased respiratory activity. And with the increase in cardiac output, there is less area for lung expansion in the chest. The recumbent position also limits adequate lung expansion.

Urinary tract. In the urinary tract, optimal functioning exists in the upright position. After a few days in the supine position, the renal pelvis becomes distended from lack of the drainage-inducing force of gravity. Urine accumulates, and there is a decrease in the voiding reflexes of the bladder. Voluntary voiding may not be initiated or bladder emptying may be incomplete. Even if voiding can be initiated, the supine position makes voiding difficult.

With the decrease in muscular activity, there are fewer acid end products excreted in the urine. The urine becomes alkaline, a condition that favors the formation of **calculi** (stones). The heightened excretion of nitrogen, phosphorus, sulfur, sodium, potassium, and calcium from protein breakdown, together with the decreased volume of produced urine (from the decreased blood volume), also favor stone development. Infection is common after a period of urinary stasis, and this, too, promotes calculi formation.

Skin. Skin breakdown and decubitus formation are seen after prolonged or excessive pressure on a body part, usually over a bony prominence. Compression causes a local **ischemia** of the part. The tissues, deprived of essential nutrients, die and slough off (see chapter 16).

Gastrointestinal. The inactive patient is an **anorexic** patient. This is thought to be due to the negative nitrogen balance, together with a decrease

Immobilization has dramatic effects on the cardiovascular system.

---

[2]H. L. Taylor et al. 1949. Effects of bedrest on cardiovascular function and work performance. *Journal of Applied Psychology* 2:223–39.

Any sustained or recurrent restriction of activity will create severe anxiety and frustration.

in psychological stimulation to the patient. An inadequate intake of food only accentuates the existing protein deficiency of catabolism.

Constipation is a frequent problem. With loss of muscle tone, the patient's defecation power is reduced. The psychological effects of the lack of privacy and the abnormal position assumed when using a bedpan contribute to the problem (see chapter 20).

Neural and psychosocial effects. In the psychosocial sphere, inactivity creates many disturbances. When activity is restricted, intellectual abilities are affected by lack of central nervous system stimulation and by changes in the psychological state of the patient. Because of altered sensory input, there is a progressive deterioration of sensory perception, intellectual function, and motor coordination. Psychologically, there is a disturbance in the patient's sense of identity as an individual and a social being. Studies in learning and motivation of immobilized or isolated individuals show that there is a decreased motivation to learn. These studies also indicate a lessened ability to retain learned material and a decrease in problem-solving ability.[3]

The normal role of the person is changed with enforced inactivity. He is no longer physically active, he no longer works, and participation in social activities is limited. His drives and expectancies are decreased, and he may find that his role of spouse or parent is reversed, altered, or eliminated.

Any sustained or recurrent restriction of activity will create severe anxiety and frustration. Emotional states expressed by immobilized patients include apathy, withdrawal, frustration, anger, aggression, and regression. Restricted activity can severely damage the person's self-image, and, in children, it can cause serious delays in development.

Planning, implementation, and evaluation for optimal motor function

Regular exercise

Regular exercise is a means of promoting optimal motor function. It has effects on all body systems, and, if sufficiently intensive, can greatly delay the various phenomena of aging. It can help avoid decreased muscle mass, decreased oxygen intake, decreased heat production, and the fall in total blood quantity. Exercise also promotes overall cerebral stimulation. It stimulates neural controls of metabolism, respiration, blood circulation, and digestion. The glands of internal secretion are also stimulated.[4]

[3]Edith V. Olson. 1967. The hazards of immobility. *American Journal of Nursing* 67:795.
[4]Kenneth L. Jones, Louis W. Shainberg, and Curtis O. Byer. 1972. *Total fitness*, pp. 47–48. San Francisco: Canfield Press.

A totally fit individual has the strength, speed, agility, endurance, and social and emotional adjustment appropriate to his age. Fitness implies the ability to function at an optimum level of efficiency in all daily living. Some activities that produce fitness are bicycling, running, jogging, swimming, and tennis. Through these exercises, the muscles grow longer and leaner, so more of the cells are closer to blood vessels. They also help in the creation of new blood vessels, and help the body to resist disease processes and some types of poisons.[5]

The amount and kind of exercise needed depend on several factors. Age is one factor. Children need more exercise than adults. In the selection of exercises for disabled or ill patients, additional factors, such as level of consciousness, state of health, amount of surgical trauma, and the degree of mobility or paralysis, must be considered.

All exercises should be adapted to the individual's tolerance level. One indication of exercise tolerance (the level at which the body responds favorably to exercise) is the pulse rate. Exercise physiologists have found that an individual undergoes favorable circulatory changes that lead to physical fitness if he works at 60 percent of his capacity. People under 30 work at 60 percent of their capacity when their pulse rate is 151 beats per minute. People over 30 work at 60 percent of their capacity when their pulse reaches 131 beats per minute. A person can check his own pulse rate after performing **calisthenics** or engaging in some sport. The pulse should be taken 10 seconds after the cessation of exercise and checked against the recommended rate.[6] Of course, people with cardiac and other limitations will have lower recommended rates. A physician always should be consulted before beginning any exercise regimen.

Exercise supervision is often one of the teaching responsibilities of the nurse. This may include teaching exercises to alert but bedfast patients, or actually performing passive exercises for the patient. In some institutions, group exercises are held for postcoronary patients, the elderly, and the disabled in preparation for crutch walking. In one nursing exercise program on an orthopedic unit, group exercises were initiated to improve appetite, decrease pain and restlessness, achieve bowel regularity, and improve social relationships.[7]

Body mechanics

Body mechanics refers to the mechanical, or physical, correlation of the various systems of the body. Special reference is made to the skeletal, muscular, and visceral systems and their neurological associations. It means working with the physical laws that govern motor activity to achieve stable,

[5] Ibid., p. 54.
[6] Ibid., pp. 74–75.
[7] Winnie Griffin, Sara J. Anderson, and Joyce Y. Passos. 1971. Group exercise for patients with limited motion. *American Journal of Nursing* 71:1742.

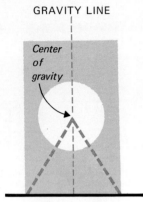

GRAVITY LINE

Center of gravity

BASE OF SUPPORT

FIG. 18-1 *Finding the center of gravity.*

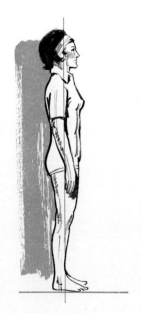

FIG. 18-2 *Good body alignment in the standing position.*

balanced, and effective movement. Good body mechanics exist when the mechanical correlation is most favorable to the functioning of the various systems.[8]

The laws of **gravity** influence motion. Gravity is the mutual attraction that the earth has for an object and the object for the earth. Activity is influenced at all times by this force, and muscle contractions supply the force for movements against the pull of gravity.

An understanding of some basic physical laws is essential here. Every object has a **center of gravity.** This is defined as the point at which all mass is centered. In a symmetrically shaped object, the center of gravity is at its geometric center. In the average standing adult, the center of gravity is inside the pelvis slightly anterior to the upper part of the sacrum.[9] An imaginary line, called the **gravity line,** passes through the center of gravity downward to the base of support of the object or individual. One basic principle of body mechanics is that the broader the base of support and the lower the center of gravity, the greater the stability of an object.

The maintenance of good posture is an example of good application of body mechanics. **Posture** is the alignment of the parts of the body with each other, and of the body as a whole. Good posture should provide minimal muscular contraction. Weight is centered at the line of gravity, and this line should pass through the center of the base of support. This illustrates another principle of body mechanics: A broad base of support and a good alignment (of the parts of the body) conserve energy and help prevent fatigue.[10]

Preventing complications from decreased mobility through proper body alignment

Providing good alignment in the supine position is one of the best ways to prevent disability and deformity.

Lying. In preventing or minimizing complications from decreased mobility when the patient is in bed, a firm mattress is necessary to permit good alignment and to promote good physiological function. If the bed sags, a firm board may be used underneath the mattress to provide level support (see chapter 16).

In positioning a patient in the back-lying **(supine)** position, the nurse should remember that the relation of the body segments to each other is essentially the same as in a good standing position. The pillow underneath the head should give enough support to relax the muscles of the head and neck, but not push the head forward. A footboard is used to prevent foot

[8]Joel E. Goldthwait et al. 1934. *Body mechanics,* p. 9. Philadelphia: Lippincott.
[9]Annetta J. Bilger and Ellen H. Greene, eds. 1973. *Winter's protective body mechanics,* pp. 1, 3. New York: Springer.
[10]Ibid., p. 10.

drop, maintain good alignment, and provide freedom of movement for the feet. The shoulder joints are supported away from the body, and the elbows are flexed. Pillows are used to support the extremities. A small roll can be placed under the knees to prevent hyperextension.[11]

When lying in this position, the patient has a tendency to rotate the hips outwardly. To correct this, a trochanter roll may be used to support the leg in a neutral position (midway between inward and outward position) or in inward rotation. Once the roll is in place, correct alignment can be checked by observing the patella. It faces directly upward when the femur is in the neutral position.

In the **side-lying** (lateral) position, the alignment of the trunk should be the same as in a good standing position. The physiological curves of the spine should be maintained, the head should be supported in line with the midline of the trunk, and rotation of the spine should be avoided.

The uppermost arm is supported on pillows so that its weight does not pull the shoulder girdle out of alignment or interfere with respirations. The arm that rests on the bed may be placed in varying degrees of shoulder flexion and rotation, the elbow in flexion, and the forearm in varying degrees of pronation and supination. The uppermost leg is supported on pillows so that its weight does not pull on the hip joint, pelvis, or low back. A footboard and sandbags can be used to support the feet.[12]

[11] Ibid., pp. 25–26.
[12] Ibid., pp. 27–28.

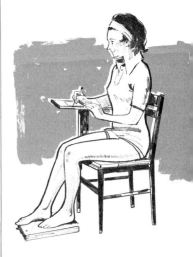

FIG. 18-3 *Good body alignment in the sitting position.*

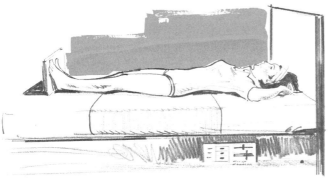

FIG. 18-4 *Good body alignment in the supine (back-lying) position.*

FIG. 18-5 *Good body alignment in the side-lying position.*

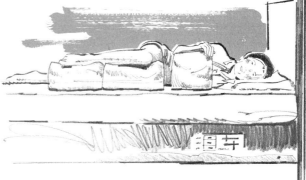

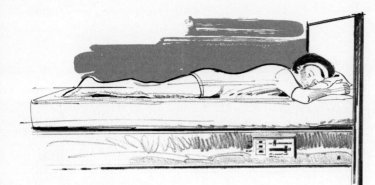

FIG. 18-6 *Good body alignment in the prone position.*

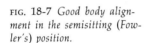

FIG. 18-7 *Good body alignment in the semisitting (Fowler's) position.*

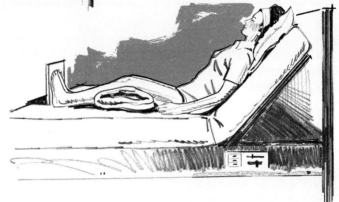

Prone. It is just as easy for the patient to have good body alignment when lying facedown as when in the standing position. The ankles should be dorsiflexed over the end of the mattress, and the arms should be abducted to permit relaxation. The pillow is used, not under the head, but under the abdomen to prevent pressure on the breasts and hyperextension of the lumbar spine.[13] A small flat pillow may be placed under the head for comfort.

Semisitting (Fowler's) position. In providing proper alignment for the patient in a semisitting position, the nurse must make sure that the supports permit flexion of the hips and knees and normal alignment of the spine. In the sitting position in bed, the knees must be flexed and the head must not be thrown forward. Not all knee gatches on hospital beds fit a particular patient's anatomy, and an improvised knee rest may be made from a soft bath blanket. Supports for the arms offset the pull of the arms on the trunk, and a pillow is placed under the head and the shoulders to prevent flexion of the neck.

Without proper attention to body alignment, the patient assumes positions that lead quickly to deformity and incapacitation. One of these positions is the "coffin" position.

[13] Ibid., p. 29.

TABLE 18-1
Effects of the Coffin Position

Causative Position	Resulting Complications
Arms along sides of body	Tight axillae with loss of arm function
Elbows flexed	Flexion contractures; impairment of circulation
Forearms and hands resting on chest	Diminution of respiration; sensation of being crowded
Wrists crossed and dropped	Loss of optimum use of wrists and hands
Hands pushed out of anatomical alignment by their own weight	Loss of use of hands and fingers
Feet dropped	Loss of controlled use of feet
Knees hyperextended	Stretching of ligaments; loss of muscle tone with resultant loss of stability and use of the knees

Standing. In assisting the patient to stand correctly, the nurse should suggest that he attempt to "stand tall." The head, upper torso, and lower torso should be in line with one another. In a properly balanced body, an imaginary straight line drawn through the body should pass through the lobe of the ear and the bump of the anklebone.[14]

Moving the patient in bed

Moving from one side of the bed to the other. To move the patient from one side of the bed to the other, the nurse begins by crossing the patient's arms over his trunk. She stands at the side of the bed, facing the patient's head, and places one leg forward so that her thigh is braced against the lower edge of the bed. She flexes both hips and knees sufficiently to place both arms under the patient, stabilizes her pelvis, and moves her trunk forward in one segment. The nurse places her arms under the patient's hips so that her forearms are flat on the bed with the palms up to support the patient's weight. She moves the patient's hips toward her as she flexes her hips and keeps her spine straight. Using the same body mechanics, she places one arm under the patient's head, the other arm under the midthoracic region of the patient, and pulls the patient's head and shoulders to the side of the bed in alignment with the hips.[15]

Moving up in bed. To move the patient up in bed, one or two workers may be needed. If the patient is able to assist, or if the patient is not extremely heavy, one nurse can complete the task. The patient should be

[14]Jones et al., p. 65.
[15]Bilger and Greene, p. 31.

343

in a back-lying position. He should be instructed to flex his knees with his heels on the bed. The nurse places one arm under the shoulders of the patient, and the other between the patient's arm and trunk, with her hand firmly grasping the underarm region. Together, the nurse and the patient push toward the head of the bed. This is easier if there are two workers, one for each side.

If the patient has the use of a trapeze, the nurse places one arm under the patient's shoulders and one arm under his thighs. The nurse, with a broad base provided by her feet, tightens her muscles, keeps her back straight, and slides the patient toward the head of the bed. At the same time, the patient pushes with his heels and lifts slightly with the aid of the trapeze.

Using a turning sheet. When two nurses are present, a turning sheet can be used. The sheet is placed underneath the patient, and should extend from the shoulders to 2 inches below the **popliteal space.** The two nurses face the patient, one on each side of the bed, and each rolls the turning sheet on her side toward the patient. Each nurse braces one thigh against the lower edge of the bed frame, flexes her hips and knees, and stabilizes her pelvis by contracting the abdominal muscles. The feet should be placed to allow movement in the direction motion will occur. The forward leg helps in the pushoff, and the back leg is used to rock back on as lifting begins. Moving her trunk forward as one segment, each nurse grasps the rolled turning sheet. At an agreed-upon signal, they both lift up and move the patient to the desired side of the bed, up in bed, or to the side-lying position.[16]

Moving the patient out of bed

Into a chair. Transferring from a bed to a chair may be accomplished by lifting the patient directly from the bed to the chair. It may also be done by assisting the patient, first to a sitting position, then to a standing position, and then to a sitting position in the chair. The choice of method depends on the degree of control that the patient possesses.

The following is a step-by-step procedure for assisting a patient who has some degree of independence.

The head of the bed should be raised so that the patient starts from a sitting position. The nurse should then face the head of the bed. She places one hand under the knees of the patient and the other hand around the patient's shoulders. She swings the patient's legs over the edge of the bed as she simultaneously helps him lift his shoulders off the bed. The patient is now sitting up with his legs over the side of the bed.

With the patient sitting squarely on the edge of the bed, the nurse

[16]Ibid., p. 32.

blocks the patient's knees with her knees. This prevents buckling of the patient's knees. The nurse then places her arms through the axillary area in order to control trunk motion while moving toward the chair. She applies counterpressure against the patient's knees and counterbalances with her own weight if the patient has trouble standing alone. The nurse should not lean backward. Instead, she should bend at the knees and hips to achieve counterbalance with the weight. The nurse then pivots the patient into the bedside chair.

If the patient has one side stronger than the other, she should make sure she is moving him toward his stronger side. He will be better able to assist with motion toward that side.[17] The patient should then be lowered slowly into the chair. He should be instructed to grasp the arms of the chair while descending.

Onto a stretcher. In moving a patient to a stretcher, the turning sheet is most valuable. One nurse stands on each side of the patient, and the other assists with the legs. The patient is instructed to keep his hands across his chest. The stretcher is put next to the bed, and, at a given signal, both nurses move the turning sheet and the patient in the direction of the stretcher. Without a sheet, a three-man carry can be used, with three people on the same side of the patient lifting and carrying the patient.

Useful mechanical devices

The **hydraulic lift,** also called a patient lifter, is used to transfer a totally dependent patient to and from a bed, a wheelchair, a toilet, a tub, or a car. Operating a lift can be complicated, and attention to the details of its operation is important to ensure a safe and efficient transfer.

The trapeze is a triangular-shaped mechanical device attached to a frame on the bed within reach of the patient. It facilitates movement and position change in bed for the partially independent patient.

The Stryker turning frame, the Foster reversible orthopedic bed, and the CircOlectric bed (see chapter 16) provide means of changing the patient to and from the facedown and back-lying positions with minimum personnel, maximum ease, and undisturbed alignment.[18] It is recommended that nursing students experience being turned and transferred in some of these devices to increase their sympathetic and instructional capacities.[19]

To maintain alignment, other mechanical devices are useful. The bed board, sandbags, and the trochanter roll have already been mentioned. A **bed cradle** is also useful in keeping the weight of the bedclothes off the patient.

[17] Georgia Foss. 1973. Body mechanics. *Nursing '73* 3:30–31.
[18] Norma G. Dison. 1971. *An atlas of nursing techniques,* 2d ed., p. 59. St. Louis: Mosby.
[19] Kerr, p. 60.

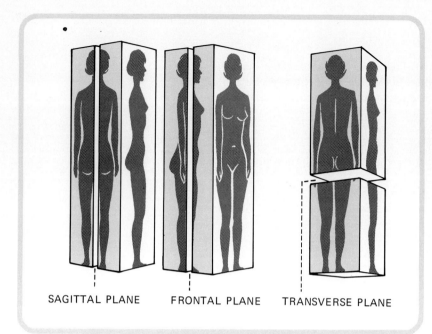

FIG. 18-8 *Sagittal, frontal, and transverse planes of the body.*

SAGITTAL PLANE   FRONTAL PLANE   TRANSVERSE PLANE

Activity

Exercises. Exercises may be performed by the patient himself (active) or by the nurse (assistive or passive). The patient should take as much responsibility as possible for his own exercises. The nurse should try to simplify them and make them interesting to increase motivation. For example, the patient can exercise his feet and ankles by lifting the heels, one at a time, off the bed, and writing the alphabet in the air.

Rhythmic exercises **(isotonic)** involve muscle contraction accompanied by a change in muscle length. Examples of these exercises are passive and active exercises of extension and flexion of the limbs. Rhythmic exercises increase muscular strength and endurance to improve circulatory status.

Isometric exercises involve a muscular contraction that occurs when the ends of muscles are fixed so that activity is evidenced by increased tension without change in muscle length.

Range of motion. **Range of motion** is the maximum amount of movement possible at a joint in one dimension of space. The dimensions of space are the planes of the body—anterior and posterior **(frontal)**, left and right **(sagittal)**, and upper and lower **(transverse).**

In doing passive range of motion exercises, the nurse should move the parts slowly and gently. Exercises done too rapidly or too vigorously can cause severe pain. The patient should attempt to lead as much as possible as each movement is initiated.[20]

[20]Ibid., p. 339.

Flexion: Movement that decreases the angle between the bones.

Extension: Movement that increases the angle between the bones.

Abduction: Movement away from the midline of the body.

Adduction: Movement toward the midline of the body.

Circumduction: Movement that combines all of the above movements in succession so that the distal end of the limb describes a circle and the shaft of the limb describes the surface of a cone.

Rotation: A revolving movement or twisting of a part of the body around the longitudinal axis of that part.

Medial rotation: Rotation toward the midline of the body.

Lateral rotation: Rotation away from the midline of the body.

Supination: Movement that places the forearm in the anatomical position (palm forward).

Pronation: Movement that turns the back of the hand forward—the radius is crossed over the ulna.

Inversion: Movement that turns the sole of the foot inward.

Eversion: Movement that turns the sole of the foot outward.

FIG. 18-9 *Classification of joint movements.*

[From *Winter's protective body mechanics,* ed. Annetta Bilger and Ellen Greene, p. 37. New York: Springer, 1973. Copyright © 1973 by Springer Publishing Co. Used by permission.]

Walking without mechanical aids. To help a patient walk, the nurse, standing at the patient's left side, places her right arm around his waist and grasps his right forearm with her left hand. If two workers assist, each may place her arm so that it interlocks with the patient's and may grasp his forearm for support. Bilateral support without clumsiness during ambulation is obtained if two workers, standing on either side of the patient, grasp the upper arm near the axilla with the arm nearest the patient. The other hand is used to grasp the wrist. The patient may tend to grasp the worker's hand. It is important that the worker control the points of support in order to utilize necessary leverage if the need arises.[21]

Walking with mechanical aids. To walk with a cane, the patient stands in normal walking position. The cane is positioned about 4 to 6 inches away from the toe of the uninvolved extremity. He moves the cane forward about the length of his foot, and moves the involved leg forward until it is parallel with the cane. The uninvolved leg is moved forward until its heel is parallel to the cane. Other methods, however, may be devised and used by the patient.

A walker is used by a fairly independent patient who only needs some assistance in walking. The patient grasps the bar of the walker with both hands, fairly spread out. He places the walker firmly in front of him, and then walks up to it.

[21] Dison, pp. 66–67.

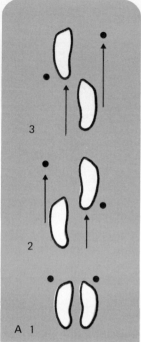

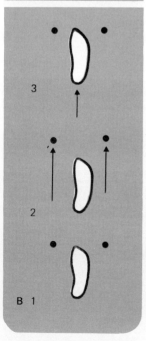

FIG. 18-10 *Two- and three-point crutch-walking gaits.*

Crutch walking. Before **crutch walking** is attempted, exercises should be started to increase muscle strength and endurance, especially in the arms, shoulders, chest, and back. Use of the trapeze should be encouraged, and active range of motion and exercises should be started as soon as the patient is able. Exercises to strengthen the quadriceps and triceps muscles should be encouraged on a regular basis.

The crutches should reach from about 2 inches below the axilla to a point about 6 to 8 inches out from the foot. The handbar should be at a level for almost complete extension of the elbow with the wrists hyperextended and the weight on the palms. There should be no axillary pressure from the crutches; this could cause arm paralysis.[22]

Someone should stay with the patient until he has learned to handle his crutches and has established a **gait.** He needs to have his mistakes corrected, but he also needs a lot of moral support.

There are three common gaits that are used to teach crutch walking:

1. When partial weight bearing is allowed, the **two-point gait** increases speed. The left crutch and the right foot are advanced simultaneously. Then the right crutch and the left foot are advanced simultaneously.
2. When bearing the weight on one extremity is permitted, the patient may use a **three-point gait.** The weight is shifted to the uninvolved extremity while the crutches are advanced. Then the uninvolved extremity is advanced. The crutches and the involved leg are moved forward at the same time. Then the uninvolved leg is moved forward.
3. The **four-point gait** is slower than the others. The right crutch is advanced, then the left foot, then the left crutch,[23] and then the right foot.

SUMMARY

At each stage of the life cycle, movement is a normal, universal drive with implications for nearly all areas of physiological and psychological functioning. Motor activity provides a means for development in many areas. It stimulates growth, language, and social behavior, and provides an outlet for the expression of frustrations. Through motor activity, the body can be developed to its optimum inherited potential.

Potentially, every organ system may be subject to dysfunction as a result of immobilization. Musculoskeletal, cardiovascular, respiratory, renal, gastrointestinal, metabolic, and psychosocial changes begin to occur within a short time. These changes may result in permanent disability or delayed recovery.

Optimal motor function can be promoted by regular exercise and

[22]Kerr, pp. 327-29.
[23]Dison, p. 70.

proper use of body mechanics in the well individual. They are best maintained by providing proper alignment and positioning in the immobilized individual. In addition, exercises for the inactive patient will help prevent disability and deformity. Active or passive range of motion exercises should be initiated as soon as possible. Creativity and imagination should be used by the nurse in devising interesting exercises (isotonic or isometric) for the patient who can perform some physical activity.

There are several mechanical aids that can be used with immobilized patients. These include the Stryker turning frame and the CircOlectric bed to facilitate position change and the hydraulic lift to transfer a patient. The trapeze may be used to assist the partially independent patient in moving. Various implements, such as the bed board, the bed cradle, sandbags, and the trochanter roll, are available for optimum positioning of the patient.

Walking can be facilitated through the use of the walker, the cane, or crutches. Prior to crutch walking, the patient should begin exercises to build muscle strength and endurance. Basic gaits for crutch walking include the two-point, the three-point, and the four-point gaits. The patient should be observed for mistakes in posture and alignment that occur when he is learning to walk on crutches. He also needs much emotional support and encouragement during this process. He should be observed to make sure that he can safely use the crutches.

STUDY QUESTIONS

1. Define physical immobilization, social immobilization, emotional immobilization, and intellectual immobilization. Describe some basic causes of each condition.
2. What are the effects of immobility on the musculoskeletal system? on the cardiovascular system? on other body systems? What are its psychosocial effects on the patient?
3. What is fitness? What are some of the factors that influence an individual's level of fitness?
4. What is body mechanics? How can an understanding of body mechanics help the nurse in her daily routine?
5. With the help of classmates, practice moving and positioning a patient as described on pp. 343–45.

SELECTED BIBLIOGRAPHY

Bilger, Annetta J., and Greene, Ellen H., eds. 1973. *Winter's protective body mechanics.* New York: Springer.
Blake, Florence G. 1969. Immobilized youth. *American Journal of Nursing* 69:2364–69.
Jones, Kenneth L., Shainberg, Louis W., and Byer, Curtis O. 1972. *Total fitness.* San Francisco: Canfield Press.
Kerr, Avice. 1969. *Orthopedic nursing procedures.* New York: Springer.
Olson, Edith V. 1967. The hazards of immobility. *American Journal of Nursing* 67:779–96.

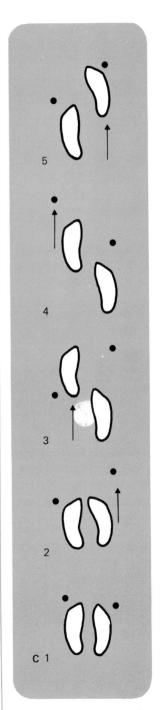

FIG. 18-11 *Four-point crutch-walking gait.*

19 Meeting nutritional needs

Upon completing this chapter, the reader should be able to:

1. Identify at least six factors that influence an individual's nutritional needs.

2. Discuss the function of each of the six components of an adequate diet.

3. Compare and contrast the signs and symptoms of an individual who is adequately nourished with those of one who is malnourished.

4. Summarize the factors that produce malnutrition.

5. Discuss six strategies that the nurse should consider in order to promote adequate nutrition.

Assessment of nutritional needs

Nutritional needs are determined by many factors. These include age, physical condition, habits, emotional responses, mental condition, and socioeconomic and religious background. An individual's food likes and dislikes, and his acceptance or refusal of food, are often reflections of his feelings about himself. They also indicate his attitude toward his illness, his family, and his environment.

Factors influencing nutritional needs

Age. The body's nutritional requirements and its ability to absorb food change with age. This is due to the effects the aging process has on hormone levels, growth patterns, and metabolism levels. Knowing basic nutritional needs for different age levels will help the nurse to better understand, evaluate, and educate. (See chapter 9 for a general discussion of the role of the life cycle.)

Before birth, the child is affected by the mother's nutritional state. The nutritional demands on the pregnant woman are enormous. She must provide nutrients not only to sustain herself but also for the growth of the fetus's bones, teeth, spine, brain, blood, and other structures and tissues.

The need for a special diet for pregnant women has long been recognized. Fewer complications in pregnancy, fewer premature births, and healthier babies have consistently occurred when the mother is well nourished. Poor nourishment, on the other hand, has generated a higher than average number of premature births, congenital defects, and stillbirths. A specific diet will usually be prescribed by a nutritionist and/or a physician in the case of a problem pregnancy.

Infancy and childhood are critical periods for proper nutrition because of the tremendous growth that occurs at this time. Eating habits are also linked to the development of personality patterns. In early infancy and childhood, food is the basis of most of the interactions between mother and child. Nutrition affects the baby's sleep habits, disposition, muscular development, and rate of growth.

The physiology of the infant includes a higher proportion of water than in older children. He also has poorly developed muscles, little subcutaneous fat, and a high proportion of skin surface to body weight. His gastrointestinal system is poorly developed, his kidneys are immature, and he has little facility for chewing. These factors determine the type of diet an infant needs. Thus, most infant diets are high in liquids, calcium, and protein and low in starches, fats, acid-producing foods, and roughage.

The rapid growth in overall size that occurs in fetal life and infancy is followed by a long period of very gradual growth. Another period of rapid growth takes place in the adolescent years. The eating of nutritionally valuable food, as well as the development of good nutritional habits, is important throughout childhood and adolescence.

The high activity level of children at this period demands a high-calorie diet (see p. 356 for an explanation of the term **calorie**). The 7- to 10-year-old usually needs about 2,400 calories daily, while the 15- to 18-year-old may require as many as 3,000 calories.[1] Foods with large amounts of **calcium** and **phosphorus** are vital during the periods preceding rapid growth. **Iron** is especially important for girls both before and during puberty.

Adequate nutrition during the childhood and teen-age years is often difficult to maintain. Children commonly use food to rebel, gain attention, assert their independence, or conform to peer-group pressures. Snacks are often so frequent and so filling (although nutritionally unfulfilling) that regular mealtimes may be ignored.

Special nutritional needs do not end with the onset of adulthood. In fact, they may become particularly acute in the years of later maturity. Many older persons have reduced incomes, physical infirmities, and other limitations on their ability to buy, prepare, and enjoy eating food. These problems, along with new and different nutritional demands made by the aging body, often lead to malnutrition.

Individual patterns and preferences. Food means different things to different people. Its meaning is influenced by psychological, cultural, religious, and socioeconomic factors. A steak, to one person, may imply status; to another, a lack of worldliness. To yet another, eating a steak would be an offense against religious beliefs.

Psychology. Food is used for "breaking the ice" between strangers and for increasing intimacy and enhancing conversation between friends. It can be used to reward or punish a child. This same child may use food to rebel against his parents. Eating may also be seen as an escape from anxiety.

Physiological and sensual reactions. Often, the eyes and nose, rather than the mouth, determine what we eat. If the sense of smell is diminished, as during a head cold, the desire to eat lessens as a result. The smell or

---

[1]Corinne H. Robinson. 1972. *Normal and therapeutic nutrition,* 14th ed., p. 293. New York: Macmillan.

sight of certain foods may cause us to salivate with pleasure. It may also cause us to gag and feel nauseated. These reactions may occur with foods we have never eaten before or with familiar foods that have been prepared in a new way or whose color is unfamiliar. The food industry, for example, has found that orange juice with an orange color sells far better than a juice with its natural yellow color.[2]

Cultural background. People eat what they have been used to eating and what has been available to them. Brown eggs are more popular in Boston, while Chicagoans purchase more white eggs.[3] Europeans consider sweet corn a food for swine, not for people.

Religion. Religious practices often dictate what a person will or will not eat, how he will prepare his food, and when he will eat it. The Jewish and Islamic religions are particularly rich in food-related traditions. Those who carefully follow the teachings of the Old Testament will not eat meat and dairy products together. Those who follow Islam celebrate religious holidays with long periods of fasting followed by enormous feasts.

Socioeconomic background. How and what a person eats is often used to link him to a particular socioeconomic group. For example, a person from a poor Italian family may be brought up on pizza, spaghetti, and bread. When he starts making a little money, his tastes change and he

Eating alone often reduces an older person's motivation to prepare an adequate meal.

[Photo by Sandor Acs]

[2]Jack Star. 1973. Why you choose the foods you do. *Today's Health* 51:34.
[3]Ibid.

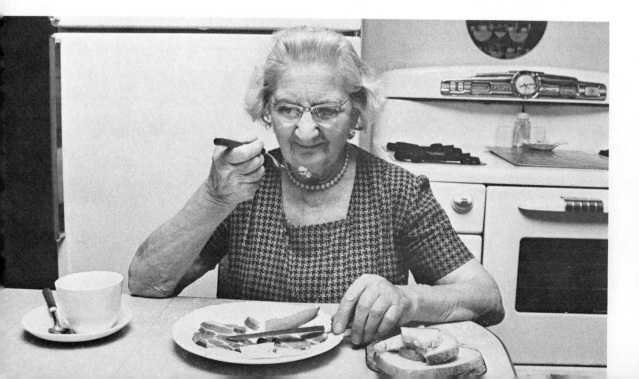

TABLE 19-1
Food Allowances for Pregnancy and Lactation

	Pregnant Woman	Pregnant Teen-age Girl	Lactating Woman
Milk	3–4 cups, whole	5–6 cups, whole	6 cups, whole
Meat, fish, poultry (liver once a week), cooked weight	4 ounces	4 ounces	4 ounces
Eggs	1	1	1
Vegetables, including:			
Dark green leafy or deep yellow	½ cup	½ cup	½ cup
Potato	1 medium	1 medium	1 medium
Other vegetables	½–1 cup	½–1 cup	½–1 cup
One vegetable to be raw each day			
Fruits, including:			
Citrus	1 serving	1 serving	1 serving
Other fruit	1 serving	1 serving	1 serving
Cereal, enriched or whole grain	1 serving	1 serving	1 serving
Bread, enriched or whole grain	5 slices	5 slices	5 slices
Butter or fortified margarine	To meet caloric needs	To meet caloric needs	To meet caloric needs
Desserts, cooking fats, sugars, sweets			
Vitamin D supplement (or use fortified milk)	400 I.U.	400 I.U.	400 I.U.
Iodized salt	Daily	Daily	Daily

Reprinted with permission of Macmillan Publishing Co., Inc., from Corinne H. Robinson, *Normal and therapeutic nutrition*, 14th ed., p. 299. New York: Macmillan, 1972. Copyright © 1972 by Macmillan Publishing Co., Inc.

begins to prefer beef and beer. When he makes yet more money, he "progresses" to steak and whiskey. Still later, after he has achieved success in the business world, his diet reflects "reverse snobbism" and he reverts to pizza and spaghetti.[4]

Hunger and appetite. The terms **hunger** and **appetite** are often used interchangeably, but actually they have very specific, different meanings. Jean Mayer, the nutritionist, has defined these terms as follows:

Appetite [is] the complex of sensations, up to a point pleasant, or at least not unpleasant, by which one is aware of desire for and the anticipation of in-

[4]Ibid., p. 35.

gestion of palatable food. Specific appetites relate, of course, to desires for specific foods.

Hunger [is] the complex of unpleasant sensations, felt after prolonged deprivation, which will impel a man to seek, work, or fight for immediate relief by ingestion of food. The passage from appetite to hunger is dependent on the duration of deprivation, the rate of energy expenditure and other factors.[5]

The degree of hunger, appetite, and **satiety** an individual experiences is regulated by an internal system that involves the hypothalamus gland, hormones, nerve cell bodies, and gastric secretions. For most people, the body adjusts the ingestion of food to meet the requirements of health, proper functioning of the body, and growth.[6] Occasionally, this homeostatic mechanism does not operate properly. This malfunction may cause excessive or insufficient hunger or appetite. In such cases, physiologically induced obesity or **emaciation** occurs.

Components of an adequate diet

The healthy body requires an adequate diet that is well balanced in many different **nutrients.** The nutrients considered vital for achievement and maintenance of homeostasis (see chapter 15) are **proteins, carbohydrates, fats, vitamins, minerals,** and **water.**

The body's requirements for various nutrients change throughout the life cycle. During periods of rapid growth, the body needs large quantities of those nutrients that contain calcium for the bones and teeth. It must also ingest nutrients that provide energy for the faster metabolism and protein for increased cell growth. An older person whose growth rate has stabilized needs smaller amounts of these nutrients. **Minimal daily allowances (MDA)** and **recommended daily allowances (RDA)** have been defined and charted for the various nutrients for infants, young children, teen-age boys, teen-age girls, pregnant and lactating women, and adults. These allowances are designed to guide the average person under normal circumstances in planning an adequate diet. The following is a brief overview of the sources and functions of the vital nutrients.

Proteins. Proteins are necessary for growth and body repair. They come in many different forms, depending on their source. Generally, they are broken down by the body into **amino acids** and then reassembled into human proteins, which serve as the body's building blocks. The best sources for proteins useful to the body are milk and milk products, eggs, fish, cereals (such as oats and rye), legumes (such as beans and nuts), and red meat. Pound for pound, children need more protein than adults, and

---

[5]Jean Mayer. 1968. *Overweight: Causes, cost, and control,* pp. 10–11. Englewood Cliffs, N.J.: Prentice-Hall. Italics in original.
[6]Ibid., p. 12.

infants need the most. During pregnancy and lactation, protein requirements are also high.

Carbohydrates. Carbohydrates are necessary for energy, for continuation
of body functions, and for the production of usable body fat. Major sources
of carbohydrates are sugars, including natural fruit sugars and cane sugar.
Most foods have some carbohydrates. In weight reduction regimens, a
restriction is often placed on the level of carbohydrate consumption rather
than on many of the other nutrients.

Fats. Like carbohydrates, fats are necessary for the body's energy needs.
Because fats contain less oxygen than other nutrients, they oxidize more
readily and release more energy. Among the most important and commonly
consumed sources of fats are butter and margarine and cooking and salad
oils. The latter are derived from peanuts, olives, soybeans, corn, linseed,
and cottonseed. Research shows that some classes of fats (the **saturates**)
may contribute to high **cholesterol** levels, arteriosclerosis, and other problems. Thus, while fats are essential in most people's diets, some patients
with potential or actual problems are advised to limit their fat intake.

Vitamins. Vitamins are a large class of distinct substances, which are
designated by the letters A, B, C, D, and E. They are necessary for such
vital metabolic processes as growth, digestion, vision, and a host of other
functions. Unlike protein, vitamins cannot be synthesized by the body,
but must be obtained from food. When one or more vitamins is lacking,
a deficiency disease results. Sometimes amounts far above the RDA for
a particular vitamin are used pharmacologically to treat physiological
disturbances. Such vitamin therapy must be carefully supervised, however,
for excesses of some vitamins can cause serious side effects.

    Vitamin A is necessary for growth, normal vision, and healthy condi-
tion of the skin and other body surfaces. Major sources of vitamin A are
dark green and deep yellow fruits and vegetables. **Vitamin B,** broken down
into four different subcategories—thiamine (B_1), riboflavin (B_2), pyridoxine
(B_6), and cyanocobalamin (B_{12})—is important for maintenance of mucous
membranes and other body surfaces. **Vitamin C,** also needed for healthy
gums and body tissues, is found abundantly in citrus fruits and green leafy
vegetables. **Vitamin D,** necessary for proper bone growth and structure
and for the efficient use of calcium and phosphorus, comes from sunshine
and enriched milks.

Minerals. Like vitamins, minerals are needed to build and maintain the
body's bones, teeth, and other systems. Minerals needed by the body fall
into two essential classes. These are the **macrominerals** (needed in amounts
in excess of about 100 mg per day) and the **microminerals,** or **trace minerals** (needed in much smaller amounts).

The macrominerals include calcium, phosphorus, magnesium, sodium, chlorine, and potassium. Most of the calcium and phosphorus in the body is present in the bones and teeth. Sodium, chlorine, and potassium are the main elements concerned with the distribution of fluids within the body (see chapter 22).

The essential trace minerals for humans are cobalt, copper, chromium, iodine, iron, manganese, molybdenum, selenium, and zinc.[7] Generally, fluorine is not considered essential for life, but it is important in the prevention of tooth decay and maintenance of calcium in the bones.[8]

Food sources for minerals include green leafy and yellow vegetables, milk and milk products (not a source of iron), eggs, and liver (a rich source of iron) and other organ meats. Also important are whole grain flours, brown rice, and iodized salt (a primary source of iodine).

Water. Water is the nutrient most taken for granted. Without adequate amounts of water, the body would begin to become severely dehydrated. Prolonged inadequacy of water can lead to disruption of the electrolyte balance in the body (see chapter 22). It can also cause digestive disorders (water is necessary to digest and absorb food properly) and circulatory problems (water is the base of blood). The quantity of water necessary for good nutritional status varies with age, but one quart per day is an average recommendation. Since all liquid foods contain high percentages of water, and solid foods have lower but varying water contents, the body's daily water consumption need not be in the pure form.

What are calories?

All foods supply a source of energy to the body in the form of calories. A calorie is "the amount of heat needed to raise the temperature of one gram of water one degree centigrade." The body needs this energy not only to engage in physical exercise but also to sustain vital body functions. Caloric requirements vary with age, body build, sex, and metabolism. During growth periods, adolescent boys often burn 3,000 calories daily. In the later years, when growth has leveled and physical exertion is often minimal, caloric requirements may drop to 1,200–1,500 calories daily. Fats and carbohydrates are generally richer in calories than foods that contain large amounts of proteins and vitamins. When intake of calories exceeds the body's energy requirements, a person tends to gain weight. Conversely, reduced caloric intake will lead to a loss of weight.

An adequate diet requires that a balanced intake of the necessary nutrients is ingested within the recommended number of calories allowed

All foods supply a source of energy to the body in the form of calories.

[7]Nina Cohen and George Briggs. 1968. Trace minerals in nutrition. *American Journal of Nursing* 68:808.
    [8]Ibid.

for a particular person. Some foods produce what are considered "empty calories." They provide low supplies of the essential nutrients but high supplies of calories. These foods, the so-called "junk foods," and sugar are low on the list of priorities in a well-balanced diet.

Adjustments in intake of any or all of the above nutrients may be necessitated by the patient's current nutritional status. Assessment of the patient thus must include not only *what* the patient eats and does not eat but *how* his body reacts to his eating habits. Basically, nutritional status falls into four broad classifications: **adequately nourished, malnourished, underweight,** and **overweight.** The nurse should rely on observation as one of the most effective and reliable tools in determining which of these categories the patient belongs in.

Adequately nourished. An adequately nourished individual can be recognized by the following signs:

1. Weight within the average range for the person's height, age, and sex
2. Good condition of skin, mucous membranes, hair, and teeth
3. Energy to accomplish movements and activities appropriate to the individual's age
4. Lack of unusual degrees of fatigue, nausea, or lethargy

An adequately nourished state implies that the person is eating and digesting an appropriate amount and mixture of the vital nutrients.

Malnourished. A person who is malnourished (poorly nourished) is eating a quantity or composition of food that is inadequate in one or several vital nutrients. Unlike adequate nutritional status, malnourishment is not always easily recognizable. It does not always present itself in the form shown in dramatic newspaper photos: emaciation, distended belly, bulging eyes. The malnourished person may, in fact, be quite obese. Furthermore, the condition is often masked by other problems, such as **alcoholism,** which actually contribute to and aggravate the malnutrition. Alcoholism frequently goes hand in hand with vitamin deficiency, because alcohol replaces food and also interferes with the absorption and conversion of whatever food is eaten.

Specific infections often interact with and mask malnutrition. This is common in groups such as the elderly who live alone, teen-agers, and food faddists. Malnutrition is higher than average among these groups.

Signs of malnutrition may appear as skin infestations, ear and eye disease, bacterial and parasitic infestation, severe anemia, listlessness, and indifference. Retarding effects on growth and mental development also have been linked to malnutrition.[9] The effects vary with the age at which the

An adequately nourished state implies that the person is eating and digesting an appropriate amount and mixture of the vital nutrients.

[9]Patience Wilson. 1972. Iron deficiency anemia. *American Journal of Nursing* 72:502.

malnutrition is experienced. The highest risk are infants who are premature, have a low birth weight, and are born to extremely anemic mothers. Also in the high-risk category are those born with hemolytic problems, such as erythroblastosis fatalis, or with severe infections, or twins or others born in multiple births.[10] In an infant under the age of 2, the effects can be reduced brain size and therefore restricted intellectual development. In a school-age child, malnutrition can reduce learning ability and responsiveness to stimuli.[11]

Overweight and underweight. These conditions are recognizable by observation, but may indicate more than just excessive or inadequate poundage and food intake relative to height, age, and sex. When these conditions exist in severe forms, malnutrition is usually also present. A diet that is inappropriate quantitatively is often also qualitatively inadequate and lacks a proper balance of vital nutrients.

Overweight and underweight and their extreme forms—obesity and emaciation—are complex phenomena with a variety of causes and consequences. Weight above or below the mean may be due to fat, bone, muscle, or fluid variations. The extremes of emaciation or obesity, on the other hand, reflect the amount of **adipose tissue.**

Both extremes endanger life and health. Even moderate obesity may tax the cardiovascular system over a long term. It complicates gall bladder disease, diabetes, and a multitude of other conditions. Extreme obesity may even disturb brain function by compromising adequate oxygen supply to the lungs and, hence, to the brain. Extreme underweight strains the body's ability to rebuild and maintain itself. It can affect all systems and even cause death.

Factors producing malnutrition

Causes of malnutrition are not only numerous but also so interrelated that they often aggravate each other to further impair nutritional status. Some factors prevent a person from eating the proper food **(ingestion),** while others prevent the food from being properly absorbed into the system **(digestion).**

Socioeconomic and education factors. These two factors are perhaps the most widespread causes of malnutrition, for they work against the means and wherewithal to get the proper food. These factors include lack of money to buy nutritious foods and lack of information or education about which foods are important. Social, cultural, or religious strictures against the intake of nutritiously balanced meals are also part of the cycle of

[10] Ibid., p. 503.
[11] Ibid.

malnutrition. It has, in fact, been shown in numerous surveys that malnutrition is inordinately high among migrant workers, lower-class blacks, and other minority ethnic groups.[12] These are people whose employment opportunities and living conditions are inadequate.

Physiological and psychological factors. These include **anorexia, nausea, general malaise,** poor condition of teeth, gums, and mucous membranes, and difficulty in swallowing.

Anorexia is the "lack or loss of the appetite for food, or . . . disinterest in the ingestion of food."[13] Its cause may be physical, as in the case of the person with a head cold, or psychological. Extreme depression or anxiety may lead to loss of appetite. In its extreme form, **anorexia nervosa,** psychologically caused anorexia may lead to emaciation and even death.

Nausea may be brought about by pregnancy, anxiety, drugs, or other factors. It may inhibit a person's desire to eat certain or all foods. If nausea persists, malnutrition may result from long-term food deprivation.

General malaise may make a person too lethargic or apathetic to eat the proper foods or to eat much of anything at all. In such cases, the appetite for food may decrease to the point where so little food is eaten that the individual's nutritional status is threatened.

A person's ability to eat properly balanced meals is also affected by the condition of his teeth, gums, and mucous membranes in the mouth. Inability to chew or pain from chewing will make a person favor foods that are soft and mushy. This means he will not be eating many of the nutritiously rich foods that have a tougher texture and consistency.

Finally, difficulty in swallowing because of throat inflammation may discourage a person from maintaining a proper diet. Pain and difficulty in swallowing may even discourage a person from ingesting anything more than liquids in minimal quantities.

Improper digestion. Once food is eaten, it must be properly digested and absorbed before the body can use the essential nutrients it contains. Proper digestion may be inhibited by decreased **gastrointestinal motility,** drugs, and **vomiting.**

Decreased gastrointestinal motility has a variety of causes. These include stomach or intestinal tract inflammations, dysfunction in gastric secretions or in metabolism, and muscle impairment from paralysis. When gastric motility is decreased, food that is eaten is not broken down into forms necessary for absorption by the body. Some of the vital nutrients may pass right through the system and be excreted without being utilized. In such cases, specific forms of malnutrition may occur, such as **protein** or **calcium deficiency.**

[12]Sarah Crim. 1969. Nutritional problems of the poor. *Nursing Outlook* 17:67.
[13]Cyril M. MacBryde and Robert S. Blacklow. 1970. *Signs and symptoms,* 5th ed., p. 370. Philadelphia: Lippincott.

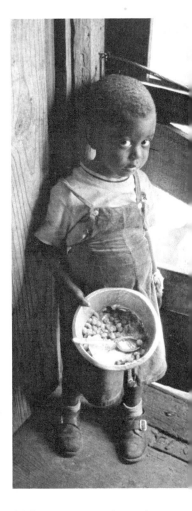

Malnutrition is a widespread problem among lower-class blacks, migrant workers, and other ethnic minorities in the United States.

[Photo by Bruce Davidson from Magnum Photos]

TABLE 19-2
Drugs Known to Cause Vitamin Deficiencies

Deficiency	Drug or Drug Class
Folic acid	Anticonvulsants, contraceptive steroids, methotrexate pyrimethamine, aspirin
B_{12}	Metformin
B_6	INH (isonicotinic hydrazide), thiosemicarbazide, hydralazine, penicillamine, L-dopa
Niacin	INH
Riboflavin	Boric acid*
C	Aspirin, indomethacin, contraceptive steroids
D	Anticonvulsants, diphosphonates?
K	Courmarin anticoagulants, cholestyramine

*Not yet documented in humans.

From Daphne Roe, Drug-induced vitamin deficiencies. *Drug Therapy*, April 1973, p. 32. Reprinted by permission of *Drug Therapy*.

Certain drugs interact with some nutrients and impair their absorption or interfere with their utilization. A person taking these drugs may suffer from specific types of malnutrition as a result. This interrelationship is caused by a series of complex biochemical reactions in which a drug influences the metabolic events in the body at the cellular level. Action at the cellular level affects the concentration of nutrients and their derivatives within the cell. It may also affect the systems essential for the transport and storage of the nutrients.[14] It is necessary, therefore, that compensations be made for those patients who do need specific vitamin-depleting drugs for other problems. See Table 19-2 for an overview of drug-related nutritional problems.

Excessive vomiting, caused by internal or external factors, can result in impaired digestion and nutritive imbalances. Vomiting may be induced by inflammations in the upper digestive tract, muscle or nerve impairments, or allergic reactions to foods.

Planning, implementation, and evaluation

Promoting adequate nutrition

The long-range goal of nutritional planning, implementation, and evaluation is to promote adequate nutrition in the patient. This is true whether the patient has a specific nutritional deficiency problem, general failing health, or relatively good health. It is always appropriate for the nurse to be concerned about and involved with the patient's nutrition.

[14]Betty Taif. 1973. Nutrition, drugs, and vitamins. *Journal of Practical Nursing* 23:16.

The goal of promoting adequate nutrition may be accomplished in several ways. These include dietary counseling, providing a pleasant eating environment, and helping the patient obtain nutritious, palatable food. For patients whose ability to feed themselves is limited by handicaps or illness, specific nursing measures can be used to promote adequate nutrition.

Dietary counseling. The nurse is the health worker most likely to be with the patient at mealtimes. What the patient receives on his tray is not necessarily what he eats. The nurse's attitude toward and understanding of nutritional concepts and principles influence whether and what the patient does, in fact, eat.

For the inpatient, dietary counseling should be planned well in advance of release. Little can be accomplished when the home diet is given just as the patient is ready to leave the hospital and is concerned about his trip home, the medicines he is to take, and his readjustment to normal activities. The process of instruction, in fact, should be part of the daily care of the patient. For example, the diabetic's tray can become at each meal a lesson in the use of the food exchange list. A complaint about unsalted food may provide the nurse with the opportunity to tell about the use of other flavoring aids. Such informal instruction, provided day by day, gives the patient an opportunity to get used to the idea of the diet, to reflect on it, and to ask questions when they occur.[15]

The patient may require guidance on choice and amounts of foods, methods of preparation, kinds of seasonings that may be used, and the number of meals and their timing.[16] Emphasis should be placed on the foods the patient can have, not those that are forbidden. In some instances, however, such as the sodium-restricted diet, it may be desirable also to provide a list of foods that are contraindicated.

Relatives of the patient may also need practical and realistic guidance in applying principles of normal and therapeutic nutrition.[17] The wife or mother of the patient may not understand the reasons for the diet. She may feel that the diet is an imposition, or may not understand how the foods are to be prepared. Therefore, she should be present at the time of instruction. For some patients, it is necessary to plan a food budget and to make arrangements for meals eaten away from home.

The nurse may find printed aids, such as a meal exchange list, useful as a supplement in counseling the patient. Illustrations, posters, and even films are helpful, particularly where group instruction is used for pregnant women, the obese, diabetics, and others.

Creating a pleasant mealtime environment. Helping to create an atmos-

[15]Robinson, p. 391.
[16]Ibid.
[17]Norma Greenler Dison. 1971. *An atlas of nursing techniques,* 2d ed., p. 171. St. Louis: Mosby.

phere that is conducive to digestion is a very basic, though often over-looked, way in which the nurse can help to promote adequate nutrition. Efforts can be made to ensure that at mealtimes the surrounding areas are clean and free of odors and esthetically unpleasant materials. Adequate ventilation should be provided and distracting activities kept to a minimum. Conversation should be pleasant. Patients who are ambulatory may enjoy eating with others. In some hospitals a dining room is provided for them. In others, food service may easily be arranged at small tables set up in the patients' lounge.[18]

The patient should be ready for his meal whether he is in bed or ambulatory. This entails mouth care, washing of hands, and the positioning of the patient so that he can eat in comfort (see chapter 16).

Satisfactory food service. While not the exclusive responsibility of the nurse, food service is yet another area in which she can become involved in order to exercise control. The appearance of the tray is very important if the patient is to eat the food given to him. The nurse can check that it conforms to some of the following basic standards for food service. There should be variations in color, flavor, and texture for sensory appeal. China, silverware, and napkins should be clean and attractively arranged. Portions should not be so large that they spill over. Food should be served at proper temperatures, with hot foods protected by a cover and cold foods served on chilled dishes. Meals should conform to the requirements of the diet order and the patient's preferences.[19]

Helping patients obtain nutritious food. For patients about to leave the hospital or outpatients in a clinic who need special nutritional consideration, the nurse may become involved in suggesting or helping to plan auxiliary food service. Many individuals with physical limitations or with temporarily disabling conditions can remain in their own homes rather than be institutionalized if some provision can be made for their meals. Services such as "meals on wheels" are available in many communities to purchase, prepare, and deliver meals to the homebound. Homemaker services, yet another alternative, adapt to the patient's home facilities in providing nutritiously satisfying meals.

Helping the handicapped patient. When the patient who is hospitalized requires assistance in eating, it is the nurse who is in the best position to provide that assistance. For some patients, it may mean cutting meat or other foods, pouring a beverage, or buttering a piece of toast. Very ill or helpless patients may have to be fed, or devices obtained by which they can feed themselves.

[From *American Journal of Nursing* 75 (April 1975):728. Reprinted by permission of Al Kaufman.]

[18]Robinson, p. 387.
[19]Ibid.

In determining how to assist the handicapped patient in eating, the nurse should consider both the individual's nutritional needs and his physical capacity. In certain situations, special attention must be given to the consistency of food required to overcome the difficulty. When self-feeding or assistance in feeding solid foods is impossible because of illness, the patient may require liquid feedings through a **nasogastric tube** or a **gastrostomy.** The nurse should give the same attention to this patient's environment and food needs as to those of the patient who is able to eat normally.

Prior to tube feeding, the nurse should give oral care to the patient to help prevent nausea. If the nurse passes the tube just prior to the tube feeding, the patient should be allowed to rest before the feeding is begun. If the tube is withdrawn following feeding, oral care may do much to promote comfort. Unless contraindicated, the patient should be encouraged to assist in the plans for and in the execution of these techniques.[20]

The **intubation** itself may be done by the physician or a skilled technician. In many cases, however, it is the nurse who carries out the procedure. Every effort should be made to explain to the patient what and why it is being done. He should know whether it is necessary for therapeutic reasons when normal eating is impossible, for laboratory studies, for irrigation or cleansing of the stomach, or for decompression of the stomach. In the case of premature or otherwise underdeveloped infants who require tube or bulb feeding because of insufficient sucking strength, reassurance to parents is important.

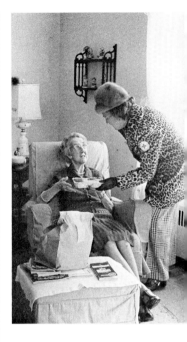

Those unable to prepare meals for themselves may be served by "meals on wheels" or similar programs. Here, a Red Cross volunteer serves an elderly homebound client.

[Photo by Sybil Shelton from Monkmeyer Press Photo Service]

Helping the patient maintain adequate nutrition

Promoting good nutrition goes beyond providing the patient with the wherewithal to eat while under the watchful eye of the nurse and other health care workers. In order for the patient to maintain adequate nutrition, his food habits must often change to some degree. Old habits die hard. Food habits, which are closely linked to culture, religion, socioeconomic background, and emotional factors, are particularly hard to alter.

The patient must have motivation, understanding, and knowledge about the purpose and characteristics of the recommended new diet. He must also have the means to adapt the new diet to past and present nutritional habits. Without a consideration of all these patient requirements, any attempt to change the patient's eating habits is bound to be unsuccessful.

Motivation. People eat for a lot of different reasons, both physical and psychological. The patient must be motivated to want to improve his

[20]Dison, pp. 171–72.

physical condition through a change in eating habits. This may involve weight loss or gain or the restriction or addition of certain foods.

The nurse may be the one person who is able to promote proper motivation in a patient, whether in the home or the hospital. The nurse's patience, tact, kindness, and firmness can become the means by which the patient accepts new food patterns.[21] The nurse must work not only to bolster the morale and motivation of the patient but those of the patient's family as well. It is they who provide the long-term support necessary for the maintenance of proper food habits.

Expanding the patient's understanding and knowledge. Many illnesses, such as infections, injuries, and metabolic disturbances, lead to nutritional deficiencies even in persons who otherwise possess good nutritional status. The individual may be unable to ingest sufficient food, or the disease process may impose greatly increased demands for most, if not all, of the nutrients.[22] Thus, during times of illness, the patient may need an enriched or regulated diet in order to help shorten the period of convalescence. In diabetes or **phenylketonuria,** a modified diet is *the* principal therapeutic agent for regulating the condition. In other cases, the diet therapy serves to support an overall therapeutic program. Not following the diet may work against whatever gains are made through medication or other therapy.

Adapting the diet to past and present nutritional habits. Cultural, religious, ethnic, and economic patterns need not be discredited in order to incorporate new food requirements into the diet. Rather, friendly persuasion and sound knowledge can help the nurse in gaining the patient's acceptance of new food habits.

New food habits may involve reducing the intake of sodium or the consumption of alcohol. Protein and vitamin consumption may have to be increased. No matter what their nature, modifications in anyone's present diet can be suggested that will not radically alter the taste or palatability of a total meal. Finding the proper food substitutes often is simply a matter of ingenuity combined with a small helping of creativity.

SUMMARY

Nutrition is an important component of total patient care. How and what a person eats determine in large measure how he feels, acts, and reacts. Nutritional needs are determined by a complex variety of factors. These include age and individual patterns and preferences based on psychological

[21]Mary Louise Manning. 1965. The psychodynamics of dietetics. *Nursing Outlook* 13. Reprinted in *Nursing fundamentals,* ed. Mary E. Meyers, p. 181. Dubuque, Iowa: Brown, 1967.
[22]Robinson, p. 382.

factors and cultural, religious, and socioeconomic pressures. Also important are hunger and appetite and current nutritional status, be it adequately nourished, malnourished, underweight, or overweight.

Adequate nutritional status is the goal to be attained, and depends on a balanced intake of the vital nutrients. A diet that is unbalanced or inadequate in one or several of the vital nutrients leads to a multitude of problems. Malnutrition may be caused by poor eating habits or problems with ingestion or digestion. These may be triggered by psychological factors or by physical problems, such as general malaise, poor condition of teeth and gums, difficulty in swallowing, or decreased gastrointestinal motility. External factors, such as the ingestion of drugs, may inhibit the proper absorption of food and result in malnutrition as well.

Nutritional planning, implementation, and evaluation for a patient with or without specific nutritional problems is aimed at promoting adequate nutrition. The nurse's role in achieving this goal involves providing dietary counseling, ensuring a pleasant environment for eating and appropriate food service, and helping a semihelpless or helpless patient feed himself. Beyond the immediate needs of the patient for attaining adequate nutritional status is the long-range need to acquire or maintain good food habits.

STUDY QUESTIONS

1. How do nutritional requirements change during the life cycle?
2. Briefly describe the factors, other than age, which influence a person's eating habits.
3. What is hunger? What is appetite?
4. What are the nutrients that make up a balanced diet? Describe the function of each.
5. How can a nurse determine if a patient is adequately nourished, malnourished, underweight, or overweight? Give a brief description of the characteristics of each condition.
6. In what ways can the nurse encourage her patients to maintain good nutritional habits?

SELECTED BIBLIOGRAPHY

Crim, Sarah. 1969. Nutritional problems of the poor. *Nursing Outlook* 17:65–67.

Manning, Mary Louise. 1965. The psychodynamics of dietetics. *Nursing Outlook* 13. Reprinted in *Nursing fundamentals,* ed. Mary E. Meyers, pp. 174–81. Dubuque, Iowa: Brown, 1967.

Mayer, Jean. 1968. *Overweight: Causes, cost, and control.* Englewood Cliffs, N.J.: Prentice-Hall.

Robinson, Corinne H. 1972. *Normal and therapeutic nutrition,* 14th ed. New York: Macmillan.

Star, Jack. 1973. Why you choose the foods you do. *Today's Health* 51:32–37.

20 Meeting respiratory and circulatory needs

Upon completing this chapter, the reader should be able to:

1. Identify six requirements for adequate respiration and the related anatomy and physiology for each.

2. Identify and describe eight criteria for respiratory assessment.

3. Relate two environmental factors that affect respiration to specific nursing interventions.

4. Discuss six measures that aid ventilation.

5. State, in order, the signs and symptoms of respiratory and cardiac arrest and identify the related resuscitation procedures for each.

Assessment of respiratory needs

Requirements for adequate respiration

Adequate **respiration** depends on several factors, which are discussed briefly below.[1]

Suitable oxygen and carbon dioxide concentrations in the inspired air. Both oxygen and carbon dioxide move by diffusion from areas of greater pressure to areas of lower pressure. The difference in pressure between **ambient** (atmospheric) and **alveolar** (lung) air determines the movement of air into the airway passages. When the lungs expand during **inspiration,** the pressure within them decreases. As a result, air moves in. When the lungs are full, the resulting rise in pressure forces the air out **(expiration).** With each breath in and out, we are using 300 to 500 ml of air. This volume is called the **tidal volume.** Inspired air contains approximately 20.95 percent oxygen, 0.04 percent carbon dioxide, and 79 percent nitrogen.

Blood entering the capillaries of the lungs has an **oxygen tension** of 40 mm Hg. (Oxygen tension is the relationship between the amount of oxygen and the pressure under which it is contained.) Since the resulting pressure is lower than that in the alveoli, the oxygen moves from the alveoli into the blood.

Normally, the carbon dioxide tension within the alveoli is 40 mm Hg. Adjustments to the carbon dioxide tension can be made by the body's homeostatic mechanisms, particularly if these adjustments can be made gradually. Among the methods the body uses to adjust the carbon dioxide tension are an increase in the rate and depth of breathing, acceleration of the heart and circulatory action, and an increase in red cell production.

Adequate ventilation. **Ventilation** is the term used to describe the exchange that takes place in the lungs between the ambient and the alveolar

---

[1]Mary Early. 1971. The gaseous exchange process: Nursing implications. In Kay Corman Kintzel, ed., *Advanced concepts in clinical nursing,* pp. 207–12. Philadelphia: Lippincott.

air. The result is that air containing a higher concentration of oxygen (ambient air) is substituted for that containing a higher concentration of carbon dioxide (alveolar air). Because the body has a very limited ability to store oxygen, adequate ventilation is vital. An inadequate supply of oxygen **(hypoxia)** can cause severe and sometimes irreparable damage to the brain, kidneys, and other vital organs. Total lack of oxygen, which leads inevitably to death, is called **anoxia.**

Permeable alveolar-capillary membranes. The exchange between oxygen and carbon dioxide takes place in what is known as the **pulmonary unit.** The membrane covering this area, which includes the respiratory bronchiole, alveolar duct, atria, and the alveolar sac, is very thin. This means that the gases in the inspired air are able to come into close contact with the capillaries, permitting easy diffusion. If the quality of this membrane is altered, the exchange process will be hampered. Among the conditions that affect the membrane are pneumonia and emphysema.

Adequate pulmonary and systemic circulation. Since both oxygen and carbon dioxide are transported by the blood, the maintenance of an effective circulatory system is essential. The circulatory system carries the oxygen-rich blood from the lungs to the heart and then throughout the body, providing nourishment for the cells. When the oxygen has been converted into energy and other elements **(oxidation),** the resulting carbon dioxide is then transported back to the lungs, to be released with the expired air.

Ability of the blood to transport oxygen and carbon dioxide between lungs and tissues. Most of the oxygen in the blood is carried by the red blood cells. The amount of oxygen that can be transported is directly related to the number of red blood cells and the **hemoglobin** level within them. When the oxygen has been used by the cells, hemoglobin then transports the resultant carbon dioxide. Any condition that lowers the number of red blood cells or the hemoglobin level will therefore reduce the amount of oxygen that can be transported to the tissues. Carbon monoxide poisoning is one such condition. In this case, the carbon monoxide combines with the hemoglobin to prevent the desired oxygen-hemoglobin combination.

Ability of the cells to use oxygen and eliminate carbon dioxide. The amount of oxygen used by the cells is dependent upon the amount available in the blood and the demands made by the body. These demands are particularly heavy during periods of strenuous exercise. The amount of oxygen given up by the blood and the resulting oxygen pressure level are regulated primarily by the hemoglobin. Too low a level can lead to starvation of the cells, while too high a level can lead to **oxygen poisoning.**

Observation is one of
the most vital tools in
the assessment of
respiratory function.

Common causes of respiratory problems

Pulmonary. As was described above, the most important function of the
pulmonary unit is ventilation, or the exchange of oxygen and carbon
dioxide. In order for this exchange to take place, sufficient air must reach
the lungs. One of the most common causes of inadequate ventilation is
a blockage in the airway. The airway may be blocked by disease or by
a bolus of food or by some other obstruction.

The capacity of the lungs to expand and contract is also a vital factor
in maintaining adequate ventilation. If he is suffering pain as a result of
thoracic or upper abdominal surgery, the patient will tend to take short,
shallow breaths **(hypoventilation).** This may result in poor ventilation.
Emphysema also affects the elasticity of the lungs. In this condition, the
alveoli remain expanded, so the patient is unable to expel a normal amount
of air from his lungs. Consequently, he is unable to take in an adequate
supply of oxygen-rich air.

Cardiovascular. The supply of oxygen to the tissues is directly dependent
upon the circulation of the blood. The amount of blood that circulates,
known as **cardiac output,** is a vital factor in respiration. Any decrease in
the cardiac output leads to a corresponding decrease in the amount of
oxygen available to the cells. Arteriosclerosis and mitral stenosis are two
conditions that lead to a reduction in cardiac output. The flow of blood
may also be impeded by the presence of a clot.

Criteria for respiratory assessment

Observation is one of the most vital tools in the assessment of respiratory function. Listed below are some of the factors the nurse should take
into account during the assessment process.[2]

Rate. Any change in the normal respiratory rate may be a sign of distress.
The normal rate of respiration for an adult is 12 to 18 breaths per minute.
Children generally take about 20 breaths per minute, and up to 44 breaths
per minute is not uncommon in infants. A faster than normal rate is known
as **tachypnea.** A slower rate is called **bradypnea.**

Type. As was stated earlier, we normally take respiration for granted. This
is because normal respiration is a passive, regular process that is virtually
effortless and noiseless. Labored or forced respiration can be brought about
by physiological or psychological causes. A common form of labored
breathing is **dyspnea.** The patient with dyspnea is acutely aware of the
process of breathing itself, finds it difficult, and has a persistent, unsatisfied
need for air. He may complain that he is "suffocating."

[2]Kurihara, pp. 68–69.

Rhythm. The principal muscle used for inspiration is the diaphragm, while the abdominal muscles play the major role in expiration. The maintenance of a normal, steady rhythm of respiration depends upon the interplay of these two sets of muscles. Also important is the ability of the lungs and the thorax to expand. This expandability is called compliance. One of the most common forms of **arrhythmia** in breathing is called **Cheyne-Stokes breathing.** This is often caused by cardiac failure. In Cheyne-Stokes, episodes of very deep breathing alternate with episodes of very shallow breathing, or even complete cessation of breathing **(apnea).**

Excursion of the chest. The **excursion** of the chest is its expansion and subsequent return to normal position. Ordinarily, these excursions are deep and even. Rapid, shallow excursions may be a sign of inadequate ventilation.

Abnormal sounds. Four common abnormal chest sounds are **rales, rhonchi, wheezes,** and **pleural friction rubs.** The sound of rales is similar to the fizzing sound of a carbonated beverage. They are heard most commonly on inspiration, and may be the result of lobar pneumonia, bronchitis, or chronic obstructive lung disease. Wheezes, which are high-pitched, continuous sounds, originate in the smaller air passages. Rhonchi, which are lower pitched, originate in the larger air passages. They may be heard during both inspiration and expiration, but are more obvious during expiration. Bronchitis and chronic obstructive lung disease are common causes. Pleural friction rubs are loud grating sounds that are heard during both inspiration and expiration. They are the result of an inflammation of the pleura.

Relationship between inspiration and expiration. In the normal adult, inspiration lasts 1 to 1.5 seconds, while expiration takes 2 to 3 seconds. In patients with chronic obstructive lung disease, such as pulmonary emphysema or chronic bronchitis, the expiration phase is lengthened. As a result, the patient's chest overexpands, trapping the air, and his breathing becomes shallow.

Color. The presence of cyanosis is an indication of respiratory insufficiency, although it may not always accompany this condition. Cyanosis is most easily observed in the lips, tongue, mucous membranes, and nail beds.

Diagnostic tests

X-ray. Of the battery of tests available for the diagnosis of respiratory function, the most important is X-ray examination of the chest. For a routine chest X-ray, no special preparation of the patient is called for. Nor is special attention needed for the patient undergoing **fluoroscopy,** a

Of the battery of tests available for the diagnosis of respiratory function, the most important is X-ray examination of the chest.

procedure that permits observation of the movements of the chest, heart, and lungs. However, for a **bronchogram,** the patient is asked not to eat breakfast, and he is given a sedative and atropine before examination.

A bronchogram involves the injection of small amounts of iodized oil into the bronchial tubes so that the outline of the tubes can be seen. In order to prevent coughing and gagging when the oil tube is inserted, the patient is given a local anesthetic in the nose and pharynx. He should receive nothing by mouth until the anesthetic has worn off.

Pulmonary function. Analysis of pulmonary function includes a wide range of studies, for example, measurement of gas volumes and capacities and chemical analyses of pulmonary and blood gases. These studies are vital in the diagnosis and treatment of cardiopulmonary diseases. Some may be carried out directly by the nurse, while in mass screening centers or physicians' offices, she usually assists only.

Direct visualization. **Bronchoscopy** is a diagnostic procedure in which a bronchoscope is inserted through the pharynx and trachea into the bronchus. It is done in order to view diseased areas and possible tumors, to obtain tissue for biopsy, and for the aspiration and study of secretions. The patient undergoing the procedure should take nothing by mouth for at least 6 hours beforehand. If he has dentures, they should be removed; then morphine sulfate or a similar drug is administered a half hour before the procedure. Afterward, he should be given nothing by mouth until the local anesthetic has worn off.

In the procedure called **thoracentesis,** chest fluid is aspirated and then subjected to laboratory studies. This procedure aids in the diagnosis of some inflammatory and neoplastic diseases of the lungs. Thoracentesis is performed with the patient in a sitting position, and sterile technique is used. A local anesthetic precedes insertion of the thoracentesis needle.

Sputum. Management of diseases of the respiratory system frequently requires collection of sputum for analysis. The sample should be taken in the morning, before the patient eats. In the procedure, the patient coughs up material from the bronchi or lungs and spits into a sputum cup. A satisfactory specimen is obtained more easily if the patient is turned to a lateral position with one arm over the head or turned on the unaffected side with the foot of the bed slightly elevated. At least one teaspoonful of sputum is needed for analysis.

Blood. Blood tests used in diagnosing diseases of the respiratory system include blood culture, sedimentation rate, blood-urea nitrogen, and uric acid. Patients undergoing these tests can eat breakfast. They should not eat breakfast before the following blood tests: icterux index, direct van Bergh, plasma protein, and nonprotein nitrogen.

Skin. There are three types of skin tests used in analysis of respiratory function: intracutaneous injection, scratch tests, and patch tests. Their purpose is to help in diagnosing pulmonary tuberculosis and to determine causes of bronchial asthma. Using the intracutaneous method, old tuberculin or purified protein derivative is injected intracutaneously. In the Mantoux test, frequently called the PPD test, a solution containing purified protein derivative is injected intracutaneously.

Promoting adequate respiration—planning, implementation, and evaluation

Environmental factors

Smoking. Smokers endanger not only their own health but also that of others (see chapter 13). Recently, it has been discovered that the effects of cigarette smoking are more lethal than those of air pollution. Indeed, the amount of carbon monoxide produced by smoking one cigarette is about 100 times greater than that found in the heaviest air pollution.[3] As was indicated on p. 367, carbon monoxide will block the ability of the hemoglobin to combine with oxygen.

Pollution. Chronic bronchitis is the main disease associated with air pollution. This condition can progress to disabling breathlessness and, ultimately, to death from respiratory or cardiac failure. Disturbances to the bronchi, bronchioles, and lung tissue produced by this disease result in impairment of the normal gas-exchange function of the lung.

People with asthma are more sensitive than others to irritants in the air. The incidence of pneumonia and other acute chest infections is greater in polluted cities than in rural areas. Chest infections recur more frequently among children living in highly polluted areas.

Physical factors

Positioning. Proper positioning of the patient is important from a therapeutic as well as a comfort point of view (see chapter 18). Many patients with respiratory disease find themselves short of breath after straining themselves, exercising vigorously, or after an acute episode of their condition. The nurse should assist these patients to assume positions and use patterns of breathing that promote adequate ventilation and encourage relaxation. Her main objective is to find a position that uses a minimum of the patient's energies for anything other than breathing.[4]

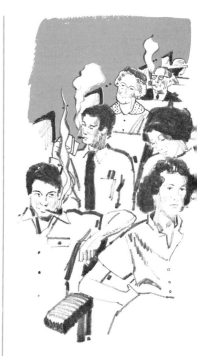

Smokers endanger not only their own health but also that of others.

[3]Stanley Freedman. 1972. Air pollution and chest diseases. *District Nursing* 15:195.
[4]Marcia Wasenius Rie. 1968. Physical therapy in the nursing care of respiratory disease patients. *Nursing Clinics of North America* 3:471–75.

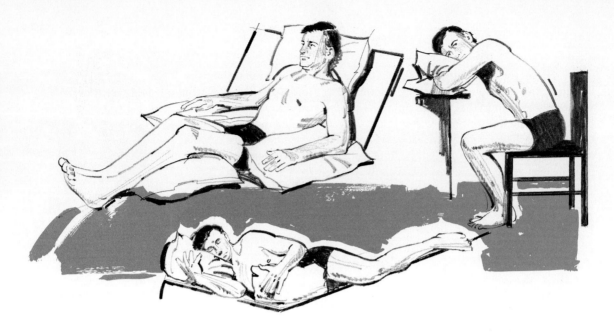

FIG. 20-1 *Relaxation positions for supervised and independent breathing exercises.*

Deep breathing. In order to encourage the patient to breathe deeply, the nurse places her hands just below the costal margin. If she exerts firm, gentle pressure on the abdominal wall, she will feel the abdomen expand as the patient inhales. If she presses her hands firmly against this same area during exhalation, she may help the patient exhale more completely.[5] The same technique will support him during coughing. Some patients will be more comfortable with a book or pillow held against the abdomen.

The nurse instructs the patient to inhale through his nose and to exhale through his mouth, partially closing his lips to maintain a small opening. During practice or controlled breathing, the inhalation phase should be slow, followed by a somewhat longer exhaling phase. When the patient is just beginning his breathing lessons and has not achieved control, the nurse might instruct him in how to pant. Panting provides a more relaxed way of breathing than does gasping for air.[6]

Coughing. An extremely important aspect of caring for the postoperative patient is to encourage him to bring up secretions by coughing. This will help him avoid such complications as pulmonary collapse and pneumonia. Unfortunately, this procedure is very painful for the patient, and so the nurse must encourage him and make him aware of the importance of what he is doing.

There are two basic techniques used in stimulating patients to cough: direct external mechanical stimulation of the trachea, and internal mechanical stimulation following prolonged exhalation. In the event these two methods fail, the physician may order **endotracheal intubation.**

[5] Norma Greenler Dison. 1971. *An atlas of nursing techniques,* 2d ed., pp. 79–82. St. Louis: Mosby.
[6] Rie, p. 475.

372

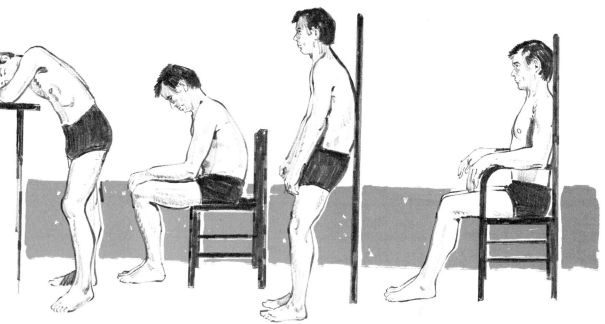

The direct mechanical technique, perhaps easiest to perform, demands firm, steady pressure during the up and down movement of the finger over the trachea. The irritation caused by this movement brings on the cough reflex. In the second technique, internal stimulation, the patient must be encouraged to expire forcefully all inhaled air slowly over a prolonged period. This technique is learned only with practice, sometimes with the aid of blow bottles or paper bags. When both methods fail, the nurse may consider endotracheal stimulation with a catheter.[7]

Splinting. If the patient has had an incision, efforts to make him cough should be preceded by **splinting** to support the incision. This may be accomplished by several techniques. It may be done manually or by placing a pillow against the area or by tightening a drawsheet over the area.

Humidification. **Humidifiers** are used to provide moisture when a patient is receiving high concentrations of oxygen by mask for extended periods. They are also needed when oxygen is administered by a catheter or nasoinhaler. The moisture they provide is necessary because oxygen is a dry gas that can irritate the mucous membranes.

Oxygen therapy

A patient requires oxygen when the oxygen in his blood cannot be maintained at an acceptable level of tension, for example, above 500 mm Hg. This lack of oxygen is corrected by the addition of oxygen to inhaled air, enabling the blood to be oxygenated more easily.

[7]Peter Ungvarski. 1971. Mechanical stimulation of coughing. *American Journal of Nursing* 71:2358–61.

A patient requires oxygen when the oxygen in his blood cannot be maintained at an acceptable level of tension.

In some institutions, administration of oxygen is the nurse's responsibility, while in others it is undertaken by an **inhalation therapist.** In the latter instance, it is still the nurse's responsibility to understand aspects of safety, comfort, and therapy so that she can give intelligent and sensitive patient care.[8]

Nasal cannula. The **nasal cannula,** or **nasoinhaler,** consists of plastic or metal tubes that are inserted about $\frac{1}{4}$ to $\frac{1}{2}$ inch into the nostrils. This procedure is used when oxygen concentrations up to 35 percent are needed.[9] The cannula is connected to an oxygen source, placed in the nose, and held in place by straps. Tubing should not block the nostrils, or else the patient will have to breathe through his mouth. This lowers the concentration of oxygen by mixing it with room air.[10]

Nasal catheter. This apparatus is used most often when concentrations up to 50 percent are needed. A **nasal catheter** makes it easier to examine the patient and to provide nursing care. The patient has more freedom of movement, too, although the catheter may irritate his mucous membranes.[11]

Before inserting the catheter, the nurse lubricates it lightly with petroleum jelly or a nonflammable lubricant. If her hands contain any oily material, she must thoroughly wash them before touching the oxygen regulator. When she can see the tip of the catheter behind the uvula, she withdraws it about 1 cm and then regulates the flow of oxygen.[12]

Mask. Use of the face mask permits high concentrations of oxygen to be reached almost at once and maintained over a long period. It is often applied in an emergency situation. Either a partial rebreathing mask or a nonrebreathing mask is used; the clinical technique is similar. When a humidifier is used, the nurse fills it with distilled water, attaches the mask to an oxygen supply, and adjusts the flow.

The mask is positioned first over the bridge of the nose and then over the mouth. The retaining straps should fit securely but not too tightly over the face. When the patient is breathing normally, the reservoir bag collapses completely. Both mask and skin should be attended to every hour or two.[13]

Face tent. When a **face tent** is used to increase oxygen concentration, it is connected to the oxygen supply with tubing. When it is used to supply

[8] Audrey L. Sutton. 1969. *Bedside nursing techniques in medicine and surgery,* 2d ed., p. 30. Philadelphia: Saunders.

[9] Ibid., p. 39.

[10] Dison, p. 90.

[11] Sutton, p. 36.

[12] Dison, p. 91.

[13] Sutton, p. 39.

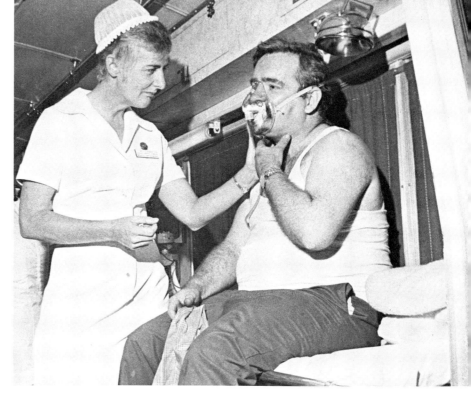

A face mask is often used to administer oxygen in emergency situations.

Photo by Tyrone Dukes, courtesy the *New York Times*

mist, the humidifier is filled with distilled water and the volume of mist flowing through the tube is checked visually. The patient may prefer to hold the face tent in place himself.[14]

Oxygen tents. The **oxygen tent** is helpful when the patient is too restless, confused, or uncooperative for other methods. Before placing the patient in the tent, the nurse must reassure him and explain the procedure. Positioning the tent near the head of the bed, she folds the top linen to waist level, turns on the air conditioner of the machine, and sets the temperature control.

After lifting the canopy carefully over the patient, she arranges the lower edge around his thighs, places a folded bath blanket over the lower edge of the tent skirt, and tucks it under the mattress. It is important to make sure the canopy is properly tucked in; otherwise oxygen will escape.

The nurse should flush the tent with oxygen for at least 1 full minute each time she administers care through the zippered openings. When the patient is under the tent for extended periods, she should move the skirt of the canopy to the patient's upper chest.[15]

Assisted ventilation (IPPB)

A respirator is either external or airway applied. The airway-applied respirator, which has many uses, is called the **intermittent positive pres-**

[14]Dison, p. 87.
[15]Ibid., p. 91.

A patient with a
tracheostomy is
especially prone to
infections.

sure-breathing apparatus, or the IPPB unit.[16] The process is referred to
as **assisted ventilation.**

There are two types of IPPB therapy, intermittent and continuous. In
intermittent therapy, inflation of the lungs is controlled while medication
or humidification is delivered at the same time. The equipment is fairly
simple to use. A number of models are available commercially, each one
varying somewhat in operation. In each, the patient sits up and breathes
into a respirator by means of a mask or a mouthpiece.

Continuous IPPB therapy is used in conditions where ventilation is
inadequate, such as respiratory arrest or severe respiratory acidosis. This
treatment is also known as "controlled" or "assisted" ventilation. A special
adjustment allows the machine to turn itself on without any effort on the
patient's part. If the unit must be used continuously for longer than one
day, the patient receives a tracheotomy tube. In this case, equipment must
be sterilized in order to prevent infection.

Intubation and suctioning

Tracheostomy. Patients with acute respiratory insufficiency may require
artificial ventilation via a **tracheostomy.** A tracheostomy is the formation
of an opening into the trachea. This procedure facilitates the aspiration
of secretions.

A patient with a tracheostomy is especially prone to infections. He
is also subject to blockage of the airway, since he is no longer able to cough
up his own secretions. The inner cannula of the tracheostomy tube must
be removed periodically for cleaning, using aseptic techniques. This prevents the introduction of large numbers of microorganisms into the airway.

A tracheostomy tube with a built-in inflatable cuff is often used now
on adult patients. When inflated, the cuff expands to fill the entire airway.
This ensures that no oxygen is lost through leakage, since the average adult
trachea is larger than the diameter of most tracheostomy tubes. (Such cuffs
are not needed for infants and children, whose tracheas are completely
filled by the tubes.) Although the cuff is valuable in sealing the airway,
the pressure it places on the wall of the trachea can lead to necrosis,
ulceration, tracheoesophageal fistula, and tracheomalacia. The pressure
therefore must be carefully monitored. One way to reduce this pressure
is to soften and stretch the cuff before it is inserted.[17]

Suctioning. Since the tracheostomy patient is not able to cough, **suctioning**
is necessary in order to remove accumulated secretions. Although the
procedure is accomplished very quickly (no more than 15 seconds per
aspiration), it is nonetheless uncomfortable and often frightening for the

[16]Sutton, p. 55.
[17]Helen A. White. 1972. Tracheostomy: Care with a cuffed tube. *American Journal of
Nursing* 72:75–77.

patient. It is important, therefore, that the nurse carefully explain the procedure to the patient before beginning work.

The suctioning procedure requires the use of a sterile catheter and gloves. The catheter is inserted into the tracheostomy tube as far as possible and then withdrawn 1 or 2 cm. Intermittent suction is applied while the catheter is rotated and removed at the same time. After no more than 15 seconds, the patient is reconnected to the ventilator or bag for several breaths. The procedure is then repeated until all secretions have been removed.[18]

When the suctioning procedure has been completed, the inner cannula is removed and soaked in a cleansing solution. It is then replaced in the other cannula and locked in place.

The skin around the tracheostomy must also be cared for to prevent irritation and infection. A bib dressing may be made by folding a 4″ × 8″ piece of gauze lengthwise and then into a V shape. Or a gauze dressing may be split to approximately $1\frac{1}{2}$ inches. The dressing is then positioned beneath the tie tapes and the flange of the tubes. It is also important to change the tie tapes when they become soiled.[19]

Postural drainage

Postural drainage is an effective technique for removing secretions from the peripheral areas of the lungs. (These secretions cannot be removed by suctioning.) The patient is first taught deep breathing techniques, stressing maximum expansion of the chest. He is then positioned according to the area from which the secretions are to be drained. Two positions are commonly used: leaning over the side of the bed or lying in a prone position on a gatch bed. Once the proper position has been assumed, there are two major techniques the nurse can use to loosen the accumulated secretions—**percussion** (clapping) and **vibration.**

Percussion (clapping). Percussion, or clapping, involves cupping the hands and then striking the chest wall over the area to be drained. When properly done, percussion produces a hollow sound. It is not painful to the patient. Percussion is generally carried on for a 2-minute period and is then followed by vibration and coughing.

Vibration. Vibration is performed while the patient exhales. The nurse presses the patient's thorax downward with the flat of her hands, after tensing all hand and arm muscles. After the patient exhales, the pressure is released and the patient then inhales. Vibration usually takes place over a period of four to five breaths. The patient should then be encouraged

[18] Ibid.
[19] Dison, p. 116.

It is important to resuscitate the patient as soon as the symptoms of cardiac arrest become evident.

to cough, thereby bringing up the loosened secretions. After a brief rest, the whole procedure is repeated until no more secretions are produced.[20]

Cardiopulmonary resuscitation

Signs and symptoms of respiratory arrest. **Respiratory arrest,** which may result from ineffective treatment or some blockage of the airway, generally begins with short, shallow breathing. As failure progresses, the patient's breathing becomes more and more labored. He appears flushed, is restless and disoriented, and feels as though he is suffocating. Eventually, his blood pressure and pulse rate fall and he will go into **cardiac arrest.** There are three major steps the nurse should take to prevent this sequence of events from taking place:

1. Maintain an open airway.
2. Assist ventilation by the use of a respirator or a self-inflating bag-valve-mask unit.
3. Call for help. If the patient's pupils become dilated, it may be necessary to begin cardiac resuscitation while waiting for the doctor to arrive.[21]

Signs and symptoms of cardiac arrest. Cardiac arrest may be the result of many factors, but the most common is anoxia. It is characterized by the absence of pulse, blood pressure, and heartbeat. Spontaneous respiration stops, and the patient's pupils dilate. Clinical death will occur within 20 to 40 seconds of cardiac arrest, but irreversible damage to the heart and brain may not take place for 4 to 6 minutes. It is therefore important to resuscitate as soon as the symptoms of cardiac arrest become evident.

Resuscitation techniques

Artificial ventilation. The goal of all resuscitation efforts is to provide adequate ventilation and effective circulation of the oxygenated blood. The following steps should be taken to restore ventilation:

1. Provide an adequate airway. The patient's mouth should be opened and the pharynx examined for obstructions. It may be necessary to suction if secretions are blocking the airway.
2. Extend the neck and insert an oropharyngeal airway, if available. The mouth-to-mouth or mouth-to-nose technique may also be used, but the artificial airway method is preferable. It is also more efficient to use a self-refilling bag, especially in cases where the patient may have an infectious disease.
3. Ventilation should be performed 10 to 15 times per minute.[22]

[20] Georgia Foss. 1973. Postural drainage. *American Journal of Nursing* 73:666–69.
[21] Kurihara, p. 72.
[22] George M. Callard and James R. Jude. 1972. Cardiopulmonary resuscitation in the cardiac care unit. *Nursing Clinics of North America* 7:571.

A technique called the **Heimlich maneuver** is especially valuable in cases where the victim has food or some other object lodged in his throat. The victim should be approached from behind. The nurse grasps him around the waist under the rib cage and makes fists with both her hands. She then hugs the victim tightly, pressing her fists sharply against his diaphragm. This forces the trapped air out of the victim's lungs. The pressure created will dislodge the obstruction in the same manner as popping a cork from a bottle.

Artificial circulation. Once the patient begins breathing on his own, the nurse should initiate **artificial circulation** by using external cardiac compression. With the patient lying on a hard surface, she places the heel of one hand over the lower half of the sternum. The other hand is then placed over the first. Keeping her arms extended vertically, she depresses the patient's sternum $1\frac{1}{2}$ to 2 inches. The sternum should be depressed for about half a second and then released. The compression procedure should be repeated 60 to 80 times per minute.[23]

SUMMARY

The respiratory system is a complicated one that depends on several factors. These include the need for suitable oxygen and carbon dioxide concentrations in the air and the ability of the cells to utilize this oxygen and eliminate the carbon dioxide.

Ventilation is the exchange between oxygen and carbon dioxide that takes place in the lungs. When ventilation is not sufficient to eliminate carbon dioxide, pulmonary complications result. Other physiological disturbances also affect respiratory function.

Both physical and environmental factors affect respiration. Smoking and air pollution are harmful to everyone, but particularly to patients with respiratory disease. The nurse can play an active role in encouraging awareness of the dangers of these pollutants.

Proper positioning is not only more comfortable for the patient but it also aids his ventilation. Deep breathing exercises are also an important part of respiratory care. The induction of coughing to bring up secretions, a painful but vital procedure, can be encouraged by several techniques. When the patient has had an incision, the incision is supported by splinting before coughing is induced.

Oxygen therapy is a form of respiratory intervention that is frequently assumed by the nurse. Oxygen can be administered in one of several ways: via nasal cannula, nasal catheter, face or oxygen mask, or oxygen tent. The purpose is to add oxygen to inhaled air, thus allowing the blood to be oxygenated more easily.

[23] Ibid., p. 576.

Assisted ventilation, or intermittent positive pressure breathing, is used in many conditions where ventilation must be aided mechanically. There are two types of IPPB therapy—intermittent and continuous. A number of equipment models are available for each.

Sometimes a patient with acute respiratory insufficiency will require a tracheostomy to aid ventilation and the aspiration of secretions. When a tracheostomy tube is used, the nurse must be extremely careful to observe aseptic procedures. When suctioning is necessary to remove accumulated secretions, sterile techniques are also observed.

Postural drainage is necessary when the patient is unable to expel secretions frequently and therefore risks infection. The procedure involves placing the patient in a suitable position and clapping him on the chest wall. With a shaking movement of the hand, called vibration, the nurse then presses the patient's thorax downward as he exhales.

Impending respiratory or cardiac arrest is recognized by a number of symptoms. The resuscitation procedure includes artificial ventilation, initially mouth-to-mouth or mouth-to-nose, then artificial circulation by external cardiac compression. Frequently, the nurse either supervises resuscitation or carries it out herself.

STUDY QUESTIONS

1. What are the essential components of adequate respiration? Briefly describe the function of each.
2. What is ventilation? Where and how does it take place?
3. Define four of the criteria used in the assessment of respiration.
4. What is oxygen therapy? Briefly describe the techniques commonly used in this treatment.
5. What is the purpose of postural drainage? Describe this procedure.
6. What are the symptoms of respiratory failure? of cardiac arrest? What should the nurse do to prevent or relieve these conditions?

SELECTED BIBLIOGRAPHY

Callard, George M., and Jude, James R. 1972. Cardiopulmonary resuscitation in the cardiac care unit. *Nursing Clinics of North America* 7:573–85.

Early, Mary. 1971. The gaseous exchange process: Nursing implications. In Kay Corman Kintzel, ed., *Advanced concepts in clinical nursing*, pp. 207–34. Philadelphia: Lippincott.

Foss, Georgia. 1973. Postural drainage. *American Journal of Nursing* 73:666–69.

Kurihara, Marie. 1972. Assessment and maintenance of adequate respiration. *Nursing Clinics of North America* 3:65.

Rie, Marcia Wasenius. 1968. Physical therapy in the nursing care of respiratory disease patients. *Nursing Clinics of North America* 3:463–78.

21 Meeting elimination needs

Assessment of fecal elimination

Appearance of stool

Among American and European populations whose diet is highly refined, the usual stool is a plastic, intact fecal mass measuring 150 to 300 g.[1] It is soft and solid, containing about 70 percent water. In those countries where unrefined grain products containing their natural fibers are the staple food, the stools are generally larger, softer, and more frequent, as a result.

Form, color, and odor are also subject to some variation as a result of dietary and bacterial influences. For most Westerners, the stool is usually olive drab or brown in color and slightly odiferous. It is shaped like a thin, medium-sized potato or segmented into pieces resembling bananas.[2]

Changes in stool color, absence of color, and the presence of unusual matter such as blood may signal obstructions or disease of the bowel, perforations, or hemorrhaging.

Changes in consistency (either much softer or harder than usual), texture, or quantity may indicate **malabsorption** or gastric imbalances in the digestive tract. Other indicators of possible problems are an increase or decrease in the quantity of stool, mucus or pus in the fecal matter, the presence of worms or parasites, evidence of undigested food particles, or a change in odor of the stool. The presence of unusual findings in one bowel movement may not necessarily indicate a serious problem, although abnormalities in the stool are often one of the first signs of a problem.

Defecation

Defecation, the process by which fecal matter is excreted, involves a complex interaction between the specialized organs composing the excre-

---

[1]Malcolm Peterson. 1970. Constipation and diarrhea. In Cyril M. MacBryde and Robert S. Blacklow, eds., *Signs and symptoms,* 5th ed., p. 381. Philadelphia: Lippincott.
[2]Ibid.

tory system. The large intestine, which receives the semiliquid waste mass, serves to absorb water and electrolytes and to temporarily store the residual waste products as feces. Storage takes place in the lower **sigmoid colon** and the rectum. As more feces collect here, the rectum is filled and the pressure on the sphincter of the anus creates the urge to open the anus and defecate. At this point, a person can voluntarily relax the anal muscles, contract the abdominal muscles, and help force the stool into the rectum. The anus then dilates widely and stool is discharged under the influence of gravity, aided by abdominal straining.

Normal bowel function for most adults includes a bowel movement every day or every few days. Only about 1 percent of healthy adults have a bowel movement less frequently than three times a week or more frequently than three times a day.[3]

Deviations from normal defecation

Distention.   **Distention** is an enlargement of segments of the intestine and spasms in the muscle layers. It is caused by **flatus** stretching and inflating parts of the intestines when **peristalsis** is reduced or absent. Distention and "gas pains" frequently occur following abdominal surgery.

Constipation.   **Constipation** is another problem caused by reduced peristaltic activity, or a hypoactive bowel. It occurs when there is undue delay in evacuating feces from the bowel. This usually results in the passage of hard dry stools, or no stool at all for an inordinate period of time.[4] With constipation, evacuation of the stools is difficult and often involves a great deal of straining of the voluntary muscles.

Impaction.   **Impaction** occurs when the rectum and sigmoid colon become filled with fecal material. After the fecal material remains in the bowel for several days, it becomes more and more compacted and contains less water. Consequently, it becomes hard and is difficult to pass through the anus.

Diarrhea.   **Diarrhea** is basically the opposite of constipation. It is characterized by the passage of loose, watery stools and an increase in the frequency of bowel movements. It may or may not be accompanied by abdominal cramping. Diarrhea occurs when excessive, strong, and frequent peristaltic action moves the **chyme** rapidly through the intestine. This reduces the amount of time available for the intestine to absorb the nutrients, electrolytes, and water.

Diet has a major effect on the elimination system.

[3] Alastair M. Connell. 1972. Physiology of the colon. In Francis A. Jones and Edmund W. Godding, eds., *Management of constipation*, p. 17. London: Blackwell.
[4] Peterson, p. 383.

Incontinence. **Incontinence** occurs when a person loses the ability to control his bowels. It arises frequently from spinal cord trauma, neurological injury, disease, lack of sphincter control, or mental disorientation.

Factors influencing fecal elimination

Diet. Diet is one of the most important factors affecting changes in the secretion and motility of the alimentary canal. It therefore has a major effect on the elimination system.

Diet also influences the type and amount of bacteria entering the digestive system. This in turn will affect the fecal characteristics. Bacteria are necessary for proper functioning of the bowel, but changes in the bulk of the diet result in rapid changes both in the number and variety of fecal flora.

Stress. Stress also affects elimination patterns. "Butterflies in the stomach" is more than just a figure of speech. In periods of stress caused by fear, grief, or anger, peristaltic activity and muscle spasms may increase or decrease. Diarrhea or, occasionally, constipation results.

Physical activity. A person's physical activity level affects the propulsive movements of the colon and, therefore, the bowels. Increased activity will stimulate the colon, while immobility or sleep will depress it. Changes in posture, such as standing up, lying down, or sitting, also affect colonic activity by influencing the amount of pressure on the alimentary canal. This in turn causes alterations in the tone of the abdominal muscles and, consequently, in the intensity of peristaltic activity within the colon.

Neurogenic conditions. Neurogenic conditions caused by traumatic lesions and organic diseases of the nervous system, such as multiple sclerosis, brain and cord tumors, and meningitis, frequently leave a person with chronic constipation. These conditions interfere with the vagus, splanchnic, and pelvic nerves, which are crucial for transmitting impulses for peristaltic contractions. When the spinal cord, because of disease or injury, is unable to recognize the presence of stool in the rectum, there is no stimulus to start the defecation reflex.

Muscular condition. Abdominal, pelvic, and diaphragmatic muscles play an important role in initiating and completing defecation. Injuries or other conditions affecting the strength of these muscles will therefore make evacuation difficult. Weakness from muscle atony may also be caused by laxative abuse or severe malnutrition.

Mechanical obstructions. Obstructions that result in an abnormal physical state of the bowel content may retard propulsion and cause constipation

Stress also affects elimination patterns.

or distention. Actual physical blockage or narrowing of the intestine's interior may be caused by neoplasms and inflammatory lesions. Hemorrhoids, fissures, and abscesses can inhibit voluntary muscle relaxation and result in constipation.

Malabsorption. Malabsorption, a common cause of diarrhea, may involve significant excess or deficiency in intake of fat, protein, carbohydrates, vitamins, or minerals.

Inflammatory disease. Inflammatory disease caused by pathogenic organisms, such as salmonella, amebas, enteroviruses, or by ulcerative colitis or by cathartics may produce diarrhea that is brief and self-limited. This type of diarrhea may be so profuse that, in extreme cases, dehydration and death will ensue.[5]

Drugs. Drugs used in the treatment of one condition often trigger side effects that interfere with elimination and cause diarrhea or constipation.

Constipation is often attributed to the neuromuscular effects of drugs, and is particularly prevalent with large intakes of morphine, cocaine, codeine, and other narcotic-forming opiates. Tranquilizers taken in large doses can also generate constipation because they tend to dull the nerves and thus lead to diminished awareness of rectal distention.[6]

Surgery. Surgery, particularly in the abdominal area, often precipitates distention and gas pains, due to the stretching of the intestines and the spasms of the muscle layers. Constipation may also occur for several days following surgery because of the effects on the body of anesthetics, as well as the emotional stress related to surgery. Another factor may be the patient's reluctance to strain in bowel evacuation for fear of pain or rupture.

Planning, implementation, and evaluation

Collecting a stool

In collecting a stool, the nurse should inform the patient and enlist his cooperation. For the patient who has bathroom privileges, a bedpan may be fitted into the toilet bowl under the seat, or it may be placed on a chair. For bedridden patients, collection should be in a commode.

A portion of the stool should be collected with a tongue depressor and approximately 1 tablespoon of the stool transferred to a specimen

[5]Peterson, p. 396.

[6]G. C. Timbury and Mary Tate. 1973. Management of constipation in psychiatric patients. *Nursing Times* 69:1050.

container. The laboratory slip, specimen container, and patient's record should be clearly and accurately marked, and the specimen should be sent promptly to the lab. Stools should be examined while still warm (at or near body temperature) and fresh. Time and changes in temperature will alter the stool. Bright red blood, for example, begins to clot, dry out, and turn dark; certain pathogens may die and thus fail to be detected.

Intervention for specific problems

Distention. Distention can be prevented or decreased through diet modification to reduce the intake of gas-forming foods, increased patient activity to stimulate the colonic movements of the small intestine, and the use of various mechanical aids. Heat applied to the abdomen, either alone or in conjunction with other measures such as the **rectal tube,** can increase peristalsis and expel flatus.

The necessary equipment for the procedure includes a lubricating cream, paper or hand towels, and the rectal tube. The patient is turned to his side and the tube is gently inserted about 4 inches. In case there is some expulsion, the free end of the tube should be placed in a folded hand towel or into a **flatus bag.** Sometimes it is necessary to anchor the tube to the buttocks with tape.

The tube should not remain in place for more than 20 minutes to half an hour.[7] Prolonged insertion can cause severe irritation of the rectal lining and spasms of the anal sphincter, which may ultimately produce relaxation of the sphincter. If the patient continues to have discomfort, the tube should be removed and reinserted after several hours. Odor control, a frequent concern of the patient, can best be maintained by air conditioning and aerosol sprays, if they are tolerated by the patient.

Colonic irrigation (also called **Harris flush**) is another procedure available for relief of distention in patients. It is also used to clean out the bowel, and is a much more extreme measure than the use of the rectal tube.[8] Colonic irrigation is a process in which the colon is alternately filled with and drained of fluid for about 15 minutes at a time, or until there is no further release of gas. A rectal tube is inserted and the rectum and colon are irrigated with fluid (usually tap water or a normal saline solution of about 105° F or 40.5° C).[9] Then, with the rectal tube still in place, the solution container or irrigating can is lowered 12 to 18 inches below the anus so that the fluid flows back into the container.

The patient should, if possible, empty the bowel before the irrigation is begun. If the patient has pain or marked discomfort during the irrigation

[7]Norma Greenler Dison. 1971. *An atlas of nursing techniques,* 2d ed.,, p. 217. St. Louis: Mosby.
[8]Thomas Hunt. 1974. Colonic irrigation. *Nursing Mirror* 139:76.
[9]This point seems to be the subject of some controversy. Many authorities cite the ideal temperature as 40.5° C. Others, such as Hunt (p. 77), prefer 35°-37° C.

procedure, the flow should be stopped by clamping or kinking the irrigation tube. The patient should be told to take deep breaths through the mouth until the cramping and urge pass. Since fecal matter as well as flatus and solution are released into the container during irrigation, the contents may become thick and offensive. They must be emptied into the bedpan and clear solution added to the irrigating container.

Constipation. Constipation can often be prevented or reduced by such nonmedical means as exercise, establishing a regular time for defecation, heeding the call to defecate, and avoiding excessive emotional stress. A well-balanced diet with sufficient **roughage** and liquids (at least 4 pints daily) is also important. High-fiber foods, such as unprocessed bran and other cereals, fresh fruit, and vegetables, are good sources for roughage. Highly refined carbohydrate foods should be avoided. Medications for easing constipation are particularly useful in prolonged or severe cases. However, dependence on medication has frequently led to reduced muscle tone and chronic constipation in habitual users. For this reason, the nurse should encourage patients instead to maintain proper diet and activity levels as a means of preventing or alleviating constipation.

When medication is necessary, several types are available. These include **stool softeners,** which are usually taken orally as liquids and serve to lubricate the fecal mass and prevent the loss of water. Some softeners, made from surface-active agents with properties similar to those of modern dishwashing detergents, will lower the surface tension in the gastrointestinal tract. These soften the feces by enabling water and fats to penetrate the stools.

Laxatives, taken orally as a liquid or solid, stimulate bowel activity by increasing peristalsis in either the bowel or small intestine. The **cathartics** cause the release of irritants that induce increased peristalsis and thus stimulate the movement of fecal matter. Of these, castor oil is the most vigorous and produces a stool within 2 to 6 hours of administration.[10] Others include senna, phenolphthalein, aloes, and cascara sagrada.

Another class of laxatives, the **bulk-formers,** contain substances that actively increase the bulk of the stools. They act by providing nondigestible, residual substances that stimulate peristalsis by reflex action and by providing bulk and lubrication when the compounds become enlarged by absorbing water. Bulk formers include the hydrophilic colloids derived from agar, psyllium (Metamucil and Serutan are trade names), and methylcellulose; and osmotically active substances such as Epsom salts (magnesium sulphate), milk of magnesia (magnesium hydroxide), and the phosphates of potassium and sodium. Bulk-producing agents are primarily used when there is an insufficient quantity of feces because of quantitative or qualitative dietary restrictions.

[10]C. H. Blenkiron. 1971. A clutch of cathartics. *Nursing Mirror* 132:45.

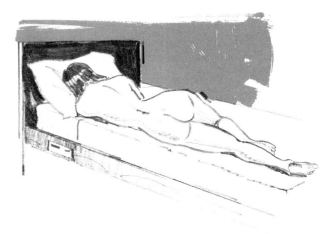

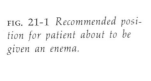

FIG. 21-1 *Recommended position for patient about to be given an enema.*

Rectal suppositories are usually cone-shaped, semisolid pellets that melt on insertion in the rectum. Some relieve pain or irritation, some contain drugs that the patient cannot take orally, and others promote bowel movements.

For proper insertion of a suppository, the nurse places the patient on a flat bed in Sim's position with his uppermost leg flexed and his back to the proximal side of the bed. Wearing plastic or rubber gloves, the nurse unwraps the foil or plastic covering the suppository. She then grasps it between the thumb and index finger of the working hand and lubricates it. The other hand draws the top gluteal fold upward and downward until the anus is exposed. After the suppository has been inserted into the anus, it should be guided by the nurse's index finger along the wall of the rectum for about 3 inches. The suppository will be ineffective if it is pushed into the fecal mass, rather than alongside it.

The nurse should instruct the patient to breathe deeply during insertion of the suppository. This relaxes the anal sphincter. He should continue to breathe deeply after insertion until the immediate urge to expel the suppository has passed. The urge to defecate fecal matter will usually occur within 15 to 20 minutes.

Enemas are fluid solutions introduced via the anus into the rectum and colon. The kind and amount of fluid used in the enema varies. The choice of enema should be determined by the age and physical condition of the patient and by the purpose of the enema.

The enema solutions most frequently used are hypertonic solutions, tap water, normal saline, soap suds, and oil. The temperature of these enema solutions (except where otherwise indicated) should be about 105° F (40.5° C), or warm to the touch. A solution which is too cold may cause cramping and usually cannot be retained, while a hot solution may damage the tissues of the rectum.

The following procedures are generally used when administering the enemas cited above.[11]

[11]Betty Tillery and Barbara Bates. 1966. Enemas. *American Journal of Nursing* 66:534. Also, Dison, pp. 211–17.

The patient is usually positioned on his left side with his right knee flexed. This position is most conducive to gravity aiding the flow of solution upwards through the colon. Other variations in the recumbent position may be used, as necessitated by the comfort or condition of the patient.

Equipment for all cleansing enemas, except the prepackaged, self-contained types in disposable packets, includes a solution container and a lubricated soft tube with side openings at the tip through which the solution can flow into the rectum. For oil retention enemas that are not prepackaged, an Asepto syringe, rectal tube or small catheter, and a small pitcher or funnel to hold the oil may be used instead.

The tube should be inserted only after all air in the tube has been expelled. If the patient strains down during insertion, the anal sphincter will relax and the tube can be inserted more easily through the anal canal and into the rectum. For cleansing enemas, insertion of about 3 inches is sufficient; for retention enemas, 6 to 8 inches.[12] Forcing or pushing the tube too far can produce injury. The pressure fluid as it enters the colon can be properly controlled by placing the fluid level in the container no higher than 18 to 20 inches above the anal canal. At this height, fluid will reach the cecum in 2 to 5 minutes, and the pressure will usually not stimulate excessive colonic contraction. Greater pressure or more rapid administration of the solution causes distention of the colon and stimulates mass peristalsis. This may cause cramping and a premature desire to defecate. Encouraging the patient to breathe through his mouth during the procedure relaxes his abdominal muscles, which in turn decreases the colonic pressure and increases his ability to retain the fluid. The fluid enema flow should be maintained for about 10 minutes at 750 ml to avoid stimulating the desire to defecate. After the tube has been removed, the patient should be encouraged to retain the fluid for 15 minutes in the case of cleansing enemas; for 30 minutes where oil retention enemas are used.

Impaction. Whenever possible, impaction should be prevented by the use of proper diet, exercise, laxatives, and suppositories. However, if the fecal mass does become impacted, the nurse can alleviate the impaction by using an oil retention and/or a cleansing enema. If necessary the mass may be removed by manual extraction. For this procedure, the patient should be placed in a Sim's position with protective pads under his buttocks. The nurse should wear rubber gloves and lubricate her index finger well. The finger is then inserted gently through the anal sphincter into the rectum. The fecal mass should be checked for consistency. Small amounts should then be dislodged, removed, and placed in a bedpan, until the fecal mass has been cleared or the patient's discomfort necessitates discontinuation. Often the stimulation of manually removing the impaction will create the urge in the patient to defecate and a bedpan should be provided. Following

[12] Dison, p. 217.

the extraction procedure, the anal areas should be cleansed, and the patient allowed to rest, for the process is very uncomfortable.

Diarrhea. This condition can often be relieved and arrested in its early stages by increased rest and changes in diet. The diet should include an increase in foods that are "absorbent" (rice, bananas, grated apple, toasted white bread) and lean (boiled chicken or other nonfatty meat). Because of the threat of dehydration, fluids are particularly important. Fatty, rich, and fried foods should be avoided, as should milk and milk products, acidic fruits and juices, and gas-producing foods. In cases of prolonged or severe diarrhea, diet modification may be combined with medications prescribed by a physician that relax the colon. Even the early stages of diarrhea should not be disregarded, however, for fluid and electrolyte balances in the body can be severely threatened by the condition (see chapter 22).

Incontinence and diarrhea can cause a great deal of discomfort, breakdown of tissue, and irritation around the anal area. The area should be kept scrupulously clean and dry, and the patient's clothing and bedding should be changed whenever necessary. A lubricant cream, spread over the anal area and buttocks, will often protect the skin from the irritating effects of moisture and fecal matter.

Patient embarrassment due to incontinence or excessive amounts of uncontrolled loose stools, as in diarrhea, can often be effectively countered by the nurse through a supportive and encouraging attitude. The patient must be made to feel that he is not "dirty" or infantile because of his lack of bowel control. In prolonged or complicated situations, a program of bowel control training should be instituted (see chapter 27).

Assessment of urinary elimination

Characteristics of urine

A well-hydrated adult, who is not losing fluid abnormally by other means such as **diaphoresis,** vomiting, or diarrhea, will excrete amounts of urine slightly higher than his daily "liquid" intake. This intake is about 1100 ml from solid foods and 1200 ml from liquids.[13]

The color of normal urine ranges from clear amber to straw. Usually the higher the specific gravity of urine, the deeper its color. The pH of urine, or the concentration of hydrogen ions, varies between 4.5 and 8, but is normally acidic at about 6. Its odor, when excreted, is mild, but after several hours it will smell like ammonia as a result of bacterial action.

It is important to remember that the composition, quantity, and appearance of urine vary from person to person because of individual differ-

---

[13] Chester Winter and Marilyn R. Barker. 1972. *Nursing care of patients with urologic diseases,* 3d ed., p. 58. St. Louis: Mosby.

ences in diet, metabolism, and so forth. Nevertheless, the nurse should always be alert for significant changes in a patient's urine, or the unusual appearance of urine in a new patient.

Structure and function of the urinary system

The process by which the body rids itself of urine in the bladder is called **micturition** or voiding. Urine accumulates in the bladder until the resulting pressure on the walls of the bladder triggers sensory nerves that make a person aware of the desire to void. When it is convenient, motor impulses cause the bladder muscles to contract and the sphincter muscles to relax. This allows the urine to flow out through the urethra.

Micturition may be an involuntary or a voluntary act. It is involuntary when the spinal mechanism operates. This action occurs in everyone who is not toilet trained or whose spinal cord is injured. It is voluntary when the sensation of the need to void is carried to the brain and the person is able voluntarily to relax the muscles of the perineum and contract the abdominal muscles to help initiate voiding.[14]

How often and how easily a person voids is as individual as bowel patterns. Urinary habits are determined by individual differences in control, which, in turn, are influenced by childhood training, physiological makeup, desire to control voluntary muscles, functioning ability of involuntary muscles and reflexes, and psychological factors. The psychological factor has often been underestimated in its effect on urinary patterns. In fact, a person's ability to absorb or tolerate stress and anxiety is often reflected in the quantity and frequency with which urine is excreted. In assessing urinary elimination status, therefore, the nurse should give particular attention to the person's individual habits and to the particular circumstances under which a person is being assessed.

Outside the range of individual differences in micturition, these are patterns and symptoms that indicate abnormalities or problems.

Frequency. A change in frequency of urination may result simply from a change in liquid intake. A decrease in frequency may also be caused by an obstruction, anxiety, or water retention within the body. An increase in frequency, with voiding often up to 30 times a day, is not necessarily accompanied by an increase in quantity. Each voiding may be only a few drops. Increased frequency may be triggered by infection, psychological stress, disease, or pregnancy.

Urgency. A feeling of constantly having to void, when in fact the bladder may be empty, often accompanies an infection of the urinary tract. It also

Increased frequency of voiding may be triggered by infection, psychological stress, disease, or pregnancy.

[14]Lorraine Delehanty and Vincent Stravino. 1970. Achieving bladder control. *American Journal of Nursing* 70:312.

occurs during pregnancy when the fetus exerts a great deal of pressure on the bladder, triggering the urge to urinate. In some cases, it may occur after surgery or after prolonged and voluntary constriction of the sphincter muscles to prevent urination. Psychological stress may be a precipitating factor.

Burning. A burning sensation upon urination, felt in the urethra as a hot, prickly liquid against the mucosal lining, often indicates the presence of infection in the urinary tract or urethral irritation.

Dysuria. Dysuria is painful or difficult urination and may occur before, during, and/or after urination. Dysuria, which is often accompanied by one or several of the above symptoms, is caused by a variety of conditions. These include traumatic injury, disease, infection, urethral narrowing, bladder neck obstruction, or some other muscular abnormality. In women, it is a common syndrome following the first few occasions of sexual intercourse (the so-called "honeymoon" syndrome).

Nocturia. **Nocturia,** or bed wetting, is an inability to control the release of urine that occurs only when the person is asleep. It may be caused by habit formation in childhood or by deformity of the urinary tract.

Retention. **Retention** of urine, a condition in which the bladder is unable to empty, may occur in any postoperative, acutely ill, elderly, or bedridden patient. Partial retention occurs when the bladder does not empty completely. Infection and even impairment of renal function may develop as a result of retention.

Incontinence. **Incontinence,** the opposite of retention, occurs when a person is unable to retain urine. This may be temporary, caused by an inflammatory condition of the bladder (cystitis). Permanent incontinence results from a more serious neurologic condition (such as paraplegia) that interferes with the mechanisms controlling the bladder and sphincters.

Stress incontinence is a form of incontinence that occasionally occurs when intra-abdominal pressure increases, as during coughing, sneezing, and laughing. It is due to a laxness of the external sphincter, a condition often occurring after childbirth because of the stretching of muscle fibers. It is also experienced occasionally by children who have not yet gained full control over their external sphincter.

Factors affecting urinary elimination

Fluid intake. Since urine is composed of 95 to 98 percent water, the amount of water in the body influences the quantity and consistency of the urine. Decreased fluid intake sometimes results in reduced urinary output. At

> Infection and even impairment of renal function may develop as a result of retention.

other times, output levels are maintained, but liquid content is reduced at the cellular level, causing dehydration.

Stress. Anxiety-producing situations influence the body's response mechanisms, reflex actions, and voluntary muscle reactions. During periods of stress, the blood pressure may rise, often causing an actual increase in urine production or in the sensation of bladder fullness.

Activity levels. Activity levels affect the body's metabolism, the quantity of waste material, and the speed with which it is produced. They also affect the muscle tone of some of the organs involved in urinary elimination and the degree to which sensations are felt. Increased activity, for example, will generally stimulate increased urine production and elimination, as well as an increased desire for fluids to replace those excreted. Reduced activity not only reduces urinary production and elimination, but the resulting decreased muscle tone may actually cause retention of urine that is produced. This is particularly true with persons who are bedridden, hospitalized, elderly, or otherwise immobilized.

Disease conditions. Disease conditions in general may aggravate fluid losses in the body and may also increase the body's water requirement by speeding up some of the bodily processes. Urinary volume may therefore be reduced, unless there is a corresponding increase in fluid intake.

A number of specific diseases can affect urinary elimination by interfering with the proper functioning of one or several of the urinary tract organs or supporting systems. Diseases that affect production of urine generally involve the kidneys, the circulatory system, and the hormonal system. Such diseases as nephritis, which causes extensive kidney damage, may reduce the amount of protein produced and increase its concentration.

Medications. Medications administered for purposes other than urinary control often cause changes in the volume and consistency of urine. Drugs causing urinary retention include those with parasympathetic depressant effects such as anti-Parkinsonism drugs, Belladonna alkaloids, and others used to reduce gastrointestinal motility. Several pain medications may depress or stimulate the central nervous system and affect smooth muscle fibers, causing urinary retention if given in large doses.[15] Other drugs that affect the body's ability to release sodium into the urine have a tendency to reduce the urinary output at the expense of water retention within the tissues (edema).

Surgery. Surgery may interfere with urinary elimination, particularly when it is localized in the abdominal area. When surgery is used to relieve

[15]Mims G. Ochsner. 1974. Acute urinary retention. *Hospital Medicine* 10:90.

abdominal trauma, the side effects of the surgical trauma may interfere with kidney functions. Most surgical patients have reduced urinary output for 24 hours postoperatively, because the body tends to retain sodium and fluids. The postoperative patient usually loses slightly larger amounts of fluid than normal as insensible water loss (perspiration and respiration), and he usually eats less solid food.[16]

Obtaining a clean-catch urine specimen

Urine samples voided into a bottle, however clean, are often not suitable for bacteriological study because of the inevitable contamination by organisms around the urethral opening. Thus **sterile voiding** or **clean-catch** specimens are frequently requested.

The male patient whose urine is to be collected should cleanse the penis thoroughly with soap and water. The first portion of the voided urine is not collected, but discarded. The next portion, the test sample, is voided into a sterile, wide-mouth bottle or large-caliber tube, which is protected by a sterile closure.

The female patient should first cleanse the vulva around the urethral opening 3 or 4 times with soapy water, each time wiping the perineum backward toward the anus, then discarding the wipe. The area should then be doused with water and the urine voided into a sterile, wide-mouth bottle.

All urine tests are ideally performed on fresh specimens, preferably from the first voiding of the day, since most urinary constituents are present in highest concentration at that time. Whenever possible, urine should be tested as soon as the sample is voided, because it becomes increasingly alkaline on standing. Bacterial contaminants also multiply rapidly, decomposing the urea and liberating ammonia. To reduce these reactions, particularly when immediate testing is impossible, the urine should be kept refrigerated. A chemical preservative is sometimes used for urine stabilization in cases of prolonged delay.

Planning, implementation, and evaluation

Intervention for specific problems

Relief or prevention of frequency, burning, urgency, dysuria, and nocturia can often be handled by the introduction of variations in the patient's fluid intake. For example, burning sensations in the bladder and urethra may be alleviated by increasing the patient's fluid intake and thereby diluting the irritants in the urine. An increase in fluid intake is,

---

[16]Winter and Barker, p. 65.

No patient should be catheterized unless absolutely necessary.

in fact, recommended for most patients with urologic disease.[17] They should, however, be warned not to take excessive amounts of fluid since this may cause water intoxication.

Control of nocturia may be achieved by having the patient avoid fluid totally 2 to 3 hours prior to bedtime. Small amounts of fluid taken frequently will often help to relieve dysuria, burning, and other common discomforts. They do so by helping the urinary system irrigate itself and preventing irritating waste materials from passing through the system in concentrated form.

Many people, particularly when they are ill, find it difficult to drink large quantities of water. The nurse should familiarize herself with the patient's preferences in terms of specific beverage and timing. She can then offer alternatives to water as a way of maintaining a patient's fluid intake without resorting to parenteral measures (see chapter 20). Fruit drinks, ginger ale, or other soft drinks may be substituted for part of the water. Juicy fruits or other solid foods with a high fluid content such as custards, ice cream, or gelatin may be more palatable than liquids for some patients.[18] Carbonated beverages or hot liquids may be better tolerated by patients who are nauseated. Care must always be taken that any substitutions for water are acceptable on the diet prescribed for the patient.

Urethral catheterization

No patient should be catheterized unless absolutely necessary. This is a procedure that carries a high risk of urinary infection. The risk can be minimized by the use of certain procedures for safeguarding the patient against infection. These include

1. Maintaining strict surgical asepsis
2. Use of a catheter that is smaller than the external urinary meatus to help minimize trauma
3. Lubrication of the catheter with an appropriate antimicrobial lubricant to reduce irritation
4. Gentle and skillful insertion of the catheter

Nonretention catheter. The nonretention catheter is used to empty the bladder in order to relieve pressure and retention. It is also used occasionally to collect a clean specimen for diagnostic purposes when it cannot be collected in other ways. It can be used to relieve retention in a postoperative or postpartum patient who cannot void spontaneously, to determine the amount of residual urine, and to protect the area postoperatively in perineum surgery.

[17] Ibid.
[18] Ibid., p. 64.

Equipment for all catheterization procedures includes a good light, a sterile field, and 2 catheters of the appropriate shape and size. Also needed are sponges, solution for cleansing the local area, a basin for the solution, cotton balls, a water-soluble lubricant, towels, gloves, and, if necessary, a specimen bottle. A drape sheet, blanket, container for urine, bed protector, and waste container should also be provided.

Prior to any physical preparation for catheterization, the procedure should always be explained to the patient. Privacy must be maintained throughout the procedure. The patient should be draped and placed in a dorsal recumbent position with protective waterproof material under the buttocks. (The lateral position may be used for female patients.) The genital area should be washed and rinsed thoroughly.

For female patients, the nurse separates the labia minor with gloved thumb and index finger to expose the meatus, maintaining this position until the procedure is completed. The exposed area is cleansed again, using fresh cotton balls and solution for each stroke. Cleansing strokes move along each labial lip from the top down toward the vagina.

The catheter tip is lubricated for about $1\frac{1}{2}$ inches, to avoid clogging the tip eye. The open end of the catheter is placed in the basin to catch the urine. The catheter is gently inserted into the meatus until the urine starts to flow, usually for a distance of 2 to 3 inches. It should not be forced or inserted beyond its usual length. The catheter is held in place until urine ceases to flow unless the amount seems excessive, more than 1000 cc. (In this case, the catheter should be removed and the patient catheterized again after about an hour.) Then the catheter should be pinched off and removed gently.

For male patients, the nurse thoroughly washes the skin of the penis surrounding the meatus. The foreskin must be pulled back for adequate cleaning, as any accumulation of mucus, urine, or stool can cause irritation and infection. A clean, solution-covered cotton ball should be used for each cleansing stroke, which goes from distal to proximal end of the penis. The cleansed portion of the penis is placed on a sterile field. One or two drops of lubricant are applied to the meatus and to the catheter tip for $1\frac{1}{2}$ to 2 inches. The open end of the catheter is placed in the basin to catch urine.

In order to insert the catheter, the penis is positioned at about a 60- to 90-degree angle in relation to the body, and the catheter is gently inserted 6 to 8 inches until urine flows. The penis should be lowered slightly after about 5 inches of tubing have been inserted. A slight rolling movement of the catheter may be helpful during insertion.

After the required specimen is collected and when the urine ceases to flow or the amount seems in excess of 1000 cc, the catheter is pinched and gently removed.

Retention (indwelling) catheter. The retention (indwelling) catheter is left in place for a longer period of time. Because the danger of infection is

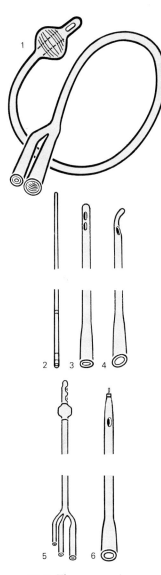

FIG. 21-2 *There are various types of catheters that may be used for urethral catheterization, including (1) two-lumen Foley, (2) Coudé—olive tip, (3) Robinson—two eyes, (4) Filiform—olive tip, (5) Owens three-way, (6) Follower.* [From Philip Cooper, Ward procedures and techniques, 2d ed., p. 122. New York: Appleton-Century-Crofts, 1967. Courtesy of the publisher.]

even greater than for the nonretention type, a retention catheter should be used with restraint and only for the following purposes:

1. To reestablish an interrupted flow of urine
2. To permit collection and measurement of urine from patients unable to cooperate adequately
3. To provide an adequate channel for drainage during surgery
4. As a last resort, to maintain a dry environment[19]

The catheter most frequently used for this procedure is a **Foley,** often of the triple-lumen type. This type allows urinary drainage through one channel, inflation of the bag with water or air through a second channel, and a continuous irrigation of the bladder through the third channel. The actual mechanism used in an indwelling Foley catheter involves a closed, sterile draining system. If the drainage tube contains a drip chamber, this will serve as an airlock and prevent bacteria from ascending from the collection container. A drainage bag that can be emptied by a valve opening at the end of the bag is most desirable.

Equipment needed for insertion of the Foley catheter includes a basin for irrigating fluid, a syringe for inflation of the catheter balloon, hemostat, forceps, waste basin, surgical towel, and sponges for cleansing the urethral meatus.

The procedure for inserting the deflated Foley catheter is much the same as that for the nonretention type. If the tubing is to be left in the bladder, it is inserted about 1 inch farther than the point at which the urine flows. If the patient experiences pain when a balloon at the tip of the catheter is inflated to retain the catheter in the bladder, the balloon should be emptied and the catheter inserted farther.[20] After balloon inflation, the catheter is pulled gently outward for a moment following anchorage to make sure that it is secure. The catheter is connected to the tubing with a sterile connecting rod and the free end of the tubing is placed in the container provided. The tubing should be anchored securely to the patient's thigh with adhesive to prevent its weight from pulling the retention bulb against the base of the bladder, damaging the sphincter. The catheter system should be checked after insertion and frequently thereafter for kinking or obstruction in the tube, and leaking or irritation in the perineal area.

To reduce the incidence of infection, the nurse should wash the perineal area and 2 to 3 inches of tubing close to the area at least twice a day with soap and water. Other measures to prevent infection include daily application of a bacteriostatic ointment to the meatus and emptying the collection bag at least every 8 hours. This is done by draining urine completely

---

[19]Julia Garner. 1974. Urinary catheter care. *Nursing '74* 4:54.
[20]Winter and Barker, p. 75.

from the bottom of the bag (the bag should never be turned upside down or raised above the patient's bladder, for this may introduce bacteria into the catheter).[21] A closed drainage system should be continuously maintained in order to prevent the introduction of even more organisms into the urinary tract.

Irrigation. Equipment for irrigations includes a small-necked bottle for the irrigating solution, a glass Asepto syringe without bulb or an aseptic funnel, a clean drainage tube, and bottle and pan for return irrigating fluid. The solution ordinarily used to irrigate catheters is sterile physiologic saline solution. The clearness of this solution makes observation of the return flow easy and it is isotonic to the body fluids.[22] Other solutions occasionally used are dilute acetic acid (0.25 to 0.5 percent) and Renacidin; and antibiotic solutions such as those containing 1 percent neomycin.

If a urethral catheter needs frequent irrigation, intermittent irrigation techniques should be used.[23] A sterile, closed reservoir flask is used to hold the irrigating solution. Sterile tubing from the flask to the catheter allows the solution to flow into the bladder upon release of the clamp on this tubing. The drainage tubing from the catheter should be clamped until the specified amount of solution has entered the bladder. The inflow tubing from the reservoir is then clamped, and the clamp is released from the drainage tubing. An accurate record of the amount of fluid used for irrigation must be kept so that the urinary output can be measured.

Constant or continuous irrigation is used when the patient is on a retention catheter and needs a continuous outflow of drainage at the same time that irrigation is taking place. Smaller amounts of solution should be introduced with the syringe (15 to 30 cc, as compared with 50 to 100 cc for intermittent) or with a drip-o-meter that allows solution to drip in at a controlled rate.

Incontinence

Regulation of fluid intake. This may help the patient who is unaware of the need to void because of muscular problems. The patient is encouraged to void at regularly scheduled intervals that are slightly shorter than the intervals between involuntary emptying of the bladder. A diuretic, such as coffee, tea, or cola, given to the patient half an hour before his regular voiding times may help to regulate the schedule. In between these times, fluid intake should be restricted.

Hygiene and comfort measures. These can be instituted by the nurse to reduce the possibility of irritation, odor, skin breakdown, and discomfort.

[21]Garner, p. 56.
[22]Winter and Barker, p. 80.
[23]Ibid.

The perineal area should be kept meticulously clean and dry. Exertion of manual pressure over the bladder may induce complete emptying of the bladder. This movement, known as the **Credé maneuver,** can be performed by the nurse or taught to the patient. A continuous, gentle but firm pressure is applied with both hands backward and downward over the lower abdomen.

Perineal exercises. These will strengthen the abdominal, gluteal, and perineal muscles, thereby increasing muscle tone and urinary control. The exercises can be explained by asking the patient to hold himself as he would if he needed to void very badly and there were no available facilities.[24] Having the patient squeeze a piece of paper or cloth in the fold between the buttocks helps to strengthen the gluteal and levator muscles. Stopping and starting the urinary stream during voiding is also helpful. Intermittent tightening and relaxing of the perineal muscles sometimes helps to relieve stress incontinence, especially in older women.

SUMMARY

Assessment of a patient's fecal and urinary elimination status is a responsibility that often falls most directly on the nurse, for the nurse is the health care professional most involved with the patient's day-to-day care. Proper assessment demands a thorough understanding of the elimination system, its functions, its problems, and the means by which these problems may be alleviated. Thus, the nurse must be able to recognize the characteristics of normal and abnormal stool and urine, the processes of normal defecation and micturition, and deviations from normal patterns. These include distention, constipation, impaction, diarrhea, incontinence, retention, frequency, urgency, burning, dysuria, and nocturia.

Fecal and urinary elimination are both affected by such factors as nutritional and fluid intake, stress, activity/immobility levels, disease, medications, and surgery. It is important that the nurse understand what effects these factors may have in regulating or altering elimination patterns.

Assessment of a patient's elimination status, particularly when problems are suspected, should be confirmed by laboratory analysis of specimens. Since it is the nurse who is frequently charged with obtaining the specimen, it is essential that the proper collection techniques be understood. Feces should be kept at room temperature, while urine should be refrigerated if there is a delay in transmitting the sample to the laboratory.

Intervention for the relief of specific elimination problems can sometimes be achieved by regulating the patient's fluid and dietary intake and activity levels. This is particularly true for distention, constipation, diarrhea, dysuria, urinary retention, and even incontinence. When these measures

[24] Ibid., p. 93.

alone are unsuccessful in relieving the problem, the nurse can use them in conjunction with more complex measures, such as medications and mechanical aids. For example, medications may be used to prevent or alleviate constipation. Mechanical aids such as catheters may be used to relieve urinary retention. Within each of these categories of medications and mechanical aids are many different types, and the choice of which to use is determined by the patient's condition, age, sex, and other factors. The one factor that is not subject to variation, however, is the need for meticulous cleanliness.

STUDY QUESTIONS

1. What are the factors that influence an individual's fecal and urinary elimination habits?
2. Name and define four common deviations from normal defecation patterns. What nursing actions should be taken for each?
3. Define dysuria, nocturia, and incontinence. What are the common causes of each? What nursing measures should be taken for each?
4. Under what circumstances should a patient be catheterized? What are the dangers of catheterization?
5. What is the procedure for inserting a retention catheter? a nonretention catheter?

SELECTED BIBLIOGRAPHY

Connell, Alastair M. 1972. Physiology of the colon. In Francis A. Jones and Edmund W. Godding, eds., *Management of constipation,* pp. 1-24. London: Blackwell.

Dison, Norma Greenler. 1971. *An atlas of nursing techniques,* 2d ed., pp. 210-30. St. Louis: Mosby.

Garner, Julia. 1974. Urinary catheter care. *Nursing '74* 4:54-56.

Peterson, Malcolm. 1970. Constipation and diarrhea. In Cyril M. MacBryde and Robert S. Blacklow, eds., *Signs and symptoms,* 5th ed., pp. 381-98. Philadelphia: Lippincott.

Winter, Chester, and Barker, Marilyn R. 1972. *Nursing care of patients with urologic diseases,* 3d ed. St. Louis: Mosby.

22 Meeting fluid and electrolyte needs

Assessment of fluid and electrolyte balance

Water

Man can live only a short time without water. There is no known substitute for it among living organisms. Water makes up 50 to 80 percent of man's body weight, and it is necessary for every major physiological function. It is the medium of all body fluids, including gastrointestinal secretions, lymph, blood, urine, and perspiration. It provides the solvent for products of digestion and metabolism, and it cushions the cells of the body. It is essential for the action of the second component of body fluid, electrolytic substances.

Electrolytes

Electrolytes are chemical substances that develop electrical charges **(ionize)** when they are placed in water. This means that an aqueous solution of these chemicals will conduct an electrical current. Some electrolytes develop positive charges and are called **cations.** Others develop negative charges and are called **anions.** Electrolytes with positive charges include sodium, potassium, calcium, and magnesium. Negatively charged electrolytes include chloride, bicarbonate, carbonic acid, phosphate, protein, lactate, and citrate. In solution, the positive and negative electrolytes are attracted to one another until equilibrium is achieved.

Sources of water and electrolytes

Water and electrolytes are taken into the body through various routes. Food and water provide both components. Water is also provided through oxidation of foodstuffs and body tissues. Hospitalized patients may receive both water and electrolytes by intravenous, nasogastric, or rectal tubes.

Requirements for water and electrolytes

To maintain a healthy state, the water taken in by a person must equal the water lost through various routes (perspiration, urination, and so forth). Under ideal conditions, with a minimum of physical activity, an adult needs

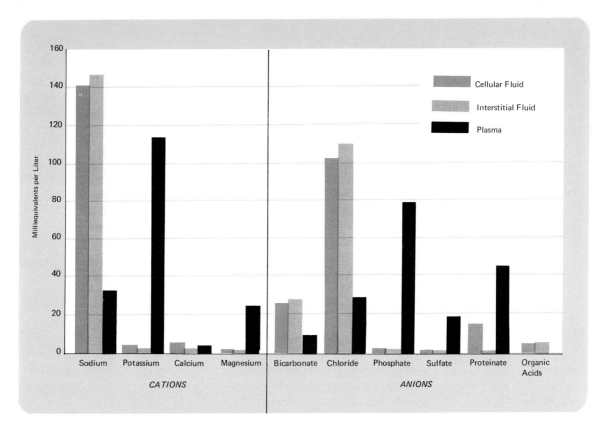

FIG. 22-1 *Electrolyte composition of normal body fluids.*

[From W. D. Snively, Jr., and D. R. Beshear, *Textbook of Pathophysiology*, p. 136. Philadelphia: Lippincott, 1972.]

about 1.5 liters of water per day. He obtains this requirement from beverages, food, and water of oxidation.[1]

Water and electrolyte requirements are different for young children. The infant exchanges approximately one-half of his extracellular volume in 24 hours. (The adult, in the same time, exchanges only one-seventh of his extracellular fluid.) Because of the infant's smaller size, his greater metabolic rate, and his larger surface area in relation to his weight, he needs more water than an adult to maintain balance. Normal infants require 150 ml of fluid per kilogram per day.[2] This is five times the normal intake for the adult.

Distribution and concentration of electrolytes in body fluid

Osmosis. **Osmosis** is an important regulator of fluid and electrolyte balance. It is a process by which water passes through a semipermeable membrane from a high concentration of water to a lower concentration of water. This continues until equilibrium is achieved on both sides of the membrane. Put more simply, water passes from a more dilute solution to a more concentrated one. Another way of understanding this is to

---

[1] National Research Council, Food and Nutrition Board. 1968. *Recommended dietary allowances,* 7th ed. Washington, D.C.: National Academy of Sciences.

[2] Paul H. DeBruine. 1972. Fluid and electrolytes. *Journal of the American Association of Nurse Anesthetists* 40:269.

remember that water goes where the electrolytes go. If blood cells are suspended in an **isotonic** solution (a solution having the same osmotic pressure as the cells), the **osmotic pressure** will remain the same inside and outside the cell. In this case, no movement occurs. If the blood cells are placed in a **hypotonic** solution (one that is much less concentrated than the cellular contents), water will flow into the cells until they swell and burst. In a **hypertonic** solution (one that is more concentrated than the cellular contents), water flows out of the cells and the cells shrink.

Diffusion. **Diffusion** is a process whereby molecules move from higher concentrations of solution to lower concentrations. Oxygen and carbon dioxide exchange in the lungs occurs through diffusion.

Active transport. **Active transport** is a mechanism, still not fully understood, whereby ions move from areas of lesser concentration to areas of greater concentration. It involves the release of energy by the action of **adenosine triphosphate (ATP).** ATP, supplying the necessary "uphill movement," enables certain substances to pass through the cell membrane. Sodium, potassium, and amino acids are probably carried through all cell membranes by active transport.[3]

Filtration. **Filtration** is related to **hydrostatic pressure** produced by the pumping action of the heart. (Hydrostatic pressure is the pressure of water or other liquids.) It involves the transfer of both solute and solvent through a permeable membrane from a region of higher hydrostatic pressure to a region of lower pressure. An example is the passage of water and electrolytes from the capillary beds to the interstitial fluid.

Pinocytosis and phagocytosis. Substances of higher molecular weight such as protein enter body cells by **pinocytosis.** In this process, the cell membrane folds inward to incorporate the substances. In **phagocytosis,** foreign particles are engulfed or digested by specialized cells called **phagocytes.**

Common sources of fluid and electrolyte imbalance

Vomiting and gastric suction. When the quantity of acidic gastric juices is reduced through vomiting or by **gastric suction,** a number of vital electrolytes are lost. These are usually hydrogen, chloride, potassium, and sodium. The total amount of fluid in the body is decreased, and the patient may develop **metabolic alkalosis** from the resulting excess of base bicarbonate. The symptoms of metabolic alkalosis include slow, shallow respiration, muscle hypertonicity and tetany, and personality changes. The patient may become disoriented or irritable and uncooperative.

[3]Norma Milligan Metheny and W. D. Snively, Jr. 1974. *Nurses' handbook of fluid balance,* p. 8. Philadelphia: Lippincott.

Intestinal suction, diarrhea, and other sources of gastrointestinal fluid loss. In a 24-hour period, 17,000 ml of fluid can be lost through diarrhea. With intestinal suction, 3,000 ml of fluid per day are lost. Prolonged use of laxatives and enemas can result in serious water and electrolyte disturbances. Gastrointestinal fluids can also be lost through **fistulas** or drainage tubes. Gastrointestinal obstruction produces fluid loss because fluids are trapped and are not able to be used by the body.

In addition to fluid volume loss, these gastrointestinal disturbances result in **metabolic acidosis** (because the intestinal secretions are primarily alkaline). Symptoms of metabolic acidosis include shortness of breath on exertion, deep, rapid breathing, weakness, malaise, and stupor progressing to coma.

Wound exudates can result in losses of protein and sodium and in a deficit in the extracellular fluid volume. Excessive perspiration can lead to abnormal losses of water, sodium, and chloride. If fluid intake of both water and electrolytes is not continued, the fluid volume and proportion of electrolytes decrease. The person may even develop sodium excess if insufficient water is ingested during a period of heavy perspiration.

"Insensible" water loss occurs through the lungs and skin. It totals approximately 600 to 1,000 ml per day in the average adult. If respiratory activity is increased, more water vapor is lost, and if there is damage to the skin, still more loss occurs. Because only water and not electrolytes is lost through the skin, water deficit and sodium excess will develop.

Hyperventilation results in respiratory alkalosis due to excessive elimination of carbon dioxide. **Hypoventilation,** which is much more dangerous than hyperventilation, causes retention of excessive amounts of carbon dioxide. This condition results in respiratory acidosis.

Factors influencing fluid and electrolyte balance

Age. From birth to about 2 years of age, a major percentage (70 to 80 percent) of the body weight is made up of water. It is thought that this extra water (20 percent more than in an adult) acts as a protective mechanism, compensating for the larger surface area in relation to body weight. Fluid is needed in large amounts to meet the infant's requirements for a more dilute urine and to satisfy his higher metabolic demands. Another difference is that in the infant, 50 percent of the body water is intracellular and 50 percent is extracellular, as compared to a 75 percent/25 percent ratio in the adult.

In the elderly also, fluid and electrolyte balance is a major point of vulnerability. Often the essential physiological systems are no longer completely adequate. Fluid imbalances may be a result of a breakdown in one or more of the following areas: respiratory, renal, cardiac, and gastrointestinal. Many of the physiological processes of aging cannot be reversed, but dangerous fluid imbalances can be avoided.

Malfunction of fluid-regulatory systems. The renal system acts both independently and in response to hormones, such as **antidiuretic hormone (ADH)** and mineralocorticoids, to excrete wastes and to conserve needed materials. When this system fails, many disturbances in fluid and electrolyte balance occur.

Integumentary. Excessive fluid and electrolytes are sometimes lost through the skin in a condition known as diaphoresis. A more profound and immediate loss comes from another disruption of the skin in burns. The degree of fluid and electrolyte loss from burns depends largely on the depth of the burn (first, second, or third degree) and the percentage of the body surface that is involved.

Respiratory. The lungs, under control of the medulla of the brain, function to maintain homeostasis. They do so by regulating oxygen–carbon dioxide exchange, controlling acid-base balance, and removing quantities of water from the body in the form of vapor. The consequences of hypo- and hyperventilation have been described previously (see p. 403).

Gastrointestinal. The most common cause of fluid and electrolyte imbalance is the loss of gastrointestinal fluids. (Gastrointestinal fluids consist of saliva, gastric juice, bile, pancreatic juice, and intestinal secretions.) Fluids can be lost, as was mentioned previously (p. 402), when they are trapped in an obstructed intestinal tract, or through gastrointestinal suction, diarrhea, fistulas, and drainage tubes. A defect in the absorptive powers of the intestinal tract can also result in fluid and electrolyte imbalance.

Endocrine. Homeostasis is maintained partially through the action of the glands of internal secretion. These are the endocrine glands, which include the adrenals, the parathyroids, and the anterior and posterior pituitary glands. A dysfunction in the endocrine system results in a major dysfunction in fluid and electrolyte balance.

Neurological. The brain's respiratory center controls the amount of carbon dioxide given off by the lungs. Here also is control of the desire to take a drink, as well as the functional ability to do so. Generally, the central nervous system influences water loss from the kidneys, the skin, and the lungs. A number of conditions, including brain tumors, infections, or trauma, can cause serious fluid imbalances.

Surgery. The first reaction to surgery is a period of fluid retention and catabolism. The activities of stress response appear to aid the body. Fluid and electrolyte retention helps to maintain blood volume, protein breakdown makes amino acids available for healing, and **gluconeogenesis** creates a ready supply of glucose.

Fluid that accumulates around the operative site just after surgery is

There is no known substitute for water among living organisms.

gradually reabsorbed and excreted during the second phase of reaction to surgery. If immobilization continues for a long time postoperatively, other metabolic changes occur (see chapter 18). Because the postoperative patient usually eats very little after surgery, a "starvation effect" takes place. This is accompanied by a negative nitrogen balance and leads to a daily weight loss of approximately one-half pound.

In this second phase, which occurs after the second to the fifth postoperative day, diuresis and anabolism begin. Water and sodium leave the body in greater amounts, and potassium is retained. Body protein is being built up, and the body regains its nitrogen balance.

Planning, implementation, and evaluation

Regulating oral intake

Increasing ("forcing") fluids. This can be accomplished by ensuring that extra fluids are supplied on the patient's tray at mealtime. He also should be offered fluids and foods between meals. If the patient has certain food or fluid preferences, these items can be secured from the diet kitchen or brought in by the patient's family. Green, leafy vegetables are approximately 96 to 98 percent water, and salads, gelatin desserts, fruits, and soups increase fluid intake in palatable ways. A pitcher of fresh water should be kept at the patient's bedside at all times.

Restricting fluids. This sometimes becomes more of a problem. The patient should be told of his limitation, in terms he can understand (that is, how many glasses allowed per day instead of how many cc's). He then should be permitted to choose the times for his fluid intake. One person may want all his fluids with his meals. Another may want to "save" his fluid ration and have a cup of tea or glass of milk at bedtime. Ice chips may go a long way toward satisfying thirst, and the total amount of actual water consumed is comparatively small. Thirst-inducing fluids, such as salty broths, should be avoided.

Intake and output

There are certain categories of patients who should automatically have all fluid gains and losses calculated. (This is done by the nursing staff and charted, usually every 8 hours.) Any patient with signs of fluid imbalance should be on intake and output (I&O) measurement (see also chapter 19).

The nurse should remember that intake includes intravenous solutions, irrigation fluids that are not returned, blood transfusions, gastric tube feedings, as well as all intake by mouth. Output includes not only measured urine but liquid stool, drainage from wounds, fluid from gastrointestinal suction, vomitus, and diaphoresis. (The amount of fluid lost in perspiration can be estimated by noting the number of changes of gowns and bed linens that are needed.)

There are certain categories of patients who should automatically have all fluid gains and losses calculated.

Intravenous therapy

If the patient cannot take fluids by mouth for any reason, intravenous fluids are given. Both water and electrolytes can be given intravenously. In general, intravenous fluids are given to maintain daily requirements for fluid and to replace past losses. Replacement should include the appropriate volume (3 liters per 24 hours in an average adult) and the correct composition of electrolytes that have been lost.

Intravenous fluids are classified according to their tonicity (isotonic, hypotonic, or hypertonic). The following is a list of some common parenteral solutions given intravenously:

1. Sodium chloride (0.9 percent, normal saline or physiological saline solution)
2. Saline solution (0.45 percent, one-half strength physiological saline solution)
3. Sodium chloride (2 to 5 percent)
4. Hartmann's lactated Ringer's solution
5. Glucose in water (5 percent)
6. Dextran

Venipuncture. Fluids are given via the vein because veins provide a direct and effective route to the extracellular fluid compartment. In some conditions, immediate medication must be given via this route. Large amounts of fluid can be given in a short time when administered intravenously.

In order to start an intravenous infusion, the nurse first assembles her equipment. Equipment includes the appropriate needle, intravenous connecting tubing, the solution to be infused, a tourniquet (or blood pressure cuff), an alcohol sponge, tape, an IV pole, and gauze. She explains the procedure to the patient, and then selects a site for the infusion.

The cephalic vein of the forearm is an excellent site for **venipuncture,** as this vein will accommodate a large needle. Also, the patient has some freedom of movement with an intravenous needle in this location.

Several kinds of needles may be used for venipuncture. A regular straight needle and a **scalp vein needle** are two common types. The scalp vein needle is approximately three-quarters of an inch long and has attached plastic wings used to hold the needle in place during venipuncture. Of the straight needles, a 19- or 20-gauge needle may be selected; an 18-gauge needle may be used for blood administration. (The smaller the gauge number, the larger the internal diameter of the needle.)

A **plastic needle** is a small plastic tube mounted on a metal needle. When the venipuncture is made, the needle is removed from the vein and the plastic tube is left in place; this is used when infusion therapy is long. An **intracatheter** is a long plastic tube inserted through a metal needle.

There are two steps to inserting an intravenous needle—piercing the skin and piercing the vein. A tourniquet is used to produce venous engorgement, and the area is cleansed with an antiseptic. The nurse (if right-handed) then grasps the extremity with the left hand so that the thumb rests on the skin approximately 2 inches below the selected site of venipuncture. She exerts tension downward toward the hand. (A location on the forearm is used in this example.) This tension minimizes the difficulty experienced when superficial veins retract or curl away from the needle point. It is helpful if the pressure is maintained until the needle is in its final position within the vein.[4]

Generally, the bevel of the needle should face upward during insertion. If a large needle is being used, however, the bevel should face downward or the needle will pierce the posterior wall of the vein.

The nurse inserts the needle through the skin adjacent to the vein approximately $\frac{1}{2}$ inch below the point at which the vein is to be entered. At insertion, the needle should be at about a 45-degree angle; after the skin is entered, the needle is lowered toward the arm. The needle is then advanced into the vein and carefully threaded upward approximately one-half to three-fourths of an inch. The tourniquet is then released. To ensure that the needle is in the vein, the nurse can lower the infusion bottle below the site of injection. A backflow of blood indicates that the needle is correctly located in the vein.

The needle is then anchored with tape and a gauze pad. If movement of the extremity is likely to dislodge the needle, an arm board or splint is applied.

In order to calculate the rate of flow, the nurse must know how many drops equal 1 ml in the administration set she is using. This varies with the types of sets made by various manufacturers. In regular administration sets, the rate varies from 10 to 20 drops delivering 1 ml. "Special" sets deliver more drops per milliliter, usually 50 to 60 drops per milliliter. The number of drops in 1 ml is called the **drop factor.**

To regulate the number of drops per minute, the nurse uses this formula:

$$\text{drops/minute} = \frac{\text{total volume to be infused} \times \text{drop factor}}{\text{total time of infusion (in minutes)}}$$

Modifying the equipment or solution. Additions to the intravenous solution frequently are ordered by the doctor. They are added directly to the solution by injecting the appropriate amount through the rubber stoppers of glass IV bottles. They may also be added by injecting the proper amount through special rubber-covered cannulas on plastic bottles. Medications most frequently mixed with infusion fluids are vitamins, electrolytes, and antibiotics. This method provides for a continuous flow of medication. The nurse should check with the pharmacist or with the manufacturer's directions for compatibility of medications.

For medications ordered in periodic doses (for example, every 6 hours),

[4]Norma G. Dison. 1971. *An atlas of nursing techniques,* 2d ed., pp. 186–87. St. Louis: Mosby.

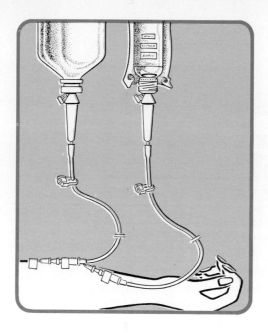

FIG. 22-2 *Setup for "piggy-back" IV.*

[Courtesy Eli Lilly and Company]

a second container can be set up alongside the regular infusion solution on the IV pole. Medication, often mixed in another infusion solution, can then be given intermittently. This may be done with an administration set with a Y-connector (one for each bottle of solution). It may also be done by attaching tubing and a needle to the bottle with medication and inserting it into a rubber stopper along the main infusion tubing. This is called a **piggyback.**

Mechanical factors influencing flow rate. There are several factors that may alter the rate of flow once it has been adjusted. These include change in needle position, height of the solution bottle, patency of the needle, and plugging of the air vent.

Blood transfusions

Two people, usually the doctor and the nurse, should check the labeling of the blood. They should make sure that the name and blood type match the name and blood type of the person to receive the blood. They should also check that the order written for the blood (whole blood or packed cells) matches the kind of blood received from the blood bank. (In teaching hospitals, the doctor administering the blood may not be the one who ordered it.) This checking is extremely important, for it appears that most mistakes of blood incompatibility are due to improper identification of blood label and patient.[5]

Before a transfusion can be given, the patient's blood is typed and crossmatched. The type determines the patient's blood group and the Rh(D) factor. The crossmatch determines whether the patient's plasma is com-

[5] Audrey L. Sutton. 1969. *Bedside nursing techniques in medicine and surgery,* 2d ed., p. 95. Philadelphia: Saunders.

patible with the donor's red cells—a measure of whether other factors in the blood are compatible. A new crossmatch is done whenever more than 24 hours has elapsed since a previous transfusion.

Blood is administered in units of 500 ml and is given via administration sets that are similar to those used for regular intravenous solutions. One difference is that a filter is attached to the blood administration set so that the blood is filtered for particulate matter as it is being given.

Once the blood is brought from the hospital's blood bank and checked for accuracy, the transfusion should be started within the hour. The unit should be hung 3 to 4 feet above the patient's heart level and given with a needle size larger than the ones used for intravenous solutions. Blood is administered along with normal saline. For the first 10 minutes, the blood is given slowly to enable the nurse or doctor to observe any untoward reactions. If no reaction occurs, the flow may be increased to as much as 120 drops per minute, unless there is some cardiac impairment. At this rate, the unit can be transfused in 80 minutes. If there is cardiovascular impairment, the rate should be slowed to about 60 to 70 drops per minute. A blood pump may be used to increase the flow in other cases.

The following possible reactions to blood transfusions may occur:

Potassium excess. When blood is stored, the red blood cells begin to break down. Potassium is released from these cells, and the longer the blood is stored, the more potassium there is. According to some research, a high incidence of cardiac arrest during surgery corresponds with the rapid infusion of large quantities of aged blood.[6] Blood stored for more than 21 days should be considered dangerous, and the nurse should check the expiration date of the blood to be given.

Calcium deficit. Calcium deficit can result from rapid administration of large volumes of blood preserved with **acid-citrate-dextrose (ACD)** solution. Citrate ions combine with the body's calcium, and signs of neuro-muscular irritability will occur because of the decreased level of circulating calcium ions.

Circulatory overload. If blood is given in massive amounts to a patient with a normal blood volume, circulatory overload can occur. It can cause not only pulmonary edema but also hemorrhage in the lungs and the gastrointestinal tract.

Cardiac arrest. Cardiac arrest during massive replacement therapy has been attributed to the administration of cold blood. When only one or two units are given, the time it takes from removal of the blood from storage (at 4° C) to actual administration (some 15 to 50 minutes later) is usually sufficient to warm the blood for safe administration.

According to some research, a high incidence of cardiac arrest during surgery corresponds with the rapid infusion of large quantities of aged blood.

[6]Metheny and Snively, p. 155.

Bacterial contamination. Bacterial contamination can be avoided if the blood is inspected for signs of bacterial growth, such as discoloration or gas bubbles.

Interaction of donor blood with the recipient's blood may cause the following:

Allergic reaction. When such symptoms as itching, **erythema, urticaria,** chills, and wheezing develop, the nurse should stop the transfusion immediately and notify the doctor.

Serum hepatitis. This can occur if the donor had this disease. Hepatitis is not an immediate reaction; the incubation period for serum hepatitis is from 6 weeks to 6 months.

Pyrogenic reactions. These reactions can result from foreign bodies in the administration set or from reaction to components of the donor blood itself. The reactions tend to occur at the end of the transfusion or even after it is completed. The predominant symptoms are fever and chills.

Hemolytic reactions. These reactions occur with blood incompatibility, with hemolyzed red blood cells, or from injections of nonisotonic solutions. Symptoms occur within the first 10 to 15 minutes of the transfusion and may include pain, fever, and chills.[7]

Hyperalimentation

For patients unable to eat or absorb nutrients through the alimentary tract, parenteral **hyperalimentation** can provide nutrients sufficient to promote tissue synthesis and anabolism. Ordinary IV solutions cannot deliver sufficient calories or nutrients to meet total body needs. One of these solutions contains 1,000 calories and 6 grams of nitrogen per liter. Electrolytes can be added to the solution. The flow rate must be slow and constant; otherwise, dehydration or convulsions can occur from **osmotic diuresis.**

Terminating an infusion

To terminate an infusion, the nurse first clamps the administration tubing to stop the flow of solution into the vein. Holding the needle firmly, she loosens the tape and any gauze. With one hand she holds a sterile dry **pledget** over the site of insertion, and with the other hand she slowly withdraws the needle or plastic tube. She then tapes the pledget to the site and applies pressure to the wound to ensure blood clotting.

[7]Ibid., p. 156.

SUMMARY

Water is a medium, a solvent, and a cushion, and it provides a solution in which electrolytes ionize. Water and electrolytes are both necessary for proper fluid balance in the body.

There are many possible sources of fluid imbalance, including decreased or increased food or fluid intake, vomiting, intestinal suction, diarrhea, hemorrhage, diaporesis, and altered respirations. All these can exhaust the body's homeostatic mechanisms and cause major fluid disturbances. The result may be too much or too little circulating fluid volume. Also possible are sodium, potassium, and calcium deficits or excesses; metabolic and respiratory alkalosis or acidosis; and abnormal shifts of fluid within the extracellular fluid compartments. Infants and older people are particularly susceptible to these disturbances.

The nurse's responsibilities in caring for patients with fluid and electrolyte imbalances include increasing or limiting oral intake of fluid and accurately calculating all fluid gains and losses. She must also regulate (and sometimes start) intravenous solutions and observe for any complications of parenteral therapy. Blood transfusions, hyperalimentation, and hypodermoclysis represent parenteral procedures that require accurate judgment and constant nursing observation.

STUDY QUESTIONS

1. What is an electrolyte?
2. Define osmosis, diffusion, and filtration. Give examples of each.
3. What are some common conditions which lead to fluid and electrolyte imbalance? How can the nurse help the patient to overcome the imbalance caused by each of these conditions?
4. Briefly describe the process of venipuncture. How does the nurse control the rate at which the solution flows?
5. What are the safety precautions a nurse should take while a patient is receiving a blood transfusion?

SELECTED BIBLIOGRAPHY

Dickens, Margaret L. 1974. *Fluid and electrolyte balance: A programmed text,* 3d ed. Philadelphia: Davis.
Dison, Norma G. 1971. *An atlas of nursing techniques,* 2d ed., pp. 184–209. St. Louis: Mosby.
Metheny, Norma Milligan, and Snively, W. D., Jr. 1974. *Nurses' handbook of fluid balance.* Philadelphia: Lippincott.
Snively, W. D., Jr., and Beshear, Donna R. 1971. Water and electrolytes in health and disease. In Kay Corman Kintzel, ed., *Advanced concepts in clinical nursing,* pp. 246–76. Philadelphia: Lippincott.
Sutton, Audrey L. 1969. *Bedside nursing techniques in medicine and surgery,* 2d ed., pp. 76–100. Philadelphia: Saunders.

Part Six

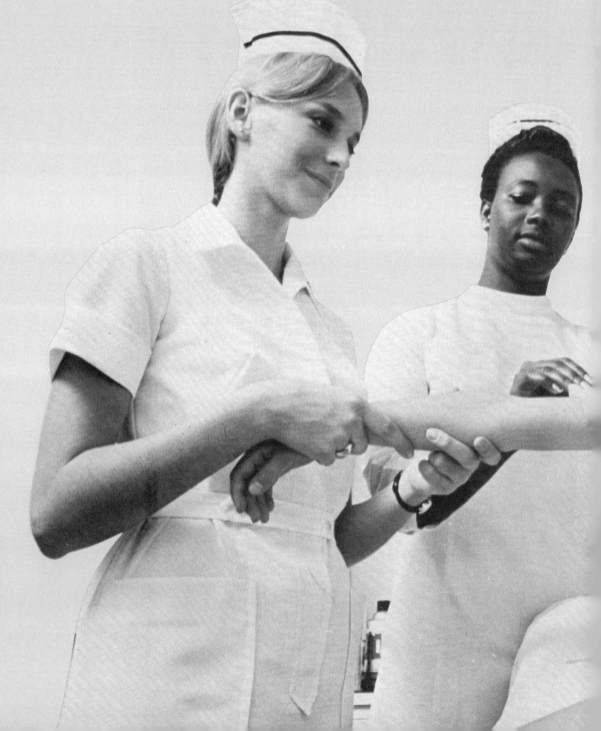

Nursing intervention in specific situations

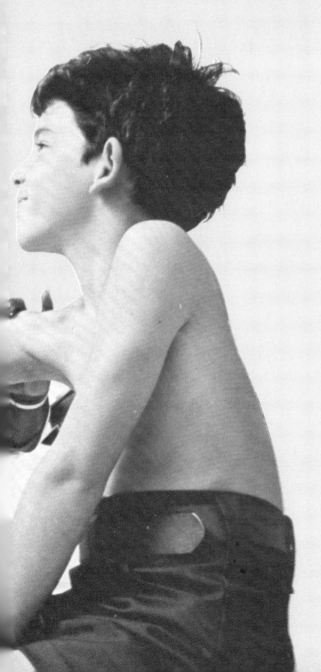

"LOCAL BASKETBALL STAR SERI-OUSLY INJURED IN CAR CRASH," read the headline in the paper the day after Steve Harrison had scored the winning points in a YMCA basketball tournament. "In a 2-car accident involving 7 local students, Steven Harrison, son of Anita and Richard Harrison, suffered extensive injuries, including a crushed chest. His brother Paul, driver of the car in which young Harrison was a passenger, escaped with minor cuts and bruises. The other passengers were uninjured."

The ambulance ride to the hospital drowned out all memories of the cheering crowd for Steve. Now he was lying in the intensive care unit of the hospital, and everything hurt. It hurt to breathe, to move. It seemed that tubes were connected to him everywhere. They gave him injections to ease the pain, but Steve found that he hurt emotionally as well as physically.

Although lots of people were constantly hovering around him, Steve had never felt so lonely or anonymous in his life. The first day in the hospital, he remembered, he had been semiconscious from the postoperative effects of surgery and the aftermath of the accident.

413

The doctors and the nurses stood in his room and talked about him as though he were a million miles away. Even his parents seemed to pay more attention to the hospital staff than they did to him. The worst thing, though, was that no one really told him what his condition was. They just concentrated on the details of his care. They explained why he was getting blood transfusions and needed to be fed through a tube. He knew that he had to be hooked up to a respirator periodically and that he must exercise his arms and legs.

But Steve wanted to know how long he'd be in the hospital and whether he'd be able to play basketball again soon. That was a question everyone, even his parents, kept avoiding. Steve felt that his brother Paul would tell him the truth, but Paul had not come to the hospital to see him. Steve wasn't mad at Paul for the accident, but he was beginning to be angry at being ignored, just when he needed someone to talk to.

The Harrisons tried to get Paul to go to the hospital, but he said he wouldn't know what to say to Steve once he got there. He did tell his parents that he thought they should tell Steve the truth about his injuries and about his having developed septicemia. Anita and Richard kept saying that they were sure that the antibiotics would pull Steve

through, that they didn't want to alarm him unnecessarily. But Steve didn't seem to be responding to treatment. Finally, Paul decided to go to the hospital.

"I'm here to talk and to listen," Paul told Steve. But now Steve turned away from him, saying, "Now *I* don't feel like talking to *you*. I'm tired of doing things when other people want them done. Just leave me alone." Steve's outburst hurt Paul greatly, but he decided to wait a couple of days and then try once more to talk to him. He realized that Steve wasn't himself, what with all the pain, the medication, and the anxiety his injuries created.

In a couple of days it was too late to talk anymore. Steve died two weeks after the accident.

What are the nurse's responsibilities in the physical care of this patient?

How can the nurse help to meet the patient's psychological and emotional needs?

What are the nurse's responsibilities toward the patient's family?

What other health team members should be involved in this situation?

23 Wound problems

Assessment of wounds

Types of wounds

Whether **traumatic** or **operative,** wounds may be classified as either clean or infected and contaminated.

Clean wounds. If traumatic wounds are treated within 6 to 12 hours, they usually close quickly and respond well.[1] However, these injuries, usually caused by a sharp object, must still be checked frequently to make sure they are not becoming infected. When the possibility of infection is considered strong, a small drain should be placed in the wound at the time it is closed up.

If an operative wound is nondraining and is not contaminated or only mildly so, little postoperative care is needed. In some cases, spray-on plastic dressings, such as Aeroplast, will be used after surgery. In other cases, ordinary gauze dressings are used. Sutures provide the main support for wound healing; adhesives should be used with caution. Deep wound disruptions should be repaired at the time they occur, unless the patient's condition makes it impossible.

It is not necessary to wear gloves in dressing clean wounds if the instruments and dressings are handled so that no part of an instrument or dressing touched by the hand touches the wound.

Contaminated wounds. Contaminated wounds include the following:

1. A traumatic wound that has been grossly contaminated or has not been cared for immediately
2. An operative wound that has been drained or left open because of significant contamination
3. An open wound in which granulations are infected or not "clean"[2]

[1]Philip Cooper. 1967. *Ward procedures and techniques,* pp. 177–79. New York: Appleton-Century-Crofts.
[2]Ibid., p. 182.

1. Discuss two types of wounds, clean and contaminated.

2. Describe the physiological process of wound healing and the factors that may complicate it.

3. Provide for the patient's psychological needs by preparing him for observations and sensations he will experience when a dressing is changed.

4. Perform the five basic procedures that are a part of sterile technique for changing dressings.

5. Apply basic bandages and binders.

Relatively rapid healing
is characteristic of
uncomplicated surgical
incisions.

Some wound infections are superficial, manifesting themselves as **cellulitis.** Others, limited to the deeper layers of the wound, lie unsuspected for long periods. This may occur when an abscess forms in a difficult-to-reach area. The treatment for both superficial and hidden wounds is heat and antibiotics. Sometimes patients with infected wounds are isolated to prevent transmission of organisms to others.

A mask and gloves are always worn by those treating an infected wound, and clothing is not allowed to come into contact with the patient's bedclothes. All contaminated materials and instruments are cleaned or disposed of according to sterile techniques.

Wound healing

Physiological processes. The healing of wounds is a complex biological process that has been fairly well understood for many years. The process is separated into three stages, according to the activities of particular populations of cells (see Fig. 23–1). One science writer uses the example of a deep skin cut to illustrate this process:

Initially, blood flows into the gap created by the cutting instrument, fills the space and clots, uniting the edges of the wound. Within several hours the clot loses fluid and the surface becomes dehydrated, so that it forms the hard scab that serves to protect the wound.[3]

As fluid enters the wound around the clot, the process of inflammation begins. At this point, the injury may become swollen and painful. Then, about 6 hours after the wound occurs, various kinds of white blood cells migrate into the wound. They then begin removing and breaking down cellular debris, bacteria, and other foreign material.

Subsequently in the dermis, or subsurface layer, the cells called fibroblasts enter the wound and build scar tissue by manufacturing collagen fibers and other proteins. Meanwhile the epidermis, or surface layer, creates a new surface similar to the old one. When this layer is almost completely formed, the scab sloughs off.[4]

Complications. Relatively rapid healing is characteristic of uncomplicated surgical incisions. In these cases, the edges of the wound are held together by sutures, clips, or strapping. This is called "healing by first intention." "Healing by second intention" refers to the healing of wounds with wide spaces between the edges. These wounds heal less quickly, and granulation tissue fills in the wound from below. In time, this granulation tissue becomes scar tissue.

[3]Russell Ross. 1969. Wound healing. *Scientific American* 220:40.
[4]Ibid.

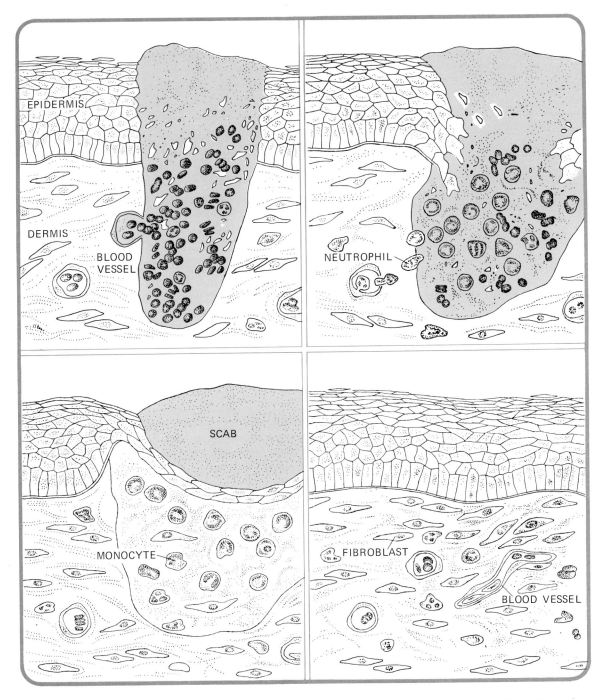

EPIDERMIS

DERMIS

BLOOD
VESSEL

NEUTROPHIL

SCAB

MONOCYTE

FIBROBLAST

BLOOD VESSEL

There are many conditions that can slow down the healing process. For example, older people tend to heal more slowly than young ones (see p. 305). In people who are anemic, malnourished, or lacking certain vitamins, tissue does not reform as quickly. Arteriosclerosis impairs circulation and prevents blood from flowing normally to the wound site. If a patient

FIG. 23-1 *Stages of wound healing.*

417

is taking steroids, an infection may go unnoticed and the wound will not heal properly. Patients on anticoagulant drugs may hemorrhage. Also, the patient who is overactive places a strain on his wound; this can prevent the edges from knitting properly, and hemorrhaging may result.

Also important is the type of dressing used and the way in which it is applied. If dressings are not applied properly, wound healing is slowed down. A dressing that does not cover the wound adequately exposes the wound to contamination. A dressing that is not changed frequently enough leaves the wound susceptible to bacterial invasion. If a dressing is changed too frequently, the healing process may suffer because of rough handling. Dressings applied too tightly can cause pressure on a wound, thus interfering with the normal blood flow to that part of the body.

Other factors that can retard the healing process include a **hematoma** (blood clot) in the wound or a foreign object, such as an item of surgical equipment, left in the wound. Local **ischemia** due to poor blood supply also slows down the healing process.

Infection is a particularly dangerous complication. Wounds caused by burns or amputation are liable to infection, as are those resulting from emergency surgery. In the latter case, proper preparation of the skin is sometimes neglected under the pressure of the situation.

Prevention of infection is an important responsibility of the nurse (see chapter 14). She must follow scrupulously the techniques for keeping the wound itself free of infection. She must also make sure that the patient's total environment is as free as possible from the hazards of bacterial infection. Despite the introduction of advanced aseptic techniques and powerful drugs, wound infection is still a major concern in hospitals.

Planning, intervention, and evaluation

Preoperative skin preparation

In order to make the patient's skin as free as possible of microorganisms, he is "prepped" the afternoon or evening before surgery. This procedure involves cleansing a wide area of the skin at the incision site and removing hair from its surface. (Hair is removed because of the possibility that microorganisms residing there will infect the wound site.)

Prep procedures vary somewhat from one hospital to another. Frequently, nothing more than soap and warm water is used for the cleansing. However, because antiseptic solutions are so effective against microorganisms, they are sometimes used instead.

Some researchers are convinced that the patient's own microorganisms, not those from the staff or equipment, are responsible for a large number of postoperative infections.[5] Guided by this philosophy, nurses at New

---

[5]Post-op infections: The patient's flora is the most likely cause. *RN* 36 (1973):OR–13.

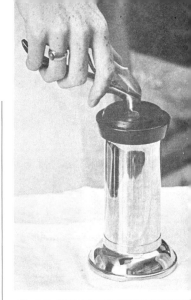

York Hospital–Cornell Medical Center prep patients by washing around the incision site for at least 3 minutes with a polyurethane sponge impregnated with a germicide. Povidone-iodine solution is used to paint the area.

In addition to skin cleansing, other measures are taken before surgery to ensure a minimum of exposure to possible sources of infection. If the patient has been in the hospital for some time and has not shampooed his hair, he should do so (or have the nurse do it) before surgery. The evening before or the morning of surgery, he should take a bath or be bathed (see chapter 16).

Handling sterile supplies

Although many sterile supplies are now available in individual packages, others must be taken from a larger supply without contamination. Some sterile equipment requires the use of sterile gloves. Often, however, the nurse will use instead a pair of forceps kept in a jar of antiseptic solution. Either way, such equipment is never touched with the naked hand.

Forceps should be removed from the solution by their handles. They should be lifted directly up out of the jar without touching the sides. The tip should always be held in a downward position so that the antiseptic solution does not spill over the instrument.

In order to prevent contamination, the lid should be held with the inside downward. The outside should be placed downward if the lid is placed on a table. When handing a sterile instrument to someone else, use the handling forceps to grasp the instrument by the tip. Sterile gauze or cotton balls should also be removed with the handling forceps. Two forceps will be necessary for removing sterile petrolatum gauze from a container. However, once the forceps have become contaminated, they cannot be used to remove a second piece of gauze.

Supplies that are enclosed in sterile packs must remain untouched. Sterile wrapping is used for such equipment as sterile dressings, towels, drapes, small basins, trays, and certain instruments. Large sterile packs must be placed on a table for opening. Usually they are held together with string, tape, or pins. The wrapper should be loosened first and then one flap at a time folded back. Fingers should never touch the inside of the wrapper.

If a package has been presterilized commercially, the nurse merely tears or peels the package at the indicated place. She then holds the package opening apart and removes the contents with sterile forceps. In order to hand the sterile article to someone else, she holds the pack with one hand and opens it with the other. Holding the pack at a distance protects the inside from contamination.

Sometimes extra sterile articles are needed after the nurse has already opened a sterile tray. This presents no problem if the tray has remained sterile. The nurse merely drops the required sterile article on the tray. When

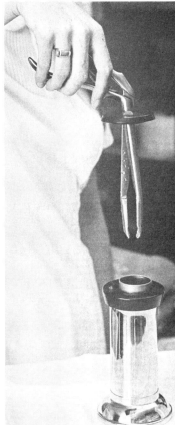

Forceps should be removed from a jar of antiseptic solution by their handles, holding the tip in a downward position.
[Photos by Dan Bernstein]

419

the article is removed, not from a sterile pack but from a disinfecting solution, it must be dropped into a sterile basin. A tray is considered contaminated when solution is spilled on the linen covering.

Pouring of a sterilized solution is another procedure which may appear simple but which requires specific techniques. When the container has a paper cap or screw top, neither the outside of the rim nor the inside of the cap should be touched.

Sometimes it is necessary—although not desirable—to open a sterile tray, add extra articles or solutions, and reclose the tray before taking it to the patient's room. In such a case, the outer wrapper is opened as described previously. The nurse grasps only a small part of the towel with the forceps, standing away from the opened outer wrapper. She then pours the sterile solution into the basin, placing the covering back over the tray with the forceps. The disinfectant solution on the tip of the forceps should not drip onto any part of the tray. To replace the wrapper, she slides her hand under the wrapper so that she is touching only the outside layer.

In certain emergency situations, a routine sterile tray is not available for the placement of equipment. When this happens, the nurse removes a sterile towel with forceps from an opened wrapper or can. She then grasps two corners of the towel, using two pairs of forceps, and unfolds the towel halfway. (The forceps should not touch the unsterile tray being used.) The towel should be double in thickness, and two must be used if the tray is large.

The nurse places the sterile articles on the towel with the forceps, as close as possible to the center of the tray. She unfolds another towel with two handling forceps, placing it double thickness over the articles and completely covering them.

All personnel handling sterile equipment must wear sterile gloves. The nurse puts on her gloves according to the procedure described in chapter 14. To assist the surgeon or other worker in putting on his, she unfolds the glove wrapper, touching only the outside surface. She shakes the powder packet toward the center of the glove folder, holding the folder so that the other worker can pick up the powder without touching the inside of the folder. She holds open the pocket first for one glove and then for the other.

In order to apply medication with a sterile applicator, the applicator must be removed from its container with a handling forceps. Insert the tip into the medication jar, without touching the sides or top of the jar. Grasping the applicator with the handling forceps, hand the applicator to whoever is applying the medication.

Psychological implications for the patient

Although the sight of a newly sutured incision is routine for a nurse, it is not routine for the patient. Unless he is prepared psychologically, he

Although the sight of a newly sutured incision is routine for a nurse, it is not routine for the patient.

may become very distressed when he sees his incision, complete with ugly black sutures. Fear of scarring or disfigurement may be very real.

In a reassuring tone, the nurse should explain that at first the incision will appear quite red and inflamed, but that gradually this inflammation will subside. If the patient's wound is extensive, draining, and/or foul-smelling, he should also be prepared for this fact. The patient's family must also be informed of what to expect.

Changing a sterile dressing

In certain situations—for example, when a patient is hemorrhaging or when there is excessive drainage—dressings should not be changed. Thus it is important to make sure that a physician has ordered a change of dressing before proceeding. In some instances a dressing should be reinforced rather than changed entirely.

Hospitals vary in the types of dressings they use for wounds, but today most prefer dressing trays or dressing packs. Except for the adhesive tape, all items are sterile, and sterile procedures are used.

Changing the dressing for a nondraining wound. The following is a list of basic items needed for this procedure:

1. Sterile towel
2. Sterile cup to hold disinfectant solution
3. One or two sterile handling forceps
4. Four to six 1″ × 1″ sterile gauze squares or cotton balls to cleanse wound
5. Sterile dressing materials—3″ × 3″ or 3″ × 6″ gauze
6. Disinfectant solution, such as 70 percent alcohol
7. Adhesive tape
8. Paper bags
9. Paper towels[6]

Items 1 through 4 or 1 through 5 may be included in a dressing tray. In cases where commercially packaged dressings are used, these items are carried separately.

After the nurse has collected all required items, she proceeds to the patient's bedside. Sometimes she will be working with several patients and will need a cart for carrying the equipment. All items are removed from the cart and placed on the bedside table.

The nurse opens the dressing tray and fills the cup with disinfectant. She then places the jar of solution on the bedside table and opens a paper bag, folding down the top slightly to keep the bag upright. Using short,

> Hospitals vary in the types of dressings they use for wounds.

[6] Audrey L. Sutton. 1969. *Bedside nursing techniques in medicine and surgery,* 2d ed., p. 126. Philadelphia: Saunders.

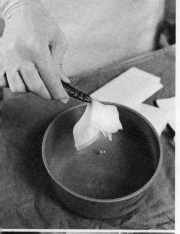

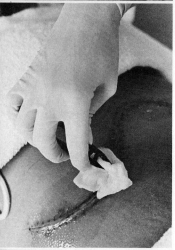

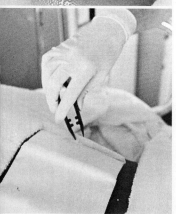

Steps in changing a sterile dressing: (1) using forceps, the nurse soaks gauze pads in a sterile solution; (2) she cleanses the wound; (3) she applies the new dressing.
[Photos by Dan Bernstein]

quick movements, she pulls off the adhesive tape, always pulling toward the wound so that the sutures do not rupture.

Soiled dressings are removed from the wound with a forceps or disposable gloves and then placed in the paper bag. Forceps should be placed on a paper towel on the bedside table and not used again. The second sterile forceps are then taken from the dressing tray and the sterile towel placed across the patient. These forceps should not touch the bedclothes.

Using the same forceps, the nurse cleanses the wound with small gauze squares soaked in disinfectant, discarding each one after use. This is the point at which sutures are removed, if that is part of the procedure. Forceps are placed on the sterile towel and the pack opened so that the physician can remove the sutures.

If no sutures are to be removed, the nurse takes the sterile dressings from the tray with forceps and positions them on the wound. When individual packs of dressings are used, she opens the pack with both hands. While opening the pack, the forceps are left on the towel and then used to take the dressings from the pack.

The dressings are then secured in place and the soiled instrument and cotton towel set on the dressing tray. After discarding soiled dressings in the paper bag, the nurse washes her hands and removes the container of disinfectant and the used tray from the bedside.

Changing the dressing for a draining wound. Basically, the same procedures and equipment hold for the care of a draining wound. However, larger sponges are used, to apply sterile water first and then a nonirritating disinfecting solution. After the patient's skin dries, the clean sterile dressing is applied. Usually, all necessary equipment is kept by the patient's bedside when his wound demands frequent changes of dressing.

Types of bandages

Circular bandage. If an arm or leg is to be bandaged, raise it to the same level as the patient's heart at least a quarter of an hour before applying the bandage. A leg that has been hanging over the side of the bed should be placed in a horizontal position 15 minutes before wrapping. The patient should be lying down during the leg bandaging procedure.

After the patient is positioned comfortably, he should be asked to raise his arm or leg slightly. The area to be bandaged should be dry and clean. Two turns should be made around the wound area first to secure the bandage. It should be held in place with the left thumb (if the nurse is right-handed) on top of the bandage and the anterior surface of the limb and the left index finger on the posterior side of the limb. The beginning and end of the bandage should not be placed directly over the wound, a bony part of the body, a part of the body the patient will lie on, or the inner side of a limb.

The bandage is then unwound toward the right, while being held not too tightly or loosely. Each circular turn is placed over the preceding turn. Only as many turns as are needed to hold the dressing in place or to immobilize the part should be used. Tape, metal clips, or a safety pin is used to secure the end of the bandage.

Spiral bandage. The procedure for applying these bandages, often used in the treatment of varicose veins, is similar to that for the circular bandage. With two circular turns, the nurse anchors the bandage at the patient's ankle. A figure-8 bandage is then used around the foot and ankle to ensure that the bandage will not slip off. Spiral bandaging then proceeds up the leg, and is always secured with a figure-8 motion across the nearest joint.

In bandaging an arm, the bandage is anchored at the wrist with two circular turns. The nurse grasps the roll in her right hand and then unwinds it downward from right to left around the arm. She then secures the bandage on the front of the arm with her left thumb and on the back with her left index finger. The part is wrapped until it is thoroughly covered.

Spiral-reverse bandage. An extremity that is thin in one place and thick in another, such as the calf, requires a different wrapping procedure. The spiral technique should be used until the bandage will no longer lie flat. The left thumb is then placed on the upper edge of the anterior turn, and the bandage is unwound 4 to 6 inches. The nurse now turns her hand downward so that the bandage is folded over her thumb in a downward direction. She continues unrolling to the right and then to the left on the underside of the leg, covering part of the preceding lap. She continues winding in the same manner and place as in the previous layers until the bandage lies flat once again.

Figure-8 bandage. This type of bandage is used to hold a dressing in place, to apply pressure or support, and to immobilize a joint. Elbows, knee joints, ankles, and wrists require this procedure.

When bandaging an elbow, the spiral reverse procedure is followed until the elbow is reached. A circular turn is made directly over the elbow. The bandage is then wrapped in a spiral upward motion just above the elbow, above the first circular turn. The next spiral turn is wrapped in a downward motion just below the first circular turn. The elbow is crossed alternately above and below until the bandage feels secure.

Recurrent bandage. A slightly different procedure is needed to hold pressure dressings in place over the tip end of a finger, toe, fist, or stump of an amputated extremity. The purpose of this type of bandaging is to prevent bleeding or swelling of the area.

The basic procedure is the same as for circular wrapping. When the area in question has been reached, the bandage roll is turned and brought

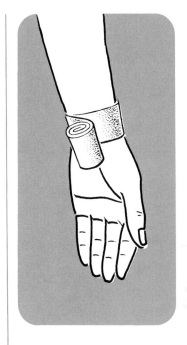

FIG. 23-2 *Application of a circular bandage.*

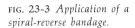

FIG. 23-3 *Application of a spiral-reverse bandage.*

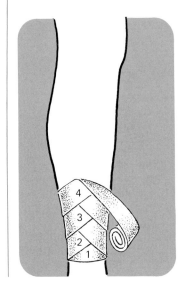

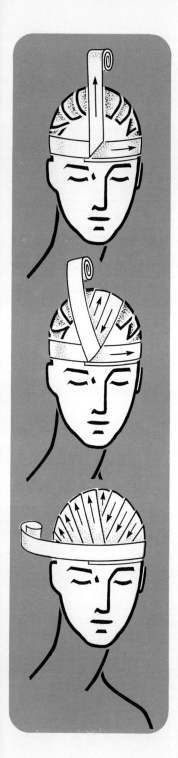

forward, over the tip of the patient's finger, for example. The bandage is then unrolled downward over the tip of the stump toward the back. Each turn is moved alternately to the left and then to the right of the first layer over the tip of the stump. Succeeding layers are held in place with the left thumb and index finger. When the stump is well covered, the direction of the roller bandage is reversed. At least two circular turns are made to cover the gathered ends.

Sling (triangular) bandage. Injured arms are the most frequent candidates for the sling bandage, which can be made from a piece of cloth 30 to 40 inches square. For a double triangle, the cloth is folded in half; for a single thickness, it is cut across the center fold.

One end of the triangle is positioned over the shoulder on the injured side. The apex (point) of the triangle is placed toward the elbow. The patient should bend his injured arm horizontally across his body with his thumb up. The other end of the triangle is brought around his injured arm and up over his injured shoulder. Tie the two ends of the triangle together with a square knot. The knot should lie to one side of the patient's neck so that he will not be uncomfortable lying down.

The apex of the triangle is folded over the elbow toward the front and secured with a pin. The height of the sling can be changed by adjusting the knot. Once the patient is wearing his sling, the circulation in his fingers should be checked often. Cold, pale fingers indicate it is obstructed.

Binders

A binder is a type of bandage usually used to provide encircling support of the chest or abdomen.

Scultetus (many-tailed) binder. This type of flannel wrapping is commonly used for patients who have undergone abdominal surgery (or who have just delivered a baby). The patient should be moved to the far side of the bed and asked to raise his hips. With the top edge at waist level, the scultetus binder is quickly slipped under his hips, with the solid part centered under his body. The bottom tail (strip) is brought across the abdomen and wrapped firmly in a spiral fashion with a $\frac{1}{2}$-inch overlap of each layer. Each succeeding tail is slanted slightly upward, and the binding proceeds toward the waist by alternating strips first from one side and then the other. The binder is secured with a safety pin.

Straight abdominal or chest binder. After the patient raises his hips or chest, the binder is slipped under him. The lower edge of an abdominal binder should come well down on the hips; the lower edge of a breast binder, to the waistline. The binder should be pulled very tightly and the lower edge fastened with a safety pin. Continuing straight up the midline, the edges are pulled tightly with about a 3-inch overlap.

FIG. 23-4 *Application of a recurrent bandage.*

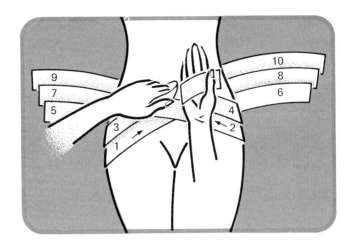

FIG. 23-5 *Application of a scultetus (many-tailed) binder.*

In order to make the binder lie flat, safety pins are used to take up the slack at various points. A "V" dart is made, starting with a large tuck at the midline. If a woman has large breasts, a pad is inserted under them before applying the chest binder to prevent irritation from perspiration.

T binder or double-T binder. The main purpose of these binders is to keep peri-pads or rectal and perineal dressings in place. After the patient raises his hips, the binder is centered under his back at waist level. The band is secured around the waist, and then a peri-pad or dressing is applied to the rectal or perineal area. The side that will touch the patient's skin should not be touched with the hands. The free end of the T is brought forward between the legs and secured at the waist.

A double-tailed binder is usually used for male patients. Each strip is brought forward between the legs. The right tail is extended to the right of the genitalia and secured to the waistband. The left tail is then brought forward to the left of the genitalia and secured.

Sometimes an embarrassed male patient may want to apply the binder himself. The nurse should certainly allow him to do so if he is able. However, she should remain on hand in case he needs help.

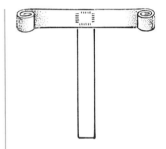

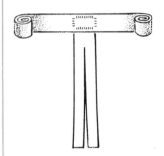

FIG. 23-6 *T and double-T binders.*

SUMMARY

Wounds are either clean or infected. Some are deep and some are superficial. Wound healing is a complex physiological process that demands careful attention to aseptic techniques. A clean wound is usually caused by a sharp object, and will heal fairly quickly unless there is a wide gap between the edges of the skin.

The rate of healing depends not only on the type of wound but also on the condition of the patient. Older people or those who are taking certain medications usually require more healing time. If dressings do not cover the wound or are not changed often enough, the healing process may be retarded and infection may result.

An important and often overlooked aspect of nursing care of wounds is psychological preparation of the patient. The patient may be shocked and distressed at the first view of ugly sutures and inflamed skin and will need considerable support from the nurse.

Sterile procedures are important not only after surgery but also before. Part of the nurse's activities include "prepping" the patient's skin for surgery. This means cleansing a wide area of skin and removing hair in order to reduce the possibility of bacterial invasion.

How often a dressing is changed depends on the nature of the wound: whether it is draining, for instance, or whether the patient is hemorrhaging. With certain variations, the same sequence of steps applies to changing a draining and a nondraining wound.

Dressings are secured with either bandages or binders. These devices serve other purposes, such as to apply pressure to stop bleeding or swelling or to immobilize an injured part. They may also be used to apply warmth to a joint or to promote circulation. A principle common to both devices is that pressure should be evenly distributed throughout the area treated. Binding that is too tight will impair circulation, while binding that is too loose may cause rubbing and skin irritation. The patient's skin should always be clean and dry.

Among the different types of bandages are circular, spiral, spiral reverse, figure-8, recurrent, and sling (triangular). Binders include scultetus (many-tailed), straight abdominal or chest, and T or double-T. Binders are generally used to provide support for the chest or abdomen.

STUDY QUESTIONS

1. Briefly outline the physiological processes involved in wound healing.
2. What is the procedure for changing the dressing on a nondraining wound? on a draining wound?
3. What are the general principles the nurse should keep in mind when handling sterile supplies?
4. Briefly outline three major types of bandages and how they are applied. Give examples of situations in which each would be used and why.
5. What is a binder? Describe the common types of binders and their uses.
6. What are some of the actions the nurse can take to relieve the patient's anxieties concerning the appearance and effects of his wound?

SELECTED BIBLIOGRAPHY

Cooper, Philip. 1967. *Ward procedures and techniques,* pp. 177–85. New York: Appleton-Century-Crofts.

Ross, Russell. 1969. Wound healing. *Scientific American* 220:40–50.

Sutton, Audrey L. 1969. *Bedside nursing techniques in medicine and surgery,* 2d ed., pp. 112–27. Philadelphia: Saunders.

Thomas, Betty, and Alexander, Carol. 1972. Psychological aspects of physical trauma. *AORN Journal* 15:45–50.

24 Administration of therapeutic agents

What is a drug?

A **drug** is a chemical substance used in treating, preventing, and diagnosing diseases.[1] Today, most drugs are made chemically, although many of natural origin are also available from plants, animals, minerals, bacteria, and fungi (antibiotics fall into this category). In all, some 25,000 drugs and drug products are now available.

Effects of drugs

Therapeutic effects. **Therapeutic effects** are those desired results for which the drug is prescribed. For example, Dramamine is often prescribed to prevent the nausea of motion sickness. The prevention of nausea is thus the therapeutic effect of Dramamine.

Side effects. **Side effects** are those effects other than the intended therapeutic effects for which a drug is prescribed. As stated above, Dramamine prevents nausea, but it may also cause drowsiness. Some side effects are minor; others are potentially dangerous. Some may even be beneficial. Known side effects should be explained to the patient so that he will be better able to cope with them. Observation of side effects is one of the most important functions of the nurse (see p. 429).

Synergistic effects (drug interaction). **Synergistic effects** are the result of taking two or more drugs at the same time. The combined effects may be very different from the effects of each drug taken alone. As in the case of side effects, the results may be either harmful or beneficial. For example, the combination of alcohol and tranquilizers or sleeping pills is potentially lethal, as the combined effects tend to depress the respiratory system. Often, a patient at home will take some nonprescription drug along with

[1] Kenneth I. Melville. 1973. Drugs and drug action. *Encyclopaedia Britannica*, 15th ed., vol. 5, p. 1041. Chicago: Encyclopaedia Britannica.

Upon completing this chapter, the reader should be able to:

1. Give examples of the three effects a drug may have.

2. Recognize that self-medication may easily result in drug abuse.

3. Compare and contrast methods for preparing and administering oral, parenteral, and topical medications.

4. Assume responsibility for the proper administration of drugs.

5. Instruct a patient in the procedure for self-medication.

427

the drug or drugs that have been prescribed by his physician. He should be warned against doing so.

Specific information on the action and administration of drugs should be sought in pharmacology texts. In addition, the nurse will find many practical reference sources in the field. The *Modern Drug Encyclopedia* and the *Physician's Desk Reference* are particularly useful.

Drug abuse

A number of drugs on the market can cause serious and sometimes fatal poisoning if used incorrectly. For this reason, the federal Food and Drug Administration has set strict controls on their use. Of course, it is customary for people to treat minor problems, such as cuts, burns, and occasional headaches, with over-the-counter medications. However, the increasing number of available drugs has produced a growing trend toward self-medication that may cause harm or may lead to addiction.

Although the term "drug abuse" is commonly associated with the misuse of narcotics, barbiturates, and alcohol, it is not limited to these substances alone. A common form of drug abuse is the overuse of laxatives, which may result in a serious fluid and electrolyte imbalance (see chapter 21). Other over-the-counter medications that are frequently overused include aspirin, antacids, and nose drops.

Drug abuse is not limited to patients alone. It is not an uncommon problem among health professionals. Doctors and nurses, in fact, have a higher than average chance of abusing one or more drugs.[2] (Demerol appears to be the most commonly abused drug among health personnel.) Not only is this abuse a serious problem and danger for the nurse-abuser, but it also represents a threat to the safety and well-being of her patients.

Responsibilities of the nurse

Proper administration of drugs

As was stated before, there are currently over 25,000 drugs in use. This number grows daily, so it would be impossible for a nurse to memorize the individual characteristics of each of the drugs she is called upon to administer. Drugs may be classified, however, according to composition, purposes, and effects, and the nurse should be familiar with the actions of groups of drugs.

Among the classifications of drugs are **antibiotics, antihistamines, hormones, narcotics,** and **depressants.** She should also seek information from any physician who orders a drug with which she is not familiar.

[2]Solomon Garb et al. 1970. *Pharmacology and Patient Care,* 3d ed., pp. 96–97. New York: Springer.

Safety

The nurse is in an excellent position to spot warnings that a drug is not working properly. As mentioned before, some side effects must be tolerated. The presence of others indicates the need for an immediate change of therapy.

Although certain side effects are associated with certain drugs, one cannot make any assumptions about the effect of a particular drug on a particular patient. Normal behavior in one patient may indicate a drug side effect in another. Thus it is important that any change in the patient's condition or behavior be reported. Symptoms frequently associated with side effects, toxic reactions, or allergies include nausea or vomiting, diarrhea, skin rash or itching, asthma, swelling, jaundice, sore throat, muscular rigidity, drowsiness or irrational behavior, changes in pulse, respiration, or blood pressure, and hematuria.

Even when a nurse was not the one who administered a drug, she is responsible for observing and reporting to the physician any suspicious consequences. A patient who has no initial reaction may have one later. For example, he may not react to an initial dose of penicillin, but may break out in a rash with a second injection. Allergic reactions are especially common in patients with asthma or allergies to particular substances.

Side effects develop for several reasons. The patient may have received too much of the medication and developed a toxic reaction. Toxic symptoms can also result from a cumulation of the drug over a long period. A patient who is sensitive to a particular drug will often develop an allergic reaction. In severe cases he may go into **anaphylatic** shock.

Sometimes a patient will develop tolerance or resistance to a drug, requiring increasing doses to produce the same initial effects. Many people dependent on diet pills are well aware of this phenomenon; in the beginning they find that one pill will cut their appetite and provide them with a mood elevation. After taking the drug for a period of months, only two pills will do.

Eventually, tolerance may lead to addiction. The addict has an overwhelming desire to continue to take the drug, usually in increasing doses. Sometimes he develops a physical dependence on the drug. It it is taken away from him, he will suffer such withdrawal symptoms as nausea, vomiting, abdominal cramps, and pain in the arms and legs.

Effectiveness

The nurse evaluates drug effectiveness by collecting data. For example, what is the patient's subjective response to his medication? The answer comes from direct questioning of the patient as well as knowledge of the patient and the particular drug.

Methods of collecting data, which should be incorporated into the

Even when a nurse was not the one who administered a drug, she is responsible for observing and reporting to the physician any suspicious consequences.

nursing plan, include the monitoring of vital signs, intake and output records, and the patient's weight. Results of laboratory tests are also helpful. Certain ones are undertaken specifically to evaluate drug response. For example, prothrombin time reflects the degree of blood coagulability and thus indicates how well certain anticoagulants are working. Other tests provide more general indications of changes in the patient's physical condition.

Specific measures will promote the effect of and/or reduce the need for each drug. For example, a nurse might assess the effectiveness of an analgesic by observing the nature of the pain and the patient's reaction to it. In order to promote the effectiveness of the drug, she might have the patient change his position in bed to relieve pressure and lessen edema. In addition, she might look for ways to divert the patient and help him to relax.

In order to make sure that a drug is given a chance to produce its maximum effects, the nurse must be aware of the demands of that particular drug. For example, antibiotics must be given at even intervals around the clock in order to maintain constant blood levels, even though the order may have been written "q.i.d." without specifying even intervals.

Legal aspects

A nurse is legally responsible for her own actions. It is not enough for her simply to obey orders unquestioningly. If the physician's order for medication is unclear or seems strange, she should question him about it. The use of the correct dosage and the proper method of administration are also her responsibility. "Twenty thousand dollars was awarded to a patient who sustained a permanent foot drop and atrophy of the calf of his leg as the result of a nurse's negligently placing an injection in the wrong area of his buttock."[3]

The nurse is also responsible for observation of the effects of medication on the patient.

If, in pursuit of her nursing assignment, a nurse notices an adverse effect of a medicine the doctor has ordered administered to a patient, she should not continue to carry out orders blindly, but should report adverse effects immediately and request further orders. Part of the nurse's duty is to observe symptoms and reactions and report them.[4]

Often a physician will delegate the nurse as his agent to dispense drugs. The American Nurses' Association has pointed out that the nurse has no

[3]Helen Creighton. 1970. *Law every nurse should know,* 2d ed., p. 120. Philadelphia: Saunders.
[4]Ibid., p. 130.

right to perform this function unless state law allows it.[5] To protect herself, the nurse should have the physician sign all verbal orders before carrying them out.

Nursing stations often include supplies of commonly used drugs dispensed by the pharmacy in stock containers. The nurse is entitled to draw from these supplies according to the doctor's prescription. The use of single-dose containers in place of stock bottles is also clearly within her province. However, "a nurse who prepares a quantity of drug greater than one dose for a patient to take away from the hospital, office, or clinic is dispensing," one specialist in nursing law points out. "In her own interest, she should avoid doing this outside her immediate area of supervised employment."[6]

Preparation of medications

Drug orders

It is the responsibility of the physician to order all medications in writing. This order may be contained in the patient's chart or on some other form designed for the purpose. The order should specify the name of the drug, the dosage, how often it is to be administered, and what method of administration is to be used. The physician must sign this order. It is also important that only recognized abbreviations be used (see Table 24-1). If the physician uses an abbreviation that is unclear or unfamiliar, it is the responsibility of the nurse to clarify what is meant. She should not proceed to give the medication if there are any questions concerning its administration.

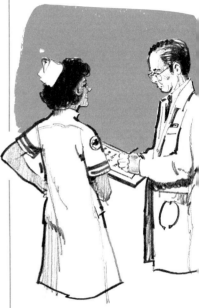

To protect herself, the nurse should have the physician sign all verbal orders before carrying them out.

The physician's written order is then transferred to a medicine card or other form devised for the nurse's use in preparing and administering the medication. All the information from the physician's original order must be transcribed accurately. The form should also be dated and initialed or signed by the nurse making the transcription.

Computation of dosage

Two systems are used to indicate the dosage of a drug, the **apothecary** and the **metric.** The apothecary system uses the **grain** as its standard of measurement, while the metric system uses the **gram.** It is possible to convert dosages expressed in grains to grams, and vice versa. A conversion system is given in Table 24-2.

It is sometimes necessary to prepare a dose of medication using a vial that contains more than one dose. To do so, the nurse must first determine

[5]Sidney Willig. 1964. Drugs—dispensing, administering. *American Journal of Nursing* 64. Reprinted in *Nursing Fundamentals,* ed. Mary E. Meyers, p. 199. Dubuque, Iowa: Brown, 1967.
[6]Ibid., p. 197.

TABLE 24-1
Common Latin Words and Abbreviations

Abbreviation	Latin	English Meaning
aa	ana	of each
a.c.	ante cibum	before meals
ad	ad	to, up to
ad lib	ad libitum	freely, as desired
agit.	agita	shake, or stir
alb	albus	white
ante	ante	before
aq.	aqua	water
aq. dest.	aqua destillata	distilled water
b.i.d. or b.d.	bis in die	twice daily
c	cibum	meals
c̄	cum	with
cap.	capsula	capsule
comp.	compositus	compound
dil.	dilutus	dilute, dissolve
elix.	elixir	elixir
gm.	gramme	gram
gr.	granum	grain
gt. or gtt.	gutta (guttae)	drop(s)
h	hora	an hour
hor. som. or h.s.	hora somni	at bedtime
m.	misce	mix
min.	minimum	minim, drop
non rep.	non repetatur	do not repeat
No.	numerus	number
o.d.	oculus dexter	right eye
o.h.	omni hora	every hour
o.m.	omni mani	every morning
o.n.	omni nocte	every night
os	os	mouth
o.s. or o.l.	oculus sinister or laevus	left eye
o.u.	oculus uterque	each eye
p.c.	post cibum	after meals
p.r.n.	pro re nata	when needed
q	quaque	every
q.d.	quaque die	every day
q.i.d.	quater in die	four times a day
q.1,2,3, h.	quaque 1,2,3, hora	every 1,2,3 hours
q.o.d.	quaque aliam die	every other day
q.s.	quantum satis	a sufficient quantity
Rx	recipe	take
rept.	repetatur	let it be repeated
s̄	sine	without
s.o.s.	si opus sit	if it is needed
ss.	semis	a half
Sig. or S.	signa	label
stat	statim	at once
t.i.d.	ter in die	three times a day
tr. or tinct.	tinctura	tincture

From Solomon Garb et al., *Pharmacology and patient care*, 3d ed., pp. 139–40. New York: Springer, 1970. Copyright © 1970 by Springer Publishing Co. Used by permission.

the concentration of the medication in the vial. That is, she must know how many grams of the medication are contained in a cc. She then divides the dose to be given by the amount per cc. In order to give a 5 mg dose of a drug from a vial containing 10 mg of the drug per cc, she would use $\frac{1}{2}$ cc from the vial (5 mg $\div$ 10 mg $= \frac{1}{2}$).

If the medication comes in tablet form and the standard tablets do not contain the required dosage, the nurse can give the correct dosage by dissolving the tablet in a solution. She then divides the prescribed dose by the available dose (the size of the tablet) and multiplies by the amount of dissolving solution. Thus, to give morphine sulfate g $\frac{1}{8}$ if the tablets are g $\frac{1}{6}$, she should dissolve the g $\frac{1}{6}$ tablet in 2 cc of solution and administer $1\frac{1}{2}$ cc ($\frac{1}{8} \div \frac{1}{6} \times 2 = 1\frac{1}{2}$).

Procedures for preparing drugs

Oral. The following are some points to remember in administering medications by mouth in either liquid or tablet form.

1. Medication cards should be compared with the Kardex and the patient's chart to make sure that the medication has not been discontinued.
2. The nurse should wash her hands (see chapter 14) before preparing the medications.
3. Medications should be prepared individually. Each bottle should be replaced on the shelf before the next medication is prepared. The label on the bottle must be checked carefully against the medication card. This should be done three times—when taking it from the shelf, when preparing the medication, and when returning the bottle to the shelf. A medication should not be dispensed from a bottle with an illegible label.
4. If a patient is receiving more than one medication, each drug should be prepared separately (more than one type of tablet or liquid should not be placed in the same container). Each medication should have a separate medicine card.
5. Pills or capsules should be shaken out directly into their individual containers. They should not be touched by the nurse's hands.
6. Liquids should be poured at eye level to ensure accurate measurement of the dosage. The top of the bottle should be wiped with a clean tissue before the cap is replaced. Liquids that have discolored or developed a strange odor should not be used.
7. The medicine card should be kept with the medication at all times.

Parenteral. In **parenteral** administration, the medication does not pass through the patient's alimentary canal. Such parenteral injections can be given **intradermally, subcutaneously, intramuscularly,** or **intravenously.**

TABLE 24-2

Metric Doses with Approximate Apothecary Equivalents

Liquid Measure

METRIC	APPROX. APOTHECARY EQUIVALENTS	METRIC	APPROX. APOTHECARY EQUIVALENTS
1,000 ml	1 quart	3 ml	45 minims
750 ml	1½ pints	2 ml	30 minims
500 ml	1 pint	1 ml	15 minims
250 ml	8 fluid ounces	0.75 ml	12 minims
200 ml	7 fluid ounces	0.6 ml	10 minims
100 ml	3½ fluid ounces	0.5 ml	8 minims
50 ml	1¾ fluid ounces	0.3 ml	5 minims
30 ml	1 fluid ounce	0.25 ml	4 minims
15 ml	4 fluid drams	0.2 ml	3 minims
10 ml	2½ fluid drams	0.1 ml	1½ minims
8 ml	2 fluid drams	0.06 ml	1 minim
5 ml	1¼ fluid drams	0.05 ml	¾ minim
4 ml	1 fluid dram	0.03 ml	½ minim

Weight

METRIC	APPROX. APOTHECARY EQUIVALENTS	METRIC	APPROX. APOTHECARY EQUIVALENTS	METRIC	APPROX. APOTHECARY EQUIVALENTS
30 gm	1 ounce	0.25 gm	4 grains	5 mg	$\frac{1}{12}$ grain
15 gm	4 drams	0.2 gm	3 grains	4 mg	$\frac{1}{15}$ grain
10 gm	2½ drams	0.15 gm	2½ grains	3 mg	$\frac{1}{20}$ grain
7.5 gm	2 drams	0.12 gm	2 grains	2 mg	$\frac{1}{30}$ grain
6 gm	90 grains	0.1 gm	1½ grains	1.5 mg	$\frac{1}{40}$ grain
5 gm	75 grains	75 mg	1¼ grains	1.2 mg	$\frac{1}{50}$ grain
4 gm	60 grains	60 mg	1 grain	1 mg	$\frac{1}{60}$ grain
	(1 dram)	50 mg	¾ grain	0.8 mg	$\frac{1}{80}$ grain
3 gm	45 grains	40 mg	⅔ grain	0.6 mg	$\frac{1}{100}$ grain
2 gm	30 grains	30 mg	½ grain	0.5 mg	$\frac{1}{120}$ grain
	(½ dram)	25 mg	⅜ grain	0.4 mg	$\frac{1}{150}$ grain
1.5 gm	22 grains	20 mg	⅓ grain	0.3 mg	$\frac{1}{200}$ grain
1 gm	15 grains	15 mg	¼ grain	0.25 mg	$\frac{1}{250}$ grain
0.75 gm	12 grains	12 mg	⅕ grain	0.2 mg	$\frac{1}{300}$ grain
0.6 gm	10 grains	10 mg	⅙ grain	0.15 mg	$\frac{1}{400}$ grain
0.5 gm	7½ grains	8 mg	⅛ grain	0.12 mg	$\frac{1}{500}$ grain
0.4 gm	6 grains	6 mg	$\frac{1}{10}$ grain	0.1 mg	$\frac{1}{600}$ grain
0.3 gm	5 grains				

These *approximate* dose equivalents represent the quantities usually prescribed by physicians using, respectively, the metric system and the apothecary system of weights and measures.

When prepared dosage forms such as tablets, capsules, etc., are prescribed in the metric system, the pharmacist may dispense the corresponding *approximate* equivalent in the apothecary system, and vice versa, as indicated in the above table.

To calculate quantities required in pharmaceutical formulas, use the *exact* equivalents. For prescription compounding, use the exact equivalents rounded to three significant figures.

NOTE—A milliliter (ml) is the approximate equivalent of a cubic centimeter (cc).
The foregoing *approximate* dose equivalents have the approval of the federal Food and Drug Administration.

From *The Pharmacopeia of the United States of America*, 17th rev. ed. New York: United States Pharmacopeial Convention, Inc., 1965.

Injections are given with sterile syringes of various types and sizes. A needle with a larger lumen is used for thicker solutions, while a longer one is needed for intramuscular injections. An intradermal injection is administered with a needle with a very small lumen. Different patients also need different types of needles: an obese person may require a longer needle for an intramuscular injection; a small child, a shorter one.

Withdrawal of medication from a vial. The most important considerations when withdrawing medication from a vial into a syringe are to maintain sterility of the medication and the syringe and to withdraw the proper dose. The following steps will enable the nurse to fulfill both of these goals.

1. The rubber stopper of the vial should be cleaned with an antiseptic solution (usually 70 percent alcohol).
2. Holding the empty syringe upright, the nurse withdraws the plunger until it reaches the mark indicating the dose she is going to use.
3. The needle is then inserted downward through the rubber stopper into the vial.
4. With the syringe still in the downward position, she pushes the plunger, forcing air into the vial.
5. The vial and syringe are now inverted and the plunger withdrawn until the desired dose enters the syringe.
6. The needle should be covered with a sterile wrapper while the syringe is being carried to the patient.

Withdrawal of medication from an ampule. Once again, the nurse must keep in mind the goals of maintaining sterility and obtaining an accurate dose. Although ampules are hermetically sealed, it is still good practice to wipe the outside of the container with a sterile solution before withdrawing the medication. The following steps should be taken when withdrawing medication from an ampule:

1. Wipe the outside with a sterile solution.
2. The top of the ampule should be tapped to make sure that all of the solution drains into the container.
3. The ampule should be opened along the break line, if one is provided. If there is not a line, the nurse should create one by scoring the constriction in the top of the ampule. It is good practice to protect the hands with sponges or pledgets before breaking the ampule.
4. If the needle is long enough, the nurse withdraws the required dosage with the syringe in the downward position. (Do not introduce air into the syringe when withdrawing medication from an ampule.) If using a short needle, the syringe and ampule should be inverted.
5. The needle should be covered with a sterile wrapper while being carried to the patient.

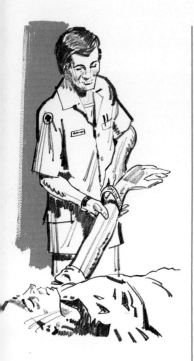

One of the most important points to remember in the administration of any medication is that the patient must be positively identified.

Topical

Topical medications include ointments, lotions, and solutions applied with wet dressings. The conditions for which such medications are commonly prescribed often cause psychological stress for the patient and his family. Skin conditions, such as eczema, pruritis, and dermatitis, may require long periods of treatment. The patient and his family may worry about his physical appearance and be concerned about the length of treatment. It is important that the nurse convey a positive attitude.

Administration of medications

One of the most important points to remember in the administration of any medication is that the patient must be positively identified. This may be done by asking him his name and checking his identification bracelet. It should not be automatically assumed that the patient in the bed is necessarily the one who is supposed to be there.

Oral

Oral medications should be taken with water. In the case of solid forms, the amount of water should be sufficient to make swallowing easy and to dissolve the medication. With liquids, the water serves to dilute the medication. In addition to being swallowed, oral medications may be held in the mouth until they dissolve. **Sublingual administration** involves holding the medication under the tongue until it dissolves. **Buccal administration** involves holding the medication between the cheek and the teeth.

Parenteral

Subcutaneous. The subcutaneous method of injection is used for a variety of drugs. Commonly called the **hypodermic,** it is effective for those medications that are easily absorbed by the tissues, such as insulin. Common sites for these injections include the upper thigh or upper arm.

As in the case of preparation of the medication, the maintenance of asepsis is important in administering any parenteral medication. Accordingly, the area of the injection should be cleansed with alcohol. The area is then pinched and the needle inserted at a 45-degree angle. The plunger should be retracted to determine that the needle has not entered a blood vessel by mistake. The solution is then injected slowly. After the solution has been injected, the needle should be quickly removed. A slight pressure is then applied to the area for a few seconds.

Intramuscular. Intramuscular injections provide for faster absorption than those given subcutaneously. They are also used for drugs such as ACTH and penicillin, which are not easily absorbed by the subcutaneous tissues or which would be irritating to those tissues.

Common sites for intramuscular-injections are the gluteus maximus or the gluteus medius muscles of the buttocks. Finding the correct site for the injection is essential in order to avoid injuring the sciatic nerve, blood vessels, or bones in the area. Figure 24-1 illustrates the area in which the injection should be given. To find the proper site, locate the iliac crest. The buttocks should then be divided in quarters, using the area above the dividing fold between the buttocks as a guide for the horizontal line. The needle should be inserted about 2 inches below the iliac crest in the upper outer fourth of the area.

As with subcutaneous injection, the maintenance of asepsis is important. Once again, the injection site should be cleansed with alcohol. This time, the skin should be stretched taut and the needle inserted at a 90-degree angle. The plunger is retracted, and the fluid is injected slowly. After all the solution has been injected, the needle is quickly removed and pressure is applied to the area.

The "zigzag," or "z-track," method of injection prevents seeping of the medication into the subcutaneous tissue. The skin is pulled to one side and the injection is given as described above. When the needle is removed, the skin returns to its normal position, leaving a zigzag track from the point of insertion.

In giving an intramuscular injection, it is important that the lumen be large enough to hold thicker preparations and long enough to reach muscle tissue.

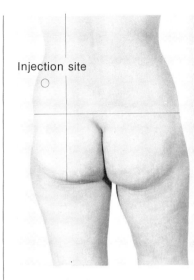

Injection site

FIG. 24-1 *Site for intramuscular injection.*
[Photo by Sandor Acs]

Intradermal. When a drug is to be absorbed very slowly, an injection may be given just under the epidermis. A very small amount of the drug is used, and the procedure leaves a small wheal on the skin.

The intradermal method also allows time to observe for any adverse reactions to the drug. If redness develops around the area of injection, the patient is sensitive to the drug, and a deeper injection is not desirable.

The inner surface of the forearm is the most common site for this type of injection. Alcohol is used to cleanse the area, which is then allowed to dry. The skin is stretched taut and the needle is inserted at a very shallow angle until the bevel is no longer visible. After the plunger has been retracted, the solution is slowly injected, producing a small wheal. The needle is then removed and the injection site is sponged with alcohol. If the injection is a skin test, an area of redness should be watched for after the prescribed time.

Topical

Ointments. An ointment should be spread on both the nurse's hands, warming it slightly. It should then be applied on the patient's skin using long strokes that follow the direction of hair growth. Most ointments require two or three applications per day. The ointment should be applied slowly but firmly, as too much or too little pressure may increase itching. After the ointment is applied, a dressing, such as cotton stockings, gloves, or gauze, is applied to keep the ointment in contact with the skin.

When applying ointments to the patient's face, the flat portion of the fingers should be used rather than the tips. When using ointment on the trunk, application should begin at the midline. For the entire anterior surface of the trunk, the nurse begins under the chin and works down to the genitals. The second stroke starts at the uppermost point of treatment adjacent to either side of the area to which the ointment was applied by the first stroke.

Application of the medication to the posterior surface of the trunk should begin at the hairline. The arms and legs are treated similarly. The patient may wish to apply lotion to his genitals, and the nurse should tell him how to do so. Heavy ointments such as Lassar's paste are spread on the skin more easily with a wooden spatula.

Lotions are applied in a fashion similar to ointments. The lotion should be shaken well so that it is thoroughly mixed.

Dressings. Wet dressings are used for several purposes. They may serve to cleanse the skin, treat infections, and reduce inflammation, edema, and pruritus. The dressing is first applied according to the methods described in chapter 23. The solution, which is usually very dilute, is then warmed to the desired temperature. It is then poured over the dressing, wetting it uniformly.

Instillations

Eye. Drugs to be instilled in the patient's eye should be at room temperature. They should always be checked for deterioration. Eye ointments contained in tubes can be warmed slightly in the hands before instillation.

After positioning the patient comfortably with his head held back, the nurse exposes the cul-de-sac by gently retracting the tissue next to the lower eyelid. She asks the patient to look up in order to protect the cornea. The dispenser should not touch the eye, nor should the medication fall on the cornea. The nurse holds a cotton pledget in the hand that retracts the lower lid to absorb or remove excess medication. When both eyes are being treated, a clean pledget should be used for each one so that organisms are not transferred.

Nose. To instill nose drops, raise the patient's shoulders with pillows and have him tilt his head back. During instillation, have the patient lower his head over the edge of the bed or hyperextend his neck if he is in a sitting position. The sitting position is mandatory when the medication

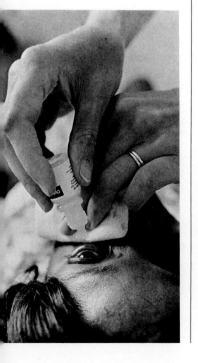

Proper procedure for instillation of drops in the patient's eye.
[Photo by Dan Bernstein]

is administered through a nasal spray. Any medicine that enters the pharynx should be expectorated.

Ear. Ear drops are instilled with the patient's head turned to the side so that the affected ear faces upward. The external ear should be gently manipulated to expose the orifice of the external canal. The medicine is then dropped against the internal wall of the canal. When a child is being treated, the external ear is gently retracted upward and posterior. For an adult, retraction is downward and posterior.

Genitourinary tract. The patient who is about to receive an instillation into the genitourinary tract should be positioned on his back. His legs should be flexed and partially spread apart. Draping the patient so that the affected area is exposed, the nurse cleanses the area with gloved hands and administers the drug. Care to prevent infection is especially important when treating this part of the body.

Bladder. Before receiving bladder medication, the patient must have his bladder drained with a catheter (see chapter 21). Afterward, the catheter remains in place and the medication is inserted slowly and gently with a sterile syringe connected to the catheter. The catheter is then withdrawn and pressure is applied to the meatus with a soft sterile sponge. The patient should not urinate for at least 20 minutes after the indicated treatment is completed.

Vagina. The patient should be asked to void before medication is applied. The nurse should then insert the applicator filled with medicated cream or jelly into the vagina to a depth of $1\frac{1}{2}$ to 2 inches. The applicator is removed while the plunger is pushed forward. If the applicator is to be used again, it should be taken apart and washed, rinsing first with cold water. A vaginal suppository may also be inserted by hand if no special equipment is available. The suppository should be held between thumb and forefinger and then pushed into the vagina to the back of the cervix. The patient should remain lying down after the medication has been inserted.

   The nurse should wear a glove on the hand she uses to expose the vaginal opening. She should wear gloves on both hands if she is inserting the medication manually.

Rectal. The patient receiving a rectal instillation should assume the side-lying position (see chapter 18). His lower leg should be extended while his upper leg is flexed. The nurse then retracts the upper buttock so that the anal area is exposed. The suppository should be lubricated if it is not self-lubricating. Wearing finger cots or a glove, she pushes the suppository forward until it passes the anal sphincter.

Care to prevent infection is especially important when treating the genitourinary tract.

The best insurance against improper self-medication is an understanding on the part of the patient and his family as to what the medication is, what it is for, and clear instructions as to how to use it.

Inhalation

The inhalation technique is used for the administration of drugs such as amyl nitrite, spirits of ammonia, and nebulized drugs. These drugs are contained in single, fragile ampules, also called **pearls.** These ampules are covered with cloth and are crushed at the patient's bedside, and the saturated cloth is held near the patient's face. He then inhales the released vapor as it passes back and forth. Drugs that are inhaled take effect rapidly so the patient should be allowed only two to three inhalations per dose.

Instructing the patient in self-medication

Often, a patient is discharged from a health care unit supplied with prescriptions for one or more medications to be taken at home. Although these may very well be the same medications he was taking in the health care unit, this is no guarantee that he will know how to take them on his own. The best insurance against improper self-medication is an understanding on the part of the patient and his family as to what the medication is, what it is for, and clear instructions on how to use it. (See chapter 11 for a discussion of teaching methods.)

A thorough understanding of the nature of the medication and how it is to be used is especially important for patients on a self-regulating program, such as that for diabetes. The patient must be aware of when to change the dosage and of the symptoms indicating incorrect dosage. His family should also be made aware of the signs of distress and how to deal with them.

SUMMARY

Drugs are one of the most powerful weapons against illness and disease. However, they must be treated with great respect, as they can be dangerous in the hands of the unskilled.

A particular concern of the nurse is the potential side effects of a drug. Although unpleasant reactions must be tolerated with certain drugs, signs of toxicity must be carefully watched for. Among the most common are nausea, diarrhea, itching, sore throat, swelling, drowsiness, and jaundice.

The nurse is also responsible for evaluating the effectiveness of a drug. Is the patient reacting as he is supposed to? If not, what type of intervention is called for? In order to answer these questions, the nurse must be familiar with the characteristics both of the drug and of the patient.

The drug abuse epidemic in this country bears witness to the fact that habit-forming drugs must be administered with great care. Prescriptions for narcotic drugs must follow special procedures outlined by law.

A nurse learns to prepare drugs for three types of application: oral, parenteral, and topical. For each, orderly methods of procedure and the observance of appropriately clean or sterile technique are mandatory. A parenteral injection is given subcutaneously, intramuscularly, or intradermally. The technique varies slightly for each type of injection, and needles of different lengths and lumen sizes may be called for. The site of injection must also be carefully selected.

Topical applications and instillations require different procedures and precautions as well. When the genitourinary tract is being treated, special care must be taken to prevent infection.

In administering medications, the nurse must make sure that she is treating the proper patient and that he is actually taking the medication. She also observes closely for side effects. Medication errors are distressingly common in hospitals. Many can be prevented if more care is taken in the administration and recording of medications.

Any successful treatment program demands the cooperation of the patient. For this reason, the nurse sets aside time for special instruction. She must make sure that the patient understands exactly what is required of him. She must also make sure that he has psychologically accepted the need for treatment. In some cases he must be prepared for a lifetime of self-care.

In administering medications, the nurse must make sure that she is treating the proper patient and that he is actually taking the medication.

STUDY QUESTIONS

1. What are the three types of effects a drug can have? Give examples of each (other than the examples given in the text).
2. How does the nurse make sure that the proper medication, in the proper dosage, is being administered to the patient at the proper time?
3. Compare and contrast the methods of administering subcutaneous, intramuscular, and intradermal injections.
4. Given the large number of drugs in use today, how can the nurse familiarize herself with their administration and effects? What sources of information should she make use of?
5. How can the nurse guard against abusing drugs herself? What should she do if she discovers that another health worker is abusing drugs?

SELECTED BIBLIOGRAPHY

Asperheim, Mary K., and Eisenhauer, Laurel A. 1973. *The pharmacological basis of patient care,* 2d ed. Philadelphia: Saunders.
Bergerson, Betty S., et al. 1969. *Pharmacology in nursing,* 11th ed. St. Louis: Mosby.
Garb, Solomon, et al. 1970. *Pharmacology and patient care,* 3d ed. New York: Springer.
Willig, Sidney. 1964. Drugs—dispensing, administering. *American Journal of Nursing* 64. Reprinted in *Nursing Fundamentals,* ed. Mary E. Meyers, pp. 197–208. Dubuque, Iowa: Brown, 1967.

25 Temperature problems and application of heat and cold

Assessment of temperature problems

Body temperature control

The maintenance of a constant body temperature is carried out by the body's homeostatic mechanisms (see chapter 15). Receptors in the skin send messages to the brain telling it that the external temperature is warm or cold. This sets off a complex series of events by which the body regulates its internal temperature at approximately 98.6° F (37° C), regardless of external temperature variations. The regulatory system essentially monitors the flow of blood to the skin surface and the rewarming of chilled blood.[1]

When the body is at rest, it is kept warm by the energy (heat) produced through the body's basal **metabolism** rate. Only in extreme conditions (see p. 444) does this fail to generate enough energy to maintain the body's normal temperature.

Factors producing increased or decreased body temperature

Although body temperature remains basically constant, slight variations will occur as a result of external conditions as well as changes in the body. The following are some of the factors that produce changes in body temperature.

Prolonged muscular contracture. Ordinary muscular exertion has little, if any, effect on adult body temperature. But activities that involve prolonged muscular contracture, such as marathon running, can cause body temperature to rise dramatically. The same effect is produced by an epileptic seizure.[2]

Time of day. Body temperature tends to be at its lowest in the morning and its highest in the late afternoon or early evening. The relative muscular

[1]L. L. Langley. 1965. *Homeostasis*, pp. 22–23. New York: Van Nostrand Reinhold.
[2]Byron A. Schottelius and Dorothy D. Schottelius. 1973. *Textbook of physiology*, 17th ed., pp. 467–68. St. Louis: Mosby.

inactivity of sleep also causes body temperature to drop at night. The opposite is true for those people who work at night and sleep in the daytime.

Age. Body temperature of young children tends to vary more than that of adults. This is due to the relative immaturity of the child's nervous system, which means that his homeostatic mechanisms are not totally effective. A child's temperature can be elevated significantly simply by a prolonged crying spell. Similar exertion on the part of an adult would have very little effect. Temperature control mechanisms may be less effective in the elderly as well.

Cold weather. Some researchers have suggested that cold weather stimulates thyroid secretion.[3] This makes it possible for the body to produce greater heat during the winter months.

Menstruation and pregnancy. The female reproductive cycle also has an effect on body temperature. At the point of ovulation, a woman's body temperature may rise as much as 0.05° C. It falls again one or two days before the onset of menstruation. (This pattern of temperature rise and fall is used as the basis of the so-called rhythm method of contraception.) Pregnancy also has an effect on temperature. The first three to four months are characterized by a slight rise. The temperature then falls slightly below normal for the remainder of the pregnancy. It returns to normal after delivery.

Signs and symptoms of temperature problems

Hyperthermia. **Hyperthermia** is a condition in which body temperature is abnormally high. It results from a disturbance of the body's heat-regulatory mechanism. As the patient's body produces more and more heat, the rate of heat dissipation falls farther and farther behind. Common examples of hyperthermia are **fever** and **heat stroke.**

The presence of fever indicates that something is wrong within the body. Mild fever leads to complaints of malaise, anorexia, headache, and slight chilliness. A more seriously ill patient may experience severe chills and his teeth may chatter. An infant or a young child may go into convulsions. Fever may produce disorientation or even delirium in the elderly.

Heat stroke is characterized by headache, nausea, vomiting, and visual disturbances or hallucinations. The victim is weak and loses muscle control. His pulse and respirations are rapid. He soon becomes delirious and comatose. Heat stroke victims often resemble stroke victims.[4]

[3] Ibid., p. 472.
[4] When the patient's problem is heat. *Patient Care* 8 (1974):45.

Hypothermia. **Hypothermia** is a condition in which the body temperature is abnormally low. It is much less common than hyperthermia. Some causes of hypothermia are prolonged exposure to cold, lowered metabolism, alcoholic intoxication, heavy sedation, and circulatory failure.[5] All of these conditions lead to a depression of body activities. As a result, the body fails to generate enough heat to maintain its normal temperature. Heat dissipation therefore exceeds heat production. Hypothermia is characterized by **shivering,** slowdown of metabolism, and a decrease in mental and muscular capabilities. The victim feels sleepy and eventually becomes comatose. A common form of hypothermia is **frostbite.** Hypothermia may also be deliberately induced (see next page).

Planning, implementation, and evaluation

Nursing intervention to relieve hyperthermia

The nurse's first concern in cases of hyperthermia is to reduce the patient's fever and chills. She is also interested in promoting his comfort and well-being.

Reducing fever and chills. Bed rest is indicated for the patient whose temperature is 100° F or above. His vital signs—temperature, pulse, and respiration—should be checked every 4 hours. It is sometimes necessary to check these signs on an hourly basis. It is especially important for the nurse to maintain close observation of a patient with a fever of unknown origin. The development of signs and symptoms in such cases may help in making a diagnosis.

If the fever is accompanied by chills, the patient should be covered by several light blankets. A cotton bath blanket placed close to his skin under the top sheet feels warmer and absorbs perspiration better than a sheet. Hot water bottles or electric heating pads may be used also, provided appropriate precautions are taken against burning (see chapter 14). These devices should be removed as soon as the episode of chills is over. Their unnecessary or prolonged use may lead to excessive sweating, resulting in loss of body fluid and sodium (see chapter 22).

The patient's fever may be reduced by sponging his body with a cool solution of water and alcohol. Ice bags may also be applied, again using the proper safety precautions. It is important that the patient's room be kept cool and well-ventilated during these procedures.

Providing comfort. An episode of high fever may lead to one or more other physical discomforts for the patient. Frequent oral hygiene is very

---

[5]Jeannette E. Watson. 1972. *Medical-surgical nursing and related physiology,* p. 70. Philadelphia: Saunders.

important, as the patient's mouth tends to dry out (see chapter 16). Cracking of the lips may be prevented by using petroleum jelly, oil, or cold cream applications.

A common side effect of fever is the development of **cold sores** or **fever blisters** around the mouth. These sores are caused by the virus **herpes simplex.** They first appear as sore, burning papules. Eventually, a scab will form. Ointments may be used to soften the scab and prevent further spread of the sores.

Promoting adequate nutrition. Anorexia is generally a problem among patients with high fevers. Because of the increase in metabolic rate brought about by the fever, it is important that the patient maintain a high caloric intake. Carbohydrates and proteins are especially vital. His fluid intake should also be increased to 2,500 to 3,000 ml in a 24-hour period. Broths and soups are valuable in maintaining this high intake level. In addition, they contain salt, which helps retain fluid.

The anorexic patient's appetite may be stimulated by offering him milk drinks or eggnog. Commercial preparations, such as Sustagen or Protinal, may be enhanced by the addition of cream, glucose, or lactose.[6]

Medications. Above-normal temperatures are generally treated with aspirin. This **antipyretic** drug lowers the sensitivity of the heat-regulating center. It also causes sweating. Adults are usually given 0.3 to 0.6 g every 3 or 4 hours. Patients who are allergic to aspirin may be treated with other antipyretics, such as Tylenol or Acetophenetidin.

Hypothermia

Therapeutic hypothermia. Sometimes a patient's condition will make it desirable to slow down his metabolic and oxygen-use rates. This is the case in certain types of surgery and following cerebral surgery or severe head injuries.[7] This slowdown is achieved by **therapeutic hypothermia.**

Hypothermia is induced by surface cooling or by the extracorporeal method. Surface cooling may be achieved by the following methods:

1. Immersing the patient in an icy bath
2. Enclosing him in large plastic sheets filled with crushed ice
3. Placing him between blankets through which cold fluid is circulated electrically
4. Applying ice bags over the body surface[8]

The extracorporeal method is used during surgery. It is accomplished by means of the heart-lung machine. This machine contains a heat ex-

[6] Ibid.
[7] Ibid., p. 71.
[8] Ibid.

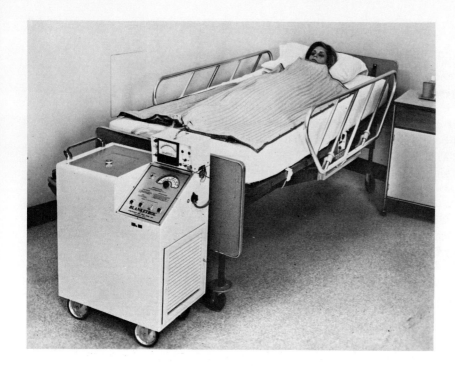

An example of therapeutic hypothermia induced by the surface cooling method.
[Photo courtesy Cincinnati Sub-Zero Products, Inc.]

changer that may be used to cool or warm the blood. This extracorporeal method enables the patient to be cooled quickly with better control of temperature during surgery than the surface method. It also permits easy rewarming of the patient after surgery.

Nursing intervention in therapeutic hypothermia. The patient treated with therapeutic hypothermia needs both physical care and psychological support. This type of treatment is understandably upsetting to many patients. Some will find it absolutely terrifying. It is always physically uncomfortable. A thorough explanation of what will happen should always be given to the patient and his family. Questions should be encouraged, as this procedure is an unfamiliar one and misconceptions are common.

Physical care of the patient undergoing therapeutic hypothermia involves care of the skin and frequent observation of vital signs. The skin should be cleansed before the cooling procedure, and is often protected with a coating of oil or lanolin. The patient should be catheterized and an intravenous infusion begun.

While the patient's temperature remains below normal, his vital signs must be checked and recorded. His skin must also be inspected hourly to guard against frostbite. He should be turned and his position changed regularly to prevent the development of decubitus ulcers (see chapter 16). Eye care is also important. It is sometimes necessary to irrigate the eyes and cover them with pads. Oral hygiene measures, including cleansing and moistening the mouth, should be carried out every 2 to 3 hours. Accumulated secretions should be removed from the nasal passages.

The rewarming period also demands regular monitoring of vital signs. These observations should continue for two to three days after the patient's temperature has returned to normal.

Frostbite. A common form of nontherapeutic hypothermia is frostbite. Frostbite results from prolonged exposure to the cold, and most often strikes the fingers, toes, and nose. To some extent, frostbite serves a protective function. When exposed to the cold, one of the body's first defensive measures is to constrict the blood vessels on the surface so that blood flow in that area decreases. This prevents the blood from becoming chilled. Frostbite represents an extreme form of this reaction, in that the vessels are so constricted by the cold that no blood flows to the extremities. This concentrates the blood flow around the vital organs, protecting them from damage.

Frostbite is best treated by immediate warming, without rubbing the affected area. This warming may be accomplished by placing the frostbitten

Hypothermia during the seven-teenth century.
[Courtesy Henry Swan, M.D.]

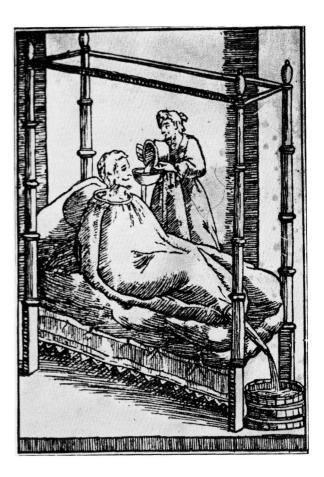

extremities in water of 110° F (if conscious) or 115°-120° F (if in a coma).[9] The extremity should be removed from the water as soon as a red flush appears. A dry gauze bandage should then be applied loosely. Rewarming may also be accomplished by body heat. The affected part may be covered with a warm hand or placed under the armpit. Serious frostbite must be treated with tetanus toxoid and antibiotics to prevent infection.

Application of heat and cold—assessment

Temperature ranges

Normal body temperature is approximately 98.6° F (37° C). A non-therapeutic drop in body temperature to 77° F (24° C), if maintained for several hours, causes death. Death also results from a rise in temperature to 113° F (45° C) or above for any length of time. (The temperature of heat stroke victims often rises rapidly to as high as 110° F.)

Transfer of heat

Body heat is lost through the skin, the lungs, and excretions. The loss through the skin accounts for about 85 percent of the total. There are four mechanisms by which this loss takes place: **radiation, convection, conduction,** and **vaporization.**

Radiation. Radiation is the process whereby heat is transferred from one object to another without direct contact between the objects. The heat is carried from one object to the other in the form of rays. The use of a heat lamp involves the transfer of heat by radiation.

Convection. Heat is lost through convection when air currents pass over a warm object, carrying its heat away with them.

Conduction. Conduction involves direct contact between objects. Heat passes from the warmer objects to the colder. This is the principle behind the rewarming of frostbite victims through body contact.

Evaporation. Evaporation of fluid on the skin results in heat loss and cooling of the skin. The more heat the body generates (as in muscular exertion), the more active the sweat glands become, thereby increasing the rate of cooling. (Heat stroke victims cease to sweat, which adds to the dramatic increase in their body temperature.) Sponging a patient with alcohol and water provides for cooling by evaporation.

Sponging a patient with alcohol and water provides for cooling by evaporation.

[9]Lucy Kavaler. 1974. How warm-blooded man adjusts to a cruel and cold, cold world. *Nursing Digest* 11:5.

The loss of body heat is influenced by external factors, including temperature and humidity. If a room is cold, body heat is lost mainly by radiation. Very little is lost through evaporation, since the activity of the sweat glands is slowed. Evaporation also becomes less effective in times of high relative humidity, since less moisture can be taken into the air.

Physiological responses to temperature changes

Application of heat. Heat causes the blood vessels in the area of application to dilate. This increases circulation of the affected area. In turn, the increase in circulation increases the oxygenation of the tissues (see chapter 20), thereby speeding up the metabolism rate. If the area to which the heat is applied is inflamed, the increased circulation will help to localize the infection.

The increase in the metabolism rate brought about by the application of heat causes the body temperature to rise. It also causes redness in the area of application and an increase in general skin temperature. Prolonged exposure to heat, or treatment with excessive heat, can damage tissues. Symptoms of tissue damage include pain, redness, and blistering.

Application of cold. The major function of cold is to lower the surface skin temperature. This causes the blood vessels in the area to constrict, slowing down bleeding or hemorrhage and encouraging the formation of clots. This constriction also reduces swelling by lessening the amount of fluid leaking into the tissues. In addition, cold lessens pain by cooling off the nerve endings.[10]

Because the application of cold decreases the circulation of blood, it also decreases the oxygenation of tissues. This lowers the metabolism rate. Prolonged exposure to cold can also damage tissues. Symptoms of damage include pain, stiffness, cyanosis of the nailbeds, mottling of the skin, redness, pallor, and blisters.

When should heat be applied?

There are no hard and fast rules for deciding when to apply heat and when to apply cold. This decision should be influenced by an understanding of the patient's immediate problem, his overall condition, and the general uses of each type of application. Basically, heat is used to

1. Reduce pain
2. Provide relaxation
3. Promote tissue healing
4. Reduce swelling

[10]Ben Merson. 1970. Ice is good medicine. *Family Health* 11:34.

The major function of cold is to lower the surface skin temperature.

Both the very young and the very old have difficulties in adjusting to changes in temperature.

The application of heat is often used for patients with inflamed joints, bursitis, or gout. It is also useful in localizing an infection in an abscess, boil, or cellulitis.

When should cold be applied?

In general, cold is applied in order to

1. Reduce pain
2. Decrease tissue metabolism
3. Reduce inflammation
4. Decrease circulation and reduce hemorrhage

There are several very common situations in which cold is applied. These include fractures, sprains, strains, muscle spasms, and stiffening of joints.

Factors affecting individual tolerance

As was indicated above, the decision to use heat or cold must take into account the individual characteristics of the patient. For some patients, such as those suffering from poor circulation, extremes of either type cannot be tolerated.[11] The patient's reaction to heat or cold will be influenced by his age, general health, disease condition, skin condition, level of consciousness, and motor response.

Both the very young and the very old have difficulty in adjusting to changes in temperature. The very young have immature nervous systems and ineffective homeostatic mechanisms. In addition, the surface area of an infant is larger in proportion to his body weight than that of an adult. This means that he tends to lose heat more rapidly. As a result, he is less tolerant of low environmental temperatures. Also, the infant's skin is thinner than that of an adult. He therefore burns more easily and damage to the underlying tissues is more likely.

In the very old, the homeostatic mechanisms, although fully developed, may be impaired. Sensitivity to pain is lessened, thereby increasing the chances of tissue damage. Like that of the newborn, the skin of the older person is very thin.

As was pointed out in chapter 14, the unconscious and the paralyzed patient present special problems in the use of heat and cold. Constant observation of these patients while undergoing heat or cold treatments is vital, as they will not be able to indicate or even realize that something is wrong.

[11] For that, you use ice . . . or is it heat? *Nursing Update* 2 (1971):1.

Planning, implementation, and evaluation

Application of heat

Heat, whether moist or dry, can be applied by various methods, depending upon the purpose of the application and the area of the body involved.

Moist vs. dry heat. Moist heat has several advantages over dry heat. It is less likely to dry or burn the skin. It also penetrates more deeply. Finally, it has less of an effect on body temperature and causes less loss of fluids through sweating.[12]

A disadvantage of using moist heat is that the compress or towel tends to cool off quickly as heat is lost through evaporation. This may be overcome to some extent by covering the compress or towel with a waterproof material and a dry towel.[13] The disadvantages of dry heat, including the use of heat lamps and heating pads, lie mainly in the safety area (see chapter 14).

Therapeutic baths and soaks. Baths and soaks may be used to treat the whole body or an individual part. For the latter, there are tubs of various designs suited to the particular purpose. The usual water temperature for such treatments ranges from 105°-110° F. Higher temperatures should not be used because of the danger of burning and tissue damage. The nurse must always regulate the temperature of the water herself, even if the patient is physically able to do so. Left on his own, the patient might inadvertently let the water get too hot.

Tub baths usually last 10 to 30 minutes, **sitz baths** 15 to 30 minutes, and foot soaks 15 to 20 minutes. The patient should be protected from drafts and chills by draping and keeping appropriate room temperature.[14]

Moist packs and compresses. Moist packs may be heated according to several methods. Two common methods are the hot water method and the **autoclave** method. The hot water method involves soaking and wringing out the pack. The pack may be wrung out by a mechanical wringer or by hand. When wringing out manually, the nurse must be careful to protect her hands. The hot water method is used when lower temperatures are required. The packs must be changed frequently, as they tend to lose heat quickly.

The autoclave method allows the pack to be heated to a higher temperature than the hot water method. The patient's skin therefore must be

> The nurse must always regulate the temperature of the water herself, even if the patient is physically able to do so.

[12]Ibid., p. 14.
[13]Ibid.
[14]Dison, Norma Greenler. 1971. *An atlas of nursing techniques,* 2d ed., p. 277. St. Louis: Mosby.

treated with oil and covered with gauze before the pack is applied. The material to be used for the pack is moistened, placed in a metal container, and then put in the autoclave. When the pressure reaches 15 pounds, the container is removed. The pack should be allowed to cool until it reaches a comfortable temperature. The pack is applied and then covered with a moisture-proof material. This covering helps to retain heat.

Moist, sterile compresses are usually applied four times a day for an hour at a time. They may be prepared by various methods, depending upon the area to be treated. One effective method of preparation involves the use of the autoclave. In this case, the prepared compresses are placed in a metal container. The container should have an opening through which a pair of forceps is inserted. The forceps and the packs are sterilized at the same time.

Hot water bottle. As was indicated in chapter 14, the temperature of the water in the hot water bottle should not exceed 125° F. After filling two-thirds of the bottle, the nurse should remove any excess air. The bottle is then tightly sealed to prevent leakage. The bottle should be covered with cloth before it is applied to the patient's skin.

Electric heating pad. The electric heating pad has the advantage of maintaining a constant degree of heat. This advantage can also be a disadvantage, however, since the danger of burning the patient's skin is increased. The pad should be tested and the cord inspected for fraying before use. The pad should not be used on unconscious or paralyzed patients. (See chapter 14 for a discussion of safety precautions.)

Heat cradle. This device is useful in treating injuries to the lower trunk and extremities. It consists of a cradle-shaped device made of metal bands with a 25-watt bulb in the center. The cradle is placed directly over the affected area. If dressings have been applied first, they should be covered with plastic and a towel before the cradle is put in place. The patient should be covered while the cradle is in use.

Application of cold

Hypothermia. See pp. 445–46 for a discussion of therapeutic hypothermia. In addition to devices for lowering the temperature of the entire body, small hypothermia blankets are also available for use on specific areas. Care of the skin around the area remains the same as that outlined for the treatment of the entire body.

Alcohol sponge bath. The alcohol sponge bath cools the patient through evaporation of the liquid from his skin. The patient's temperature should be checked before and after the sponge bath in order to monitor the

The alcohol sponge bath cools the patient through evaporation of the liquid from his skin.

effectiveness of the treatment. As with any bathing procedure, the patient should be draped and covered to ensure privacy and to prevent chilling. The alcohol and water solution should be tepid, rather than cold. (A cold solution would stimulate shivering, which raises body temperature.) It is sometimes helpful to place cloths soaked in the solution on the patient's groin and axilla.

The sponge bath treatment should be discontinued if there is a change in the patient's respiration, if his lips and nailbeds become cyanotic, or if his pulse is rapid and weak.

Moist compresses. Moist compresses are made by soaking precut gauze or other material in ice water. The material is then wrung out to remove excess moisture and applied to the skin. The compresses should be changed frequently as the heat of the body warms them. Placing an ice bag on top of the compress keeps it cold longer.

Ice bags. Ice bags are available commercially or may be made from plastic bags. Care must be taken with the latter to see that they are properly sealed. After the bag is half filled with ice, the excess air is removed. The bag is then sealed and covered with flannel. Treatment should be discontinued if there are signs of redness or swelling or if the patient complains of numbness or pain.

SUMMARY

By a complex series of regulating processes, the human body is able to maintain an internal temperature of 98.6°F despite a wide range of external conditions. Even when overheated from vigorous exercise, the temperature of the body rises only slightly, if at all.

Hyperthermia, or elevated body temperature, is a pathological condition that demands immediate medical attention. The most common form of hyperthermia is fever. Heat stroke is also a form of hyperthermia. Nursing care of the patient with fever includes frequent observation of temperature, pulse, and respiration. Also important are measures to reduce the chills that often accompany the elevated temperature. Attention must be paid to the patient's oral hygiene, as his mouth tends to dry out and fever blisters are common. The patient's diet, which must contain adequate fluid and calories, is also important.

The opposite of hyperthermia is hypothermia, or subnormal body temperature. Various physiological conditions can lead to hypothermia, and it is also induced therapeutically in certain cases. Many techniques have been devised for bringing the patient's temperature down below normal. An important nursing measure is to relieve any anxieties the patient may have about the procedure.

Frostbite is one form of accidental hypothermia that is well known

By a complex series of regulating processes, the human body is able to maintain an internal temperature of 98.6° F despite a wide range of external conditions.

to people living in cold climates. Treatment must be immediate and includes immersing the affected part in hot water or warming it by body contact.

Both heat and cold are applied therapeutically for a wide range of medical conditions. Heat is used to reduce pain, promote relaxation, absorb bleeding and swelling, and to localize infection. Cold is used to reduce pain, inflammation, and hemorrhage. It does so by constricting the blood vessels, thereby decreasing circulation and tissue metabolism.

Heat can be applied in a variety of ways. These include therapeutic baths and soaks, moist compresses and packs, hot water bottles, electric heating pads, and heat lamps. Moist heat is generally preferred over dry, as it is more penetrating and less likely to dry or burn the skin. Cold may be applied through therapeutic hypothermia, alcohol sponge baths, moist compresses, and ice bags. In applying either heat or cold, the nurse must observe the patient closely for signs of impending tissue damage.

An important consideration in the use of heat and cold is the tolerance of the individual patient. This tolerance is influenced by the patient's age, disease condition, general health, level of consciousness, and motor response.

STUDY QUESTIONS

1. What factors influence man's body temperature? By what means is this temperature regulated?
2. What is hyperthermia? What nursing measures should be taken to treat a patient suffering from hyperthermia?
3. How can accidental hypothermia be recognized? How is it treated?
4. What is the purpose of therapeutic hypothermia? What nursing measures are needed during this form of treatment?
5. Define the four means by which body heat is lost. Give examples of each.
6. What are the physiological effects of heat on the body? of cold? Given these effects, what are the general situations in which heat or cold is applied?

SELECTED BIBLIOGRAPHY

For that, you use ice . . . or is it heat? *Nursing Update* 2 (1971):1, 11–15.
Kavaler, Lucy. 1974. How warm-blooded man adjusts to a cruel and cold, cold world. *Nursing Digest* 11:3–11.
Langley, L. L. 1965. *Homeostasis*, pp. 22–33. New York: Van Nostrand Reinhold.
Watson, Jeannette E. 1972. *Medical-surgical nursing and related physiology*, pp. 66–73. Philadelphia: Saunders.

26 Managing pain

What is pain?

The practice of good nursing is inseparable from the knowledge of how to comfort and relieve the patient in distress. One physician has defined **pain** as a

psychological experience of events occurring within the patient's body, always unpleasant and associated with the impression of damage to the tissues. This blend of physiological and psychological events has to pass through the patient's powers of expression and speech before being described and made comprehensible to a nurse or doctor.[1]

Another proposed definition is that "Pain is a basically unpleasant sensation referred to the body which represents the suffering induced by the psychic perception of real, threatened, or phantasied injury."[2]

Although this definition implies the ideas of injury and suffering, it does not mention actual physical injury. "The idea of injury as well as the need to suffer may lead to pain, just as may a real lesion or injury," the author points out. "Similarly, the need to suffer or not to accept the fact of injury may render a 'painful' injury painless." Doctors and nurses do not deal with pain itself, but with the patient's verbal and nonverbal statements about his pain.

Unlike almost all other observations of a patient, the observation of pain depends mainly on the patient himself and not on the nurse, this author points out. Pain is the result of a complex series of events occurring between a noxious stimulus and the brain. Thus, the patient's manner of behaving and speaking is the end result of many stages of processing of the original stimulus.

Pain is usually classified as acute or chronic, mild or severe. **Acute pain** includes the sensation that results from a broken tooth or a sharp stab in the arm. It is felt at once, and gradually diminishes either of its

---

[1]Kenneth D. Keele. 1972. Pain: How it varies from person to person. *Nursing Times* 68:890.

[2]George L. Engel. 1970. Pain. In Cyril M. MacBryde and Robert S. Blacklow, eds., *Signs and symptoms*, 5th ed., p. 45. Philadelphia: Lippincott.

When a person experiences pain, he is not undergoing an isolated physiological event.

own accord or after treatment. **Chronic pain** may develop so gradually that the person is not sure when it began. It comes and goes, often over a period of years. Sufferers from chronic maladies such as bursitis or angina are all too familiar with it.

Is there any purpose to pain? In healthy people, pain serves to protect by forcing them to withdraw from sources of harm. For example, a child may not know the meaning of fire until he burns his hands. Pain can also secure for sick people the rest that they need in order to become well.

Types of pain

Neurophysiological. Bodily pain generally occurs through mechanical, chemical, electrical, or thermal stimulation of receptors located in almost every tissue of the body. A painful stimulus can draw an immediate response or reflex action, such as rapid pulling away from the source of stimulation. Or it can draw a delayed response or cortical action, such as physical activity to avoid further stimulation.[3] Both immediate and delayed reactions are skeletal muscle reactions.

Another kind of reaction to pain is the autonomic response, which can also be either immediate or delayed. In an autonomic reaction, the pain sensation travels via the afferent nerves to the central nervous system.[4]

Psychosociocultural. When a person experiences pain, he is not undergoing an isolated physiological event. His current experience is closely entwined with his previous pain experiences, cultural attitudes, and his preexisting physiological and psychological status. His reaction to pain can be influenced by any of these factors.[5]

A psychic reaction such as anxiety adds to the patient's perception of pain by lowering the pain threshold and thus intensifying the response to pain. This intensified pain experience also increases the psychic reaction, thereby initiating a vicious cycle. Some women enter the labor room with such anxiety that every contraction of the uterus seems utter agony. Other women, who have either conditioned themselves through prenatal classes or who are less anxious by nature, are able to accept the experience without fighting. Consequently, it is less painful.

One of the early functions of pain is to help the child realize that his body is a separate part of his environment.[6] If he grabs a knife and cuts himself, he learns that it is his own body that is enduring the pain. Early pain experiences also serve to condition the way we react in later life.

Another important attitude we learn toward pain in our childhood is its association with guilt. When we are naughty, our parents spank us.

---

[3] Pain, part 1: Basic concepts and assessment (programmed instruction). *American Journal of Nursing* 66 (1966):1092.
[4] Ibid., p. 1095.
[5] Pain, part 1, p. 1097.
[6] Engel, pp. 50–51.

In adult patients, this attitude often takes the form of lamentation, "What have I done to deserve this?" People who have been punished often as children are sometimes able to endure more pain. They see suffering as the inevitable prelude to reconciliation with a loved one and the lifting of a sentence of guilt.

Attitudes toward pain and methods of dealing with it also vary from one culture to another. For the nurse, it is important to understand how a patient's background may affect his response. In some cultural groups, crying and moaning are considered natural and acceptable reactions. In others, the sufferer is expected to withhold expressions of anguish. Of course, there are no rules. One cannot simply assume that a person who belongs to a "temperamental" Latin race will wince at the sight of a needle, while a stoical Swede will always withhold his complaints.

Certain kinds of pain appear to originate entirely in the individual's mental or psychological state.[7] This type of pain, as real as that originating from neurophysiological conditions, is often termed psychogenic or psychoneurotic. Three examples are **hysteria**, hypochondriasis, and **phantom pain**. In each condition, the sensation of pain does not originate with a physical stimulus, but rather in the past experience of the person. The stimulation of memories of past experience does not lead to painful emotions, but rather to localized sensations of pain.

Components of the pain experience

Initiation. For a long time it was thought that pain occurred when a pain stimulus was perceived by a pain receptor and was transmitted along pain pathways to a pain center in the brain. Today, neurophysiologists discount that theory, which they say implies that stimulation of receptors must always bring forth pain. Such a model, they point out, confuses the psychological experience of sensation with physiological function.[8]

A theory currently accepted is Melzack's **gate-control theory**. This theory holds that

when an input, whether coming from the body, the environment, or from the mind (fantasy), is interpreted as signifying injury, the movement of impulses to the areas of the brain mediating avoidance and internal adjustment is facilitated, and the total complex of pain as behavior and subjective experience is elicited.[9]

Perception. In understanding the mechanisms of pain, it is important to remember the concept of perception. Perception is the process through which we understand something new by making it a part of our previous knowledge and experience. The experience of pain involves interpreting

It is important to understand how a patient's background may affect his response to pain.

---

[7]Margo McCaffery. 1972. *Nursing management of the patient with pain*, p. 3. Philadelphia: Lippincott.

[8]Engel, p. 46.

[9]Ibid.

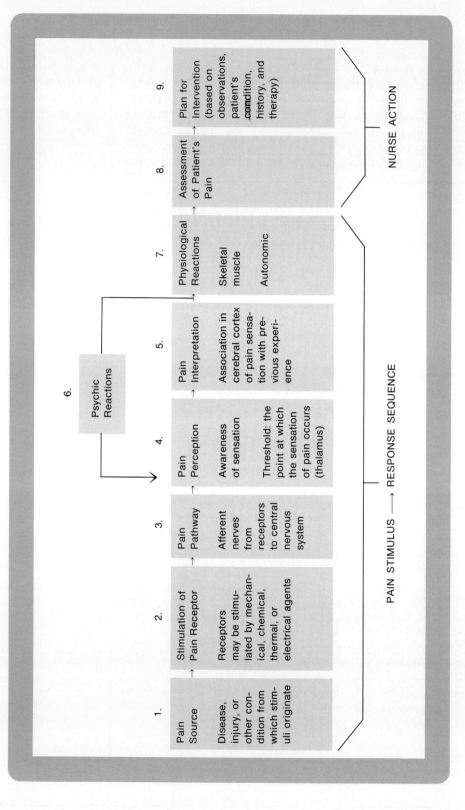

FIG. 26-1 *Pain stimulus and response.*
[From Pain, part 2. *American Journal of Nursing* 66 (1966):1346. Reprinted by permission of the American Journal of Nursing Co.]

the sensory input in terms of previous experience, and the end result is influenced by current and past psychological experience. For this reason, two people can react differently to one stimulus, and the same person can react differently at two different times.

In fact, a person can feel pain without even being actually injured. As one author explains, "pain is not a perceptual fact until and unless psychological processing of underlying physical events in the nervous system has taken place."[10]

According to the gate-control theory, small-diameter fibers carry the pain signals. At the same time, large-diameter cutaneous fibers **(afferents)** may inhibit the transmission of these pain impulses from the spinal cord to the brain.[11] This is accomplished by a gating mechanism that regulates the afferent patterns before they influence the central transmission cells in the posterior (dorsal) horn of the spinal cord (see Fig. 26-2). The patient perceives pain and responds to it when the output of the central transmission cells reaches or exceeds a critical level. The gating mechanism thus balances the stimulus due to pain signals against the inhibitory signals and conveys the net result to the brain. If the activity in the small fibers is greater than that in the large, pain is felt. If the activity in the large fibers is greater, the pain stimulus in the smaller fibers is overcome.

Fiber activity is not the only influence on the transmission of impulses. Brain activities set in motion by the afferent patterns in the dorsal column systems are also important. This means that present and past experiences also affect the system. The input is evaluated in terms of its physical properties as well as its meaning to the individual. Then it is felt as sensation.

Interpretation. The challenge to both nurse and physician is to interpret what a patient means when he reports himself in pain. Complaints may reflect one or more of the following:

1. The presence of local tissue injury or of a peripheral stimulus approaching the threshold of tissue injury.
2. A local afferent input that has become associated in the mind with the threat of injury or disease, so that a sensation not previously felt as painful is felt and reported as pain. For instance, a man who fears he has an ulcer may report a slight stomach upset as pain.
3. Peripheral or central nervous system damage that interferes with the normal modulation of small fiber afferent input (e.g., the neuralgias, causalgia, and "central" pain).
4. An unconscious psychological need to suffer or to be punished or to assume the role of sufferer.
5. A deliberate attempt to deceive others (malingering).[12]

[10] Ibid., p. 45.
[11] McCaffery, p. 33.
[12] Engel, p. 51.

The challenge to both nurse and physician is to interpret what a patient means when he reports himself in pain.

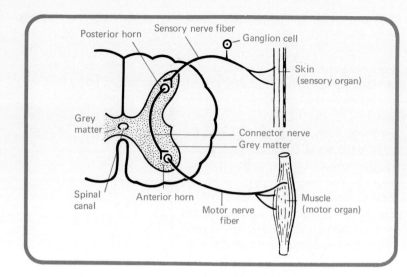

FIG. 26-2 *Transmission of pain sensations to the spinal cord.*

[From Evelyn Pearce, *Anatomy and physiology for nurses,* 15th ed., p. 346. London: Faber, 1973. Reprinted by permission of Faber and Faber, Ltd.]

What is the case when the patient says he feels no pain? Most obviously, he has suffered no injury, tissue damage, or peripheral stimulation. On the other hand, his receptors or pathways may be damaged, or the tissue or structure involved may have no afferent nerve supply capable of transmitting impulses into the dorsal root system. Possibly there is not enough stimulation to activate the receptors, fibers, or connections of the dorsal root system.

It is also possible that the patient reports no pain because his level of consciousness or attention is dulled. For psychological reasons, he may reject the notion of injury or suffering, and therefore does not feel pain or does not wish to report it.

Types of pain

The sensory discriminative system operates in such a way that pain is always associated with a particular place in the body.[13]

Superficial somatic. These areas are well supplied with receptors and fibers. As a result, pain sensations are likely to be well localized. **Superficial somatic** structures include skin and subcutaneous tissue; fascia and fibrous tissue encasing the limbs and trunk; and the periosteum, ligaments, and tendon sheaths.

Deep somatic and visceral. These structures, for example, the heart, have fewer fibers. Pain experienced here is thus more diffuse and less well localized. Pain from the deeper structures is often "referred" rather than felt in the affected area.

Sometimes past or concurrent pain affects the location of present pain. A patient suffering an attack of angina pectoris may feel the pain in his right arm if he has recently injured it.

[13]Ibid., pp. 52–53.

460

The term **radiating** is often used to describe pain from the deep structures and especially from the **viscera.** Pain in the gall bladder feels as if it originates in the right hypochondrium and radiates to the angle of the scapula. Because different disorders are identified fairly often with specific patterns of radiation, these patterns are very useful in diagnosing illness. Sometimes the direction of the radiations is toward the focus of the illness rather than away from it. This is called inverse radiation.

Neurogenic. In **neurogenic** pain, the input is so modified by damage to the peripheral or central nervous system that the patient experiences any sensation as pain.[14] The patient may be undergoing abnormal processing of normal afferent activity or paroxysmal activity originating within the nervous system itself. The degree of pain is unrelated to the stimulus.

Psychogenic. This type of pain can arise from a variety of sources, including fantasies, wishes, needs, or impulses. Frequently, the patient is obsessed with associations between pain and injury, punishment, atonement, or suffering. Psychogenic pain is produced through psychic mechanisms, such as symbolization (conversion) and simulation (malingering).

Assessment

Patient's verbal reports of pain

Because pain is such a subjective experience, the nurse must rely to a large extent on the patient's ability to describe it. She must also observe his nonverbal reactions (see chapter 10 on communication).

Location. The location of pain can affect the quality of the sensation as well as the patient's physiological and physical responses to it. For example, cutaneous pain is often described as bright and pricking, and tends to result in a "fight or flight" response.[15] (See p. 155 for a general discussion of fight or flight.) Fight or flight, also called **activation,** is the immediate response the patient has to pain.[16] He may feel anger (the desire to fight) or fear (the desire to flee). His reaction usually takes place immediately after a sudden, intense pain sensation. The physiological changes prepare the victim either to escape or to defend himself. The fight or flight response is reflected not just physiologically but verbally.[17] The patient may scream or shout angrily. He may strike out at the cause of his pain or withdraw from it, shielding the area of pain.

[14] Ibid., p. 60.
[15] McCaffery, p. 39.
[16] Ibid., p. 14
[17] Ibid., p. 39.

Because pain is such a subjective experience, the nurse must rely to a large extent on the patient's ability to describe it.

In contrast, visceral pain, which arises from within, has an aching quality that seems to depress most behavioral responses. Because it is almost impossible to run away from an attack that comes from inside, the patient usually makes no outward response. He may moan and groan, however.

Cutaneous pain is usually caused by an external stimulus, while visceral pain is internally induced. Even so, a patient's reaction may be influenced by other factors. For example, if he blames his internal pain on a person rather than a pathological process, he may respond more demonstratively.

Intensity. Given the same external stimulus, one patient may report himself in moderate pain, while others will call the same sensation either mild or unbearable. Normally, there is a sound relationship between intensity of stimulation and severity of pain. However, if the patient is in a lowered state of consciousness—for example, in shock—he may report much less intense pain. If he is alone, he may feel worse than when someone is with him. The patient who is immobilized in a body cast is also more likely to report severe pain.

Concentration is another important consideration. If a patient is listening to music he likes or is involved in an interesting conversation, he may not express as much pain as he would if undistracted. If a patient—for example, a woman in labor—is instructed to breathe deeply from time to time while feeling pain, she often requires less narcotic relief. Psychologically, she responds to being told that the breathing will relax her muscles and decrease pain.

The severity of pain can also be influenced by the patient's expectations. If he is anxious and fearful of what will happen, he may report even the slightest pressure as discomfort. Often a patient becomes more tolerant of pain as he gains confidence in his health care workers.

Many patients have a need to assume the role of sufferer, sometimes in order to expiate themselves from guilt and other times in order to manipulate those around them. Consciously or unconsciously, these patients often act as if they are in great stress when people important to them are in the room.

Others may minimize pain in an effort to appear tough or to overcome the fear of serious illness. If such a patient suffers a mild coronary, he may ascribe his sensations to "indigestion." After recovering, he may confess that he was actually in severe pain. Other patients, particularly children, are apt to deny pain in the hopes of avoiding further treatment or of pleasing the physician.

Sometimes distorted reports of pain are based in pathological processes. Patients with peripheral or central nervous system lesions that interfere with the gate-control mechanism may feel excessive pain response to minor stimulation.

Given the same external stimulus, one patient may report himself in moderate pain, while others will call the same sensation either mild or unbearable.

Chronology (onset and duration). Normally, the rise and fall of a pain corresponds with the rate of stimulation.[18] For example, if a person suddenly falls to his knees, he will feel a sharp pain almost immediately. The pain will then subside and persist for a short time. On the other hand, pain associated with nerve or root injury is often not felt immediately, yet the sensation is more intense after the peak moment.

A patient who endures a brief pain of low intensity may not make any sign of the fact that he is in pain. However, a brief pain of high intensity, such as touching a hot iron, often causes the victim to withdraw.[19]

Pain of brief duration, whatever its intensity, is usually forgotten. However, when a person, particularly a child, is exposed to brief pain repeatedly, the cumulative effect is that of chronic pain. Chronic pain is not an isolated but an all-consuming event. The patient becomes very tired. He talks and moves less, and he seems unable to concentrate on anything other than the source of pain.

Qualitative characteristics. When the patient is describing the quality of his pain, he must be allowed to use his own words. If he merely nods assent or disagreement to the nurse's or physician's words, the truth may not come out.

A patient's ability to describe pain depends first on his vocabulary and fluency with language. Often he will speak in terms of past experience, such as receiving an electric shock. He may use similes, such as "It felt like my skin was being burnt off" or "I had the feeling something was exploding inside me."

Some patients will describe their sensations with dramatic gestures, others in flat tone. If the nurse pays close attention to the patient's choice of words, she may also find major clues to his problem. One patient with a herniated intervertebral disc said that his pain "was like a dog would bite you," and then, "as if somebody lit a match and went down the back of the leg with it."[20] The dog imagery described the sudden onset and ensuing muscle spasm, while the match simile referred to the radiation of burning pain along the root distribution.

Sometimes a patient is incapable of describing the quality of his pain simply because he has never experienced anything like it before. This is particularly true of pain originating from injured nerves or from lesions involving the mediating system. Often the terms knotting, cramping, crushing, or burning are used to describe such experiences.

Previous experience, treatment, and effect. How a patient reacts to pain will depend to no small extent on conditioning from past experience.[21]

> How a patient reacts to pain will depend to no small extent on conditioning from past experience.

[18]Engel, p. 55.
[19]Ibid., p. 56.
[20]Ibid.
[21]McCaffery, p. 54.

Frequently, the only place where the patient shows he is suffering pain is in his face.

A patient who has just undergone surgery may complain that his arms are sore, for example, simply because his arms were sore after a previous operation. Other patients may report pain relief simply because a particular drug brought them relief previously. Adults who have had a number of painful experiences as children are likely to be more susceptible to pain.

Whether the nurse considers the patient's distress real or imaginary, she must remember that it is real to him. To be an effective judge, the nurse must try to rid herself of her own prejudices—for example, that acute pain is always accompanied by groaning or gestures.

Patient's nonverbal behavior. Frequently, the only place where the patient shows he is suffering pain is in his face.[22] He may clench his teeth, compress his lips tightly, open his eyes widely or shut them tightly, wrinkle his forehead, bite his lips. Intensity of pain can often be judged by the frequency and duration of facial expressions.

Four types of body movement are associated with pain: immobile, purposeless or inaccurate, protective, and rhythmic or rubbing. By analyzing the frequency and duration of these movements, one can usually find clues to the severity and meaning of the patient's distress.

People often immobilize themselves in a particular position in an attempt to minimize discomfort. Sometimes the patient will maintain whatever position he was in at the time of injury. Other times he will choose a position that seems comfortable. When a patient immobilizes only a small part of his body, he is usually giving a good indication of the location of pain. Generalized lack of movement can also be significant. For example, a patient who has undergone thoracic surgery may stop moving entirely to keep from breathing deeply or rapidly and thus avoid pain of moving the chest wall.

Some patients have learned that muscular relaxation minimizes pain, but the majority will react by tensing muscles, for example, clenching their fists. Purposeless or inaccurate body movements are an expression of the patient's frustration at being unable to help himself. He may thrash his arms or kick his legs, accidentally knocking something over. Or he may react with a protective movement, such as involuntarily pushing away the nurse who is causing him pain. Such reflex movements are a natural component of the flight reaction.

A person who is suffering may go through a number of behavioral changes in an attempt to find relief.[23] He may try resting, changing his position, eating more or less food, or attempting to throw up, urinate, or defecate. He may try to apply heat, cold, massage, compresses, or pressure. He may try to medicate himself.

Generally, the person in pain will first turn to measures that had

[22] Ibid., p. 20.
[23] Engel, p. 58.

provided relief in the past. For example, the person who has found that aspirin relieves headache pain may take aspirin in an attempt to relieve the pain of a foot injury, to no avail. Sometimes a person who fails to find relief will turn to dangerous or irrational activities. Patients with acute myocardial infarction have been known to try doing pushups to relieve their pain.

Environmental factors

Physical aspects. Pain can intensify in healthy as well as sick people as a result of certain environmental conditions. These include extreme cold, wind, high altitudes, air pollution, and solar radiation.[24] Skin conditions can be rendered more painful by exposure to the sun's rays or strong winds. In patients with second-degree burns, even a slight draft can cause wincing.

The excessive sodium loss that follows strenuous exercise in hot weather may cause heat cramps. Extreme cold may cause painful frostbite, especially in people whose circulation is poor. Arthritis is aggravated by cold weather; in fact, many arthritics claim they can predict changes in the weather by the increase in joint pain. Patients with inflamed respiratory tracts may find that low humidity irritates the condition. Others find that breathing is more difficult in warm air.

The sensory restriction that accompanies hospitalization can also increase a patient's sensitivity to painful stimuli and decrease his ability to withstand discomfort (see chapter 17).

Particular incidents or continuing stress. Both physical and emotional circumstances can influence a patient's perception of and reaction to pain. Fatigue resulting from lack of sleep, physical exertion, or emotional weariness may throw reactions off balance. A person who is worn out has less energy and an impaired mental ability for utilizing such techniques as distraction or fantasizing to deal with pain. He may begin to have horrible visions of the effects of his illness, thus increasing his subjective reaction to pain. He may cry out for medication rather than try to bear with his discomfort.

Family and social history. As has been discussed, individual and cultural patterns of pain perception and response are crucial in interpreting a patient's pain experience and planning effective intervention (see page 457).

Age and sex. In America, little boys are expected to repress expressions of pain, while little girls are not discouraged from crying. Adult women are permitted more expression of pain than adult men, although elderly men are expected to react more vocally.

[24]McCaffery, p. 40.

> Both physical and emotional circumstances can influence a patient's perception of and reaction to pain.

Planning, implementation, and evaluation

Anticipate and prevent painful stimuli

The nurse has a number of means of cutting off or alleviating the source of pain.[25] The technique she chooses will depend on the pathology of the patient's disease and the variety of his personal characteristics, which she must assess individually for each patient.

As discussed, various elements in the patient's environment can cause pain and should be controlled as far as possible. For example, the patient with extensive burns should be kept away from drafts, as even a very mild air current will stimulate the exposed nerve endings. Patients with sickle cell anemia should be careful to climb stairs slowly, while the patient with lung disease should get an air conditioner if he lives in a polluted region.

Often the patient's pain is manageable until he starts making certain movements. He usually knows which activities are painful, and the nurse can help him figure out ways of avoiding them. Pressure on an injured area can be related to nearby organs, or it can be caused by contraction of surrounding muscles. Upper abdominal pain of visceral origin, for example, may be increased by the pressure of the diaphragm. When this is the patient's problem, the nurse might urge him to pull his shoulders back and hold his arms away from his body to allow for lateral expansion of the lungs. When muscle contraction is causing the pain, the nurse might recommend a splint.

A number of simple measures can reduce pain associated with various procedures and wound dressings. In order to avoid discomfort of adhesive tape, which pulls at skin and hair, the nurse should use a binder or an elastic nonadhesive material to hold the dressing in place and to provide support. When adhesive tape is used, she can minimize the irritation that accompanies removal by moistening it with warm water. The remaining adhesive substances can then be cleaned off with mineral oil or olive oil rather than stinging alcohol.

To minimize the pain during the dressing procedure, she should work as quickly as possible. Also, it is important to remember that the patient's pain will not be increased when several areas are dressed at once rather than one at a time.

Relieve pain source. The circuit from pain source to pain reactions can be interrupted or modified at any point if the proper actions are taken.[26] The first consideration is to break the circuit of pain at its source. For example, if a patient with prostatic hypertrophy is suffering from a distended bladder, the nurse might try to help him void by asking him to

Various elements in the patient's environment can cause pain and should be controlled as far as possible.

[25] Ibid., pp. 176–79.
[26] Pain, part 2: Rationale for intervention (programmed instruction). *American Journal of Nursing* 66 (1966):1355.

stand up. This stimulates sensory nerves that bring about reflex contractions of muscles of the bladder wall.

Topical anesthetics can also be used to decrease the transmission of noxious stimuli that accompany some painful procedures.[27] For example, a local anesthetic will relieve pain in an open wound or ulceration.

Occasionally, certain foods will either relieve or bother a patient, even though they are not specifically recommended or contraindicated for his condition. A glass of milk will often relieve burning sensations in the stomach. Intestinal cramps associated with diarrhea can be alleviated if the patient drinks less coffee, eats smaller amounts of food at a time and chooses foods low in residue. A glass of prune juice will relieve abdominal discomfort and headache related to constipation. Burning urination will often diminish when the patient drinks larger amounts of water.

Decrease pain stimulus. Sometimes it is simply not possible to relieve pain at its source. For example, a middle-aged woman is in a cast from her toes to her midthigh because of a fractured left tibia and fibula.[28] The nurse notices that her bed covers are disarranged, and that she is perspiring and restless. Her left leg is unsupported and poorly aligned, and she is complaining of a burning pain in her toes. The nurse asks the patient to bend her toes, but she can only flex them, not extend them.

Possibly the patient's source of pain can be relieved, possibly not. The nurse should elevate the leg at once and position it so that no pressure is being exerted by the cast edges. She should then call the physician and ask if he would like to have the cast bivalved.

The following is an example of a situation where it is not possible to relieve the source of pain. An elderly man has advanced osteoporosis with compression of vertebral bodies causing pressure on spinal nerve roots. Because of advanced anatomical changes, the nurse cannot possibly alter the source of pain. However, she may be able to reduce the intensity of the stimulation of pain receptors by maintaining and supporting the spine in the best possible alignment. She can also support the weight of extremities on pillows and provide emotional support.

Block pain pathway. In the preceding case, it may also be possible to interrupt the pain pathway with surgery, such as nerve block or cordotomy, or injection of a drug to inhibit transmission of nerve impulses.

Decrease pain perception, modify pain interpretation, decrease pain reaction. Another way that the nurse can relieve the suffering patient is to decrease his perception of pain by raising the threshold of pain perception. This can be done by analgesics, hypnosis, or distraction. One patient with severe back pain might need a small dose of morphine, while another might be relieved by the diversion of a good movie and a mild anesthetic.

[27] McCaffery, p. 179.
[28] Pain, part 2, p. 1356.

Generally, environment, state of mind, and bodily condition act in concert to intensify the pain experience.

Once a barrage of impulses from a diseased or injured part of the body has activated pain circuits between the thalamus and the cerebral cortex, disturbing sensations other than actual pain will tend to cause pain to be perceived as more intense.[29] Suffering can also be intensified when the patient's pain threshold is lowered as a result of activation of the thalamocortical pain circuits.

If a patient is anxious, angry, bored, or lonely, for example, his pain threshold will be lowered. If he is hungry, thirsty, or tired or if he needs to defecate or urinate, his pain threshold will also be reduced. And if his environment is distressing—glaring lights, unpleasant odors, excessive noise—he will tolerate pain less easily.

Generally, environment, state of mind, and bodily condition act in concert to intensify the pain experience. For example, Mrs. A., who has just had abdominal surgery, is resting quietly, trying not to notice the dull, aching pain in the area of her incision.[30] Suddenly she hears a loud argument in the corridor between the woman who is sharing her room and the woman's husband.

The couple become apologetic once they are aware of the disturbance they are causing. However, Mrs. A. is no longer able to rest. She feels angry, her muscles are tense, she is getting a headache, and the abdominal pain is more intense. Her pain is intensified initially as a result of an environmental disturbance. However, her state of mind after the argument adds to her pain, as do her bodily changes.

But not all influences on the pain experience are negative. The nurse who takes the patient's hand and conveys a sense of concern is directly intervening to alter his state of mind. She can also alter this state by distracting his attention, for example, with a newspaper or with dinner.

Apparently, the cerebral cortex is unable to sustain more than a certain amount of circuit activity at a given time. Also, it is able to react selectively to stimuli. For example, an elderly woman with a sprained ankle is distracted with a new photograph album of her grandchildren. This stimulation tends to arouse cortical activity that is strong enough to take precedence over the pain circuits in the cerebral cortex and to raise her pain perception threshold. Her perception of pain and her suffering diminish.

Drugs play an important part in interrupting the pain pathway. Narcotic analgesics given in the presence of existing pain generally act only at the cortical level to modify pain interpretation or decrease pain reaction. The same drugs given before pain occurs tend to act at both the cortical and thalamic levels to decrease pain perception.

General anesthetics, such as ether or nitrous oxide, decrease pain perception. Local anesthetics, such as alcohol or procaine hydrochloride, block the pain pathway by interfering with the transmission of nerve

[29] Ibid., p. 1359.
[30] Ibid., p. 1360.

impulses. Tetracaine, benzocaine, and other topical anesthetics block pain reception and thus decrease the reception of pain stimuli. Hypnotics, such as phenobarbital, both modify pain interpretation and decrease pain reactions when given in small doses. On the other hand, pain perception is decreased by the administration of large-dose hypnotics, such as sodium tilpental and amobarbital, which act as general anesthetics.

Tranquilizers, such as reserpine and chlordiazepoxide, decrease pain reactions, as do mild sedatives or hypnotics. However, chlorpromazine and related phenothiazines decrease both pain perception and pain reactions through their action at the thalamic and hypothalamic levels. They may also act at efferent nerve endings. Muscle relaxants, such as mephenesin, block the efferent skeletal muscle pathways and thus decrease skeletal muscle reaction. Antibiotic drugs, such as penicillin, relieve pain at the source.

SUMMARY

Dealing with pain, in all its physical and psychological aspects, is an important function of the nurse. In many cases, it is she more than any other professional who can relieve what to the patient is the focus of his illness—the personal discomfort.

Physiologically, the components of the pain experience are complex. The source of pain is provided by disease, injury, or other conditions that stimulate pain receptors. This process can be mechanical, chemical, thermal, or electrical. The pain sensation is carried by the afferent nerves from receptors to the central nervous system. It is then perceived in the thalamus and interpreted in the cerebral cortex. Physiological reaction to the pain sensation can take the form of skeletal, muscle, or autonomic response.

Pain is classified according to where it is perceived in the body. Superficial pain, felt in areas such as the skin and subcutaneous tissue, is well localized. Pain in the deep somatic and visceral structures, such as the bladder, is more diffuse. Neurogenic pain originates within the nervous system, while psychogenic pain arises from a disturbed psyche.

How a patient experiences pain depends not only on physiological processes but also on his physical condition, previous experiences, cultural attitudes, and emotional needs. All of these must be taken into account when the nurse assesses his description of pain. A skier who yearns to get back on the slopes may deny that his broken leg hurts him. The elderly man who feels neglected may report the pain of a cut finger as intolerable.

In assessing a patient's pain, the nurse elicits his own report of where the pain is located, how intense, when it began, how long it lasts, and how it feels. If he is in a state of lowered consciousness, he may not feel pain as intensely. If he is fearful or anxious, the slightest ache may be distressing. The patient who is trying to marshal sympathy may exaggerate his pain, while the one who wants to appear heroic may minimize it.

Studies have shown that background weighs heavily in a patient's reaction to pain. Some people come from cultures where expressions of pain are readily accepted, while others have been taught to repress them. Women may also feel more free than men to verbalize distress. In making her assessment, the nurse must try to set aside her own preconceptions. She must remember that whether a patient's pain is physical or emotional in origin, it is real to him.

There are many ways in which the nurse can interrupt the pain pathway and provide the patient with relief. Her first consideration is to anticipate and prevent any obvious sources of discomfort. The patient with serious burns should be kept well out of air currents, while those with muscular injuries should be taught ways of avoiding certain movements. Wound dressings can be applied and removed with a minimum of discomfort.

Often seemingly minor measures, such as changing a patient's diet, can provide him with relief. And one of the most effective pain relievers is distraction. A patient who concentrates on nothing but himself is bound to feel worse. The nurse might provide him with a magazine, turn on the radio, or simply chat with him for a few minutes.

Drugs are invaluable aids in pain relief, and the nurse must be thoroughly familiar with them. However, their use can be minimized by intelligent nursing care.

STUDY QUESTIONS

1. What factors, physical, psychological, and sociocultural, influence an individual's reaction to a pain stimulus?
2. What is the "gate-control" theory of pain?
3. What are the major types of pain? How can the nurse differentiate between them?
4. In what ways does a patient indicate that he is in pain? What methods can the nurse use to help him describe his pain more fully and accurately?
5. What actions can the nurse take to relieve a patient's pain? Explain the principle behind each action.

SELECTED BIBLIOGRAPHY

Engel, George L. 1970. Pain. In Cyril M. MacBryde and Robert S. Blacklow, eds., *Signs and symptoms*, 5th ed., pp. 44–61. Philadelphia: Lippincott.

Keele, Kenneth D. 1972. Pain: How it varies from person to person. *Nursing Times* 68:890–92.

McCaffery, Margo. 1972. *Nursing management of the patient with pain.* Philadelphia: Lippincott.

Pain, part 1: Basic concepts and assessment (programmed instruction). *American Journal of Nursing* 66 (1966):1085–108.

Pain, part 2: Rationale for intervention (programmed instruction). *American Journal of Nursing* 66 (1966):1345–68.

27 Rehabilitation

What is rehabilitation?

Rehabilitation is the continuing, cooperative process of restoring the individual to optimal functioning in all areas of his life. Its goal is to maintain, as far as possible, the person's ability to live a productive, ego-satisfying life in his home and community environment. The following considerations are central to the concept of rehabilitation.

The nurse's role

Rehabilitative nursing is not a specialty limited to the particular agencies or settings. It is a vital part of nursing in the patient's home, the hospital emergency room, nursing home, clinic, and any and all settings in which health care is provided. Temporary or nonphysical conditions can cause situations that require the same kind of rehabilitative treatment that long-term disabilities do. This is the case with the immobility of the mental patient who is allowed to sit for overlong periods of time or the subcritical burn patient who lies too long unturned.

In working with the patient with a long-term disability, the nurse's attitude is especially important. Understanding, encouragement, and flexibility continue to be important. Also crucial are firmness and, above all, patience. It takes time and practice to learn new techniques, but if the patient is to achieve maximum independence, he must be supported and not pushed. The nurse must know the patient's background as well as his medical history. He must be treated in the context of his psychological reactions, economic situation, family relationships, and availability of community resources.

Sociocultural aspects of disability

At the heart of the disabled person's ability to come to terms with his new role is his reaction to society's concept of that role. Depending upon the extent of his disability, he may feel deprived of any or all of the assets by which his peers measure success or, at minimum, acceptability. These include physical attractiveness, sexuality, the ability to earn one's own way, social acceptance without special consideration, and so forth.

Upon completing this chapter, the reader should be able to:

1. Discuss the importance of beginning the rehabilitation process at the onset of the disability.

2. Identify three factors that affect an individual's response to a disability and the rehabilitation process.

3. Relate the nature of the disability to the type of rehabilitation methods the nurse should employ.

4. Identify the relationship between patient independence during and following the rehabilitation process and such factors as community resources, health team cooperation, and family goals.

Much of the patient's ability to adjust will depend upon his age. The younger the child at the onset of the illness or accident, the easier the adjustment to a more limited body image. The older child can recognize in his friends his own uncomfortable reaction to a disabled person. The adolescent, with so much of his life colored by a growing awareness of sexuality, is deeply affected by any bodily change that lessens his confidence in his sex role. The adult adds to these concerns those of his ability to function as a marriage partner and parent, to provide an income for a family or maintain a household, and to keep from becoming a burden. The older person, perhaps already fighting the feeling of being a burden, already lonely and without interest in the future, may simply give up.

Assessment

The patient's physical condition

The kind of disability that requires rehabilitation may be as uncomplicated as a leg fractured in a skiing accident. It may be as complex as the effects of hemiplegia resulting from a cerebrovascular accident. In assessing the patient's potential for rehabilitation, the nurse must take a variety of factors into account. These include such general aspects as overall physical condition and stability, motor and sensory deficiencies, level of functions, and limitations of mobility. She must also be aware of the presence of related or unrelated conditions ranging from pressure sores to cardiac or respiratory problems and other chronic medical conditions. Also important is an understanding of the patient's psychological, sociological, and cultural background and their probable effects upon his condition and its treatment. The patient's understanding of his disability and his goals must also form a part of this assessment.

Psychological and cognitive condition

Accurate assessment of the patient's emotional state enables the nurse to anticipate potential problems. It will also indicate the most effective attitude to take in responding to the patient. Depending upon the patient's personality and the extent of his disability, his psychological reaction may range from mild tension and depression to severe anxiety and anger. The patient who shows *no* specific outward reaction should be of equal concern to the nurse. Fear, anger, and depression are normal reactions to a disability, and their absence indicates an unhealthy repression of normal emotion or denial of reality. (See chapter 28 for a discussion of loss and grief.)

Even acceptance needs to be regarded critically by the nurse. As a positive force, it is beneficial, but it might instead be a negative force. For example, the patient receives no psychological support from the kind of acceptance that is actually a surrender to guilt. The patient may feel that he is being punished for wrongdoing, so he must give up and take the worst. What appears to be acceptance may also be a disguised fear of failure. It may also reflect satisfaction in paying back a supposedly uncaring family member. This is the "I'll hold my breath till I turn blue and then you'll be sorry" reaction. Acceptance needs to be realistic without being pessimistic. Ideally, it combines a minimum of self-pity with a maximum concern for those others, family members in particular, who are affected by the patient's changed condition in life.

Cognitive state is also a crucial factor for anyone suffering from a neurological disability. Physiological effects may be accompanied by memory lapses, weak attention span, instability, and poor perception of spatial relationships. These factors affect the patient's ability to comprehend what he is taught or told and to retain and act upon it. Thus, they affect his overall chances for optimal rehabilitation.

Extent and nature of disability

Adjustment to a disability is always influenced by various factors in the patient's sociocultural background and personal psychology. These factors present complications enough in the case of a simple permanent disability. When the disability is multiple in nature, adjustment is even more difficult and complex. A final complication is added when the disability is not static, that is, when its status is subject to change, for better or for worse. In particular, the patient with a progressive disability may lack even the comfort of certainty and the resultant incentive to plan for optimum rehabilitation and accomplishment.

Multiple sclerosis presents a typical picture of a nonstatic disability. It is neither temporary nor altogether permanent, in that while there is no cure now known, there exists the possibility of regression and remission. It is a complex disability, exhibiting a variety of symptoms. These include loss of balance, double vision, weakness in the extremities, slurred speech, and headaches. It may be a very mild case, undiscovered throughout the patient's lifetime, or severe enough to cause fatal complications.

Environment

Home and community. If the patient's family has been included in planning his rehabilitation and discharge programs, they can be solidly supportive. The family that has not adjusted to the situation or has not taken part in the program planning can be as much a disability as the patient's physical condition. Guilt feelings are often a factor in the unadjusted family. They may feel responsible for the disabling accident, if any, or for unintended feelings of resentment toward the one who has upset their lives and drained their financial resources. They may also feel guilty over an inability to maintain as high a level as they might wish of concern and contribution to the patient's welfare. Like the patient, they, too, may interpret the family's suffering as punishment for wrongdoing.

The nurse must determine what community facilities are available

> Acceptance needs to be realistic without being pessimistic.

to assist both patient and family. Such facilities will range from the purely medical to the financial. Among the areas in which community help may be available are education, family counseling, vocational training, housing, child care, legal advice, and transportation. There also may be resources for financial management advice, mental health counseling, and English as a second language classes.

The purely physical aspects of the patient's home and community environment also need careful study. At least one site visit to the patient's home (and, if possible, his job) should be made. The health care team needs to be aware of its location in terms of availability of transportation and condition of roads and sidewalks and steps. Also important are its nearness to shopping facilities, jobs, schools, and relatives and friends. On the basis of the data gathered, arrangements can be made to order special equipment and make whatever structural changes are practical. It may be necessary to modify the program to adapt to physical situations that cannot be changed.

When satisfactory arrangements cannot be made within the home environment, other solutions may be found. A patient who is unable to bathe independently may be assisted by a visiting nurse or rehabilitation team member. When the preparation of food is a problem, "meals-on-wheels" may be the answer. Service organizations connected with churches, Boy or Girl Scouts, schools, etc., may be able to provide a range of special services. These include shopping for the patient, getting books at the library, taking care of pets, or just having someone come in to talk.

Specialized rehabilitation center

The patient who convalesces in a specialized rehabilitation center is already past the most traumatic part of the onset of his disability. He knows what his condition is and should have a fairly good idea of what it will be and how it will affect his life-style in the future. He may gain a feeling of satisfaction from being part of a situation in which the entire program is geared to him and his problem. The patient is not competing for time and attention with others whose situations are completely unrelated. There is reassurance in knowing that he is dealing with professionals who are specialists in his particular condition and that they are all directly concerned with him. He is in surroundings with which he will have time to become familiar, to which he can add personal touches. There will be time enough to get to know the staff and to make friends with other patients, who will understand his problem and not be distressed by it or uncomfortable with him. There will be time simply to come to terms with his problem and to learn how to cope with it. He feels that he is ceasing to be an invalid and is becoming a self-determining individual again.

Since such a center—whether for rehabilitation of cardiac, neurological, musculoskeletal, tubercular, emotional, or other conditions—is set up for

The patient may gain a feeling of satisfaction from being a part of a situation in which the entire program is geared to him and his problem.

the longer-term patient, both physical surroundings and programs can be more informal. More individual variation is possible and a greater range of activity can be provided, as a general rule. Visits by family and friends are encouraged. There are even a few new rehabilitation centers in which the whole family takes up residence and is treated as a unit. Many more are completely family-oriented without actually involving residence.

The patient should never be allowed to overexert or overtire himself.

Planning, implementation, and evaluation

All rehabilitation programs, for no matter what disability, share a certain number of basic assumptions. Two of the most basic assumptions are that

1. The successful program is the one that makes the patient the expert.
2. The program should never become routine or fixed but must remain dynamic, always adapting itself to the changing needs and abilities of the patient.

It is important that teaching sessions be kept as consistent as possible, held at the same time and by the same person. The patient should never be allowed to overexert or overtire himself. Such strain can lead both to muscle injury and to failure, which can be as damaging to the patient's progress and mental state as actual injury. The patient who has achieved optimum function will sometimes pressure his therapist to extend treatment beyond the point where nothing else can possibly be accomplished. Such pressure must be resisted or the patient will be encouraged to believe that there may be, after all, hope for further restoration of function, thus finding it that much harder to accept his disability realistically.

Neuromuscular training

The patient with motor dysfunction caused by damage to the nervous system, specifically to the cervical spinal cord, needs to accomplish several goals in his rehabilitative program. Active exercises work toward improving his strength. Passive stretching develops coordination, helps prevent contractures, and counteracts spasticity.

In **hemiplegia** resulting from a cerebrovascular accident, the patient faces several problems in addition to motor impairment. He may have spasticity or flaccidity of the affected limbs, sensory loss, vision and speech impairment, and loss of sphincter control. But neither the hemiplegic nor the paraplegic, with the upper half of the body functional, faces the same threat to independence as does the quadriplegic. The degree of function remaining in the upper body in quadriplegia depends upon the point of injury to the spinal cord. The higher up the spine the injury, the greater the loss of motor function.

Bowel and bladder training

The patient whose disability involves the function of bowel or bladder faces a psychological disruption of a particularly difficult nature. To the frustrations and anxieties already present is added the fear of becoming personally offensive. It is wise to wait until he has begun to come to terms with his disability before starting any training program, since his full understanding and cooperation are essential to any measure of success.

Achievement of bowel and bladder control depends upon the cause of loss of control, the extent of brain damage, and the existence of other complications, such as infection. In planning each individual program, the nurse has three primary functions:

1. To become fully familiar with the patient's present and previous bowel and bladder habits and condition
2. To take whatever measures are necessary to ensure the patient's physical and psychological comfort until his future regimen can be determined
3. To plan, along with the patient, a long-range, specific program to ensure the maximum possible rehabilitation

Bowel training. The goal of the patient whose excretory system has not been surgically changed is to gain control over his bowel movements without the use of medication or mechanical means. Maintaining a stool that is fairly firm but soft through proper diet and high fluid intake is essential. Loose stools are difficult to control. Too firm a stool may result in constipation and, over a period of time, hemorrhoids. Physical activity is also important to sustain muscle tone.

Both patient and nurse must be aware that a daily bowel movement is not absolutely necessary. For some persons, a movement every two or three days is normal. Some patients, attempting to create a daily habit, develop a dependence upon laxatives that must be overcome before a proper training program can begin.

The choice of toilet equipment is necessarily guided by the patient's relative mobility. Since the squatting position is most desirable, a toilet should be used whenever possible. If necessary, support can be provided by backrest, safety belt, handrail, or raising the toilet. A commode with similar support features can also be used. If a bedpan must be used, the patient must be assured both privacy and comfort, and pressure sores must be guarded against. A patient should not be allowed to remain on the bedpan, toilet, or commode for more than 20 or 30 minutes.

It is necessary, in setting up a program, to select a specific time of day, usually after the morning or evening meal. The interval selected should be based upon the patient's previous habits.

Peristalsis is helped by a fluid intake of $2\frac{1}{2}$ to 3 quarts of fluid daily, plus a glass of warm liquid before a meal or just before defecation. Foods such as those that provide roughage and certain fruits and juices are also useful. It is always important to consider the patient's preferences.

There are two basic types of bowel management programs: those requiring medication for effectiveness and those using mechanical methods. In the former, use is made of such medications as suppositories, laxatives, or bulk-forming compounds. The latter two medications are rarely recommended on a permanent basis. Suppositories have been the traditional means of promoting bowel management, as they can be used on a permanent basis if necessary. Proper insertion is essential. The suppository should rest against the rectal wall beyond both internal and external sphincters.

Mechanical methods—enemas and digital stimulation—have been demonstrated to be more consistently effective than those using medication. They provide less delay in response, fewer accidental evacuations, and a higher percentage of success.[1] These methods are recommended in particular where anal sphincter muscular tone is defective, although in these cases it is necessary to provide a means of retention of fluid when an enema is given. Generally speaking, enemas are recommended only in the early stages of a program when there has been a delay in defecation or an impaction, a hard concentration of the stool. Patients with advanced multiple sclerosis may also require them on a more regular basis.

If the spinal cord injury occurred above the sacral nerve roots and the patient has retained the **reflex arc,** digital stimulation of the anal sphincter will help defecation. This simple procedure brings about the reflex response causing evacuation. It involves inserting a gloved, lubricated finger 1 to $1\frac{1}{2}$ inches into the rectum and stretching the anus slightly through a circular or back-and-forth motion. After a few times it may become possible to identify a certain area that causes relaxation promptly upon being touched. The patient can help by breathing deeply and, if possible, bearing down. The process should last anywhere from $\frac{1}{2}$ minute to no more than 5 minutes. Results should occur within 30 minutes, but can be much more prompt.

The patient who has undergone a **colostomy** faces an entirely different problem. With the surgical removal of the rectum, a new anus is created on the abdominal wall by making an opening directly into the large bowel. The protrusion of the bowel forms a **stoma,** a budlike opening through which the stool is removed. The goal of a colostomy control program is to have fecal material expelled only during irrigation. To achieve this, the patient must be familiar with his bowel physiology, equipment, dietary needs, irrigation procedures, as well as how to regulate them. He must also learn that the colostomate can live a normally active life.

---

[1]Sudie A. Cornell et al. 1973. Comparison of three bowel management programs. *Nursing Research* 22:321–28.

One of the patient's first jobs is to learn to change the temporary **ostomy bag.** The area around the stoma is gently wiped, washed with warm, soapy water, and patted dry. It is then coated with an ostomy cream or tincture of benzoin as a protective measure against skin irritation. Karaya gum powder or karaya gum rings are an additional protection. These can be applied directly to the skin and the bag (which has an adhesive facing) fixed over them. The opening of the bag should be about $\frac{1}{8}$ inch larger than the stoma, which changes in size according to the patient's position.

After the initial period following surgery, a colostomy can be regulated and the patient no longer has to wear a bag over the stoma. The irrigation procedure, which lies at the heart of colostomy control, should be learned as soon as possible. It is performed daily at first, until control is established, and then every other day. The time of day depends upon the patient's daily schedule, his previous habit pattern, job, uninterrupted access to toilet facilities (the procedure requires about an hour), and so on. An hour after the big meal of the day is usually best, since the bowel will be full.

In performing an irrigation, several rules must be remembered:

1. The reservoir must not be hung too high (above shoulder height).
2. Approximately 2 quarts of warm, never hot, water is usually enough.
3. The catheter should be inserted only about half its length, some 4 to 8 inches, with a rotating motion and moved slowly back and forth while the water flows. It should never be forced; to do so could cause perforation.

The patient must be taught to recognize and avoid problem foods that cause gas and odor, diarrhea, or constipation. Offenders in the first category are spicy foods, carbonated drinks and beer, onions, peas, beans, cauliflower, cabbage, pork, and nuts. Diarrhea can be caused by green leafy vegetables, uncooked fruits, fruit juices, spicy or irritating foods, and large quantities of liquids, especially beer. The patient can lessen the effect of eating these foods if he is careful always to chew his food well, eat slowly, and keep his mouth closed while chewing to avoid swallowing air. Additional peace of mind is available through some commercial odor-restricting products provided by ostomy supply services.

Bladder training. In a bladder training program, the goal is the control of urination, without a catheter, if possible. (Prolonged use of a catheter causes infection and eventual kidney damage.) Control implies both a predictable voiding pattern and adequate bladder emptying.

Bladder problems take two opposing forms: incontinence and retention. In the case of the neurogenic, or cord, bladder resulting from a spinal cord injury or lesion, the type of training needed depends upon the location of the lesion. When the lesion is *above* the second, third, or fourth sacral segment (the upper motor neuron lesion), the reflex center is intact. This permits the bladder to be emptied sometimes by reflex, and training is aimed at making this reflex emptying more efficient. If the external sphincter as well as the detrusor muscle is spastic, adequate emptying may be prevented. When the lesion is at the second, third, or fourth sacral segment (the lower motor neuron lesion), there is injury to the reflex center. As a result, the bladder muscle loses its normal tone, and the patient cannot void by reflex emptying. In both situations, the patient is unaware of the need to void and cannot do so without training.

When incontinence is caused by other factors—disease, brain damage, infection, congenital deformity, psychological regression, etc.—awareness may be present without control. Loss of control may be either temporary or permanent in such cases. Control is unlikely ever to become possible in the case of patients with sphincter damage, fistulas, advanced multiple sclerosis, multiple myeloma, high-level quadriplegia, and severe brain damage. If catheter use must be continued for these patients, it is essential to maintain a program of high fluid intake, asepsis in catheter care, and bladder irrigation to fight infection. Where possible, use of the catheter should be replaced by an external urinary appliance for men or protective clothing for women.

As soon as a patient's physical condition is stable and he can sit upright, a trial of voiding is attempted to determine if he is able to void without a catheter. The usual procedure for this begins with breakfast. The patient receives 200 cc of fluid every hour for about 3 hours until the bladder has accumulated some 300 cc. The catheter is then removed and the patient encouraged to void on a toilet or commode at regular intervals. A record is kept of the amounts voided and of any incontinence between voiding. The bladder is also checked for residual urine. If, after 3 or 4 hours, the patient has not voided, the catheter should be reinserted and the program postponed for a week or so. If voiding has begun, the hourly intake of fluid and 2- to 3-hourly attempts to void should be continued throughout the day.

When the actual training program begins, the patient will be receiving some 3,000 to 4,000 cc of fluid per day. This usually takes the form of an average glassful every hour between 7 A.M. and 8 P.M. Intervals between voiding are increased from 1 to 2 hours, then to 3, and even, in some cases, to 4. Fluid intake and output are recorded meticulously, and evaluations and adjustments are continued until a satisfactory pattern is established.

Voiding may be stimulated by various means. For the patient with complete upper motor neuron bladder, these include stimulation of "trigger areas" on the thigh, abdomen, or genitalia; anal and rectal digital stimulation; tapping the abdomen; or doing push-ups while sitting in a chair. The lower motor neuron lesion patient may try inward and downward stroking pressure over the bladder **(Credé's technique)**, straining (as in **Valsalva's maneuver**), or, if possible, contraction of the abdominal muscles. There are also various drugs that provide certain assistance in treating incontinence.

As the patient absorbs emotional and social stimulation through the attempt to reach him on the level of his senses, his responses tend to open out.

Two other important aspects of any bladder training program are cleansing and the fluids that constitute the daily 3,000-cc intake. It is essential that the patient be kept clean and dry, both for esthetic reasons and to prevent damage to the skin. Within the fluid diet, it is wise to be moderate in the intake of the following:

1. Fruit juices (they are alkaline and can cause problems in bowel consistency)
2. Milk (its high calcium content helps stone formation)
3. Carbonated fluids (which tend to irritate the bladder)

Acid-based drinks like cranberry juice help to prevent the formation of stones in the urinary tract. A special effort should be made to keep the fluid intake varied and to include to the extent possible those fluids the patient particularly likes.

Sensory rehabilitation. Any program of sensory rehabilitation reaches out to the patient on a particularly instinctive level. If he is suffering from the forgetfulness, confusion, and disassociation that characterize senility, he may withdraw deeply inside himself. Withdrawn into his own more comfortable past, he may not be willing to emerge into a world he cannot even sense very well, much less keep up with.

Organic brain syndrome and senility are not completely irreversible. With care and close attention, even the severely brain damaged can show an increase in sensation, understanding, and coordination. As the patient absorbs emotional and social stimulation through the attempt to reach him on the level of his senses, his responses tend to open out. This creates a circle of stimulation—response—greater receptivity—increased awareness of stimulation, and so forth. Personal contact is an essential part of the development of this responsiveness. Closeness to another person is reassuring to someone who has been increasingly alienated from both the physical world and the people in it because of the lessening receptivity of his senses. Apart from any other aspect of sensory rehabilitation, the very fact of having someone else's attention concentrated upon him lessens the patient's feeling of personal insignificance.

Psychological and cognitive factors

The immediate psychological impact of an accident-caused disability can be greater than that resulting from illness. In the latter case, there is apt to be more time for the patient to adjust, although a different kind of anxiety can accompany his awareness of the progress of the disease.

It should be borne in mind that personality problems frequently precede disability, instead of being caused by it. Any problem is exaggerated by the disability and, in turn, can seriously affect the patient's eventual adjustment.

Psychometric tests and aptitude tests can help to bring forth unsuspected interests and abilities in a disabled patient. He may well be experiencing his first uncommitted "leisure" time without family or peer-group pressure to spend it in some accepted manner.

Assisting the patient's "grief work." Anyone who has lost an ability to function normally undergoes a grief reaction. This mourning for the loss of the former, whole self is similar to the reaction of terminally ill patients and their families. The nurse needs to recognize that the patient must be allowed to grieve. Her support of him and of his right to mourn will be a strengthening factor in his progress toward a healthy acceptance of his disability (see chapter 28).

Maintaining patient motivation. In helping the patient maintain his motivation, two basic considerations should be kept in mind:

1. Although competition can be helpful, a patient should never be goaded into better performance by unfavorable comparisons with another patient. Building in chances for small successes in his program will accomplish the same end much more effectively.
2. The daily exercise and therapy routine may be tedious to the point of discouragement, if not actually painful. The patient needs to know the nurse is concerned about his discomfort and to know that his efforts are really accomplishing something.

Reality orientation is a special rehabilitative technique for working with acutely confused patients. This procedure helps such patients to become reoriented to their immediate surroundings and to relearn the basic activities of daily life. Its underlying goal is to reawaken their interest in themselves and their environment. This is accomplished through constant reminders to the patient of who and where he is and what he is doing and why. Activities are structured as simply and unchangingly as possible. Sensory training is conducted and the patient is kept in touch with the outside world and encouraged to be independent.

Promoting optimal independence

Activities of daily living. The **activities of daily living (ADLs)** are generally considered to include eating, bathing, personal hygiene (washing, brushing teeth, shaving, hair, nails, makeup), dressing, and toilet activities. Also important are sitting up and changing position in bed, transfers (between bed, toilet, and car), driving, and ambulation or operating a wheelchair independently. There are many devices available to the nurse for helping patients with eating, dressing, and hygiene.

Family members must be taught that the patient does not wish always to be helped, that he would rather take 10 minutes to put on his wristwatch

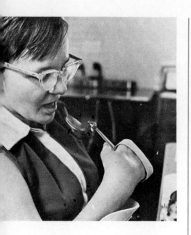

Many devices are available to help the handicapped patient with such activities as eating.

[Photograph by Dan Bernstein]

but do it himself. Both patient and family must guard against his trying to do too much, however. Progress can only occur with adequate rest, proper diet, and correct exercise.

Whenever possible, the rehabilitation nurse should visit the home of the patient. This will enable her to assess more accurately the difficulties that may or may not occur as he shifts from a planned, professional situation into an unfocused one. (See the comments on environment on pp. 473–74.) If a home visit is not possible, the family should do their best to supply floor plans, pictures of rooms, measurements of doorways, etc. They should also be asked for the details of any other relevant situation (steps leading to a family room, for instance).

When the visit has been made, the nurse can draw upon all her ingenuity in adapting the physical situation to the patient's home-care/self-care program. Are there many plants in the patient's room? Using the tools required for indoor gardening may provide excellent physical therapy for hand dexterity. Is there a pool table in the family room? Get him back in the game; it provides excellent eye-hand coordination practice. Is the kitchen full of cookbooks? Get the rolling pin back in the patient's hand. Activities such as these have the added value of being independently initiated. They are not therapeutic "exercises" that the patient is required to do, but leisure pastimes that he can choose to do, and thereby feel less a patient and more a person.

In helping the disabled person to learn any of the techniques that will carry him through his ADLs, the nurse must always move slowly. Procedures must be accomplished one step at a time, making sure that everything up to that point is absolutely clear before the next step is taken. Goals should be realistic and generous praise should accompany each small success. With help of the right kind of adaptive equipment, the disabled person can manage to do a remarkable number of things, and do them independently.

Vocational rehabilitation. Vocational rehabilitation presents problems on another level. Retraining for a different kind of work requires an investment of pride not needed for learning a new tooth-brushing technique. Failure to succeed in a new occupation is particularly damaging to the disabled person's self-image. The occupational therapist should assess the patient's physical and mental abilities, his educational background, and any special aptitudes. Following the assessment, the goal of the vocational rehabilitation can be established. The patient may be able to return to his former occupation. He may have to learn another kind of work or go into sheltered work. The underlying goal of any such program is to coordinate the needs for financial help, occupational satisfaction, and self-respect.

Cooperation among members of the health team. The membership of the health care team may vary during the course of rehabilitation. The nurse may be a public health or visiting nurse, an extended care nurse, or a nursing home nurse. Other members include the physician/surgeon and the physical therapist. The team may also include an occupational therapist, speech therapist, psychologist or other guidance personnel, and a community social worker. The patient and his family are the most vital members of the health team.

Relations among members of the team may depend, to a certain extent, upon whether the individuals are directly connected with a hospital or with a community health agency. The primary factor will be one of attitude. If the team is to be optimally effective, it must work as a whole. To do so, the members must be prepared to treat each other as professional colleagues, with respect for their competency and without regard for petty questions of status. They must be willing to learn from each other and to share their insights. This calls for the establishment of close working relationships. Once members of the health team have the desire to cooperate, the lines of communication can be worked out. They will ordinarily fall into two categories: direct/dynamic and indirect/stable. The first is the conference, with all members present and the whole program open to reemphasis or redirection and reassessment. The second is the written documentation. Coordination of activities and cooperation among members

A visit to the patient's home is important in formulating a realistic rehabilitation program.

[Courtesy Veterans' Administration Prosthetics Center, New York, N.Y.]

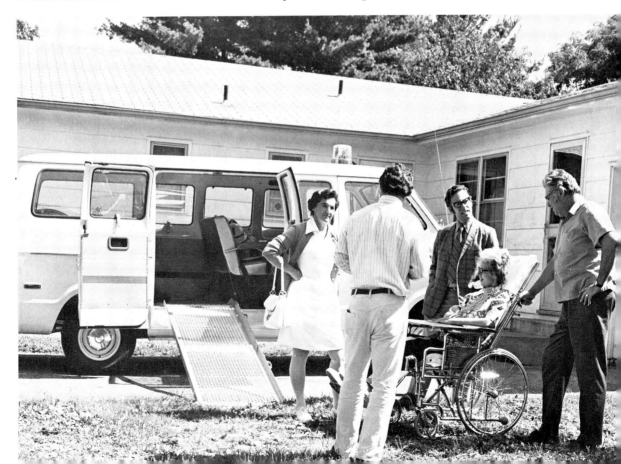

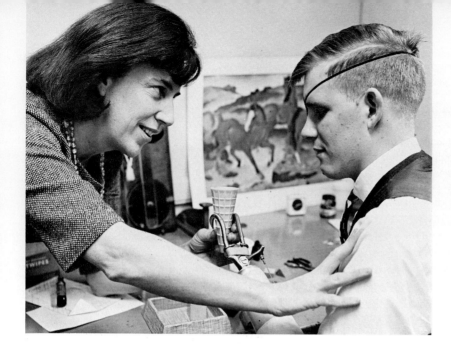

Members of the health care team can together devise a plan for helping the patient with the activities of daily living.

[Photo courtesy the ICD Rehabilitation and Research Center]

are possible only if everyone is working with the same understanding of the situation.

SUMMARY

Rehabilitation is a dynamic process that begins with the onset of a disability and continues throughout its existence. It considers the whole patient—physically, socially, and economically—not just the affected part of his body. It has as its goal the restoration of the patient to the maximum independence of which he is capable.

In its various phases, it may take place in a hospital, in extended care or nursing setting, or a specialized rehabilitative institution. It may also take place in the home, with access to community facilities. Wherever or whenever it takes place, the patient and his family must be part of the program's planning and implementation. They are the most important members of the rehabilitation team. The rehabilitation team may consist of a number of professionals from different areas. The nurse's role as coordinator is especially important. She is also the member of the team with the primary responsibility for setting into motion the various decisions reached as a result of team-conference agreements.

Part of rehabilitation involves teaching new ways to perform the various activities of daily living. The nurse carries the main responsibility for teaching these techniques to both the patient and his family. She will help them find devices to aid in accomplishing these activities. She will also assist them in creating new techniques and devices to fit new conditions and situations.

A large part of rehabilitating the patient involves helping him to adapt to his disability. He will be concerned about what others think of him in his changed state, particularly how his family will react. He will be worried about finances and how he will manage in his day-to-day life. He will also be concerned as to how his disability will affect his overall life-style. The younger the patient, the easier his adjustment will probably be. The more unexpected the disability, the more traumatic the shock.

The nurse must let the patient work through his own period of grief, as this is part of the rehabilitation process. She must try to provide the patient with consistent understanding, strength, friendliness, and positively oriented realism. A thorough knowledge of the patient and his health and personal history is essential if the nurse is to help meet all his needs.

The patient is prepared to return to daily living through various means. He is trained to function as effectively as he is able. If possible, he is put in touch with others who have learned to deal with problems similar to his. His home and community environments are studied carefully so that any inherent problems can be planned for in advance. Vocational possibilities are investigated and arranged for when appropriate.

The disability that requires rehabilitation may be simple or complex. It may be temporary or permanent, static or changing. Its effect upon the person's psychological state may be severe or mild. A disability is an impairment; a handicap is the way in which a person is diminished by his disability. The goal of rehabilitation is to remove the handicap from the disability.

STUDY QUESTIONS

1. What are some of the major factors that enter into the concept of rehabilitation?
2. Define three factors that must be considered when assessing a patient's rehabilitation status. What is the role of each?
3. Why are home visits important in a rehabilitation program? What information do they provide?
4. What methods can be used to promote communication between members of the rehabilitation team?
5. In what general ways would a rehabilitation program for a multiple sclerosis victim be similar to that planned for a stroke victim? How would they differ?

SELECTED BIBLIOGRAPHY

Heidell, Beth. 1972. Sensory training puts patients "in touch." *Modern Nursing Home* 28:39–43.

Motivating the unmotivated patient. 1974. *Nursing '74* 4:31–36.

Riffle, Kathryn L. 1973. Rehabilitation: The evolution of a social concept. *Nursing Clinics of North America* 8:665–71.

Snowden, Myrtis J. 1972. Rehabilitation: The chronic long term illness patient. *AORN Journal* 15:59–62.

Stryker, Ruth Perin. 1972. *Rehabilitative aspects of acute and chronic nursing care.* Philadelphia: Saunders.

28 Loss, death, and grief

Assessment of loss, death, and grief

Types of loss

Loss is described as a state of being deprived of or of being without something one has had.[1] It may be sudden or gradual, traumatic or nontraumatic. Four kinds of loss are

1. The loss of a significant loved or valued person
2. The loss of an aspect of the self
3. The loss of external objects
4. Developmental loss, or the loss occurring in the process of growth and development

Loss of a loved or valued person can occur through death, divorce, or separation. An aspect of a person, such as a special quality or personality, can be lost through illness. The loss of a person can be total or partial, permanent or temporary.

A person can lose part of his self, that is, part of his totality of experiences and images of himself. He may lose his health and feel significantly changed in the process. He may lose bodily function; the power of his senses (hearing, sight, smell) may be diminished; or he may even lose a part of his body through surgery or trauma. His social role as a worker, family member, and community participant may be lost. Attitudes about his normal way of relating to the world may be altered, and changes in his bodily drives create marked psychological consequences. In other words, any negatively perceived change in the individual's accustomed way of relating to the world can be considered a loss of self.

The loss of external objects, such as possessions, money, or a home, constitutes the third form of loss. Inanimate objects have symbolic meaning for human beings, and their loss can result in powerful emotional reactions.

Developmental loss occurs in the process of normal human growth and development. Birth is a sudden loss of a comfortable intrauterine

[1]David Peretz. 1970. Development, object-relationships, and loss. In Bernard Schoenberg et al., eds., *Loss and grief*, p. 4. New York: Columbia University Press.

environment. Changes in the body, as well as changes in a family situation, are all considered developmental losses. Infancy, childhood, and old age—stages of human development in which there are many marked changes—represent particularly vulnerable times in which loss occurs.

Reactions to loss

Grief is a type of bereavement that is temporary and requires no specific medical advice or treatment. It is experienced by people who are losing or have lost anything significant in their lives. With support and time, the grieving person can return to his normal level of functioning and feeling state. Other bereavement states, such as **depression, hypochondriasis,** and **acting-out** reactions, are considered states of maladaption to loss. They do not run a course to recovery, and are destructive of the bereaved, his family, and friends.

"Normal" grief is characterized by a number of predictable stages. They have been identified by Dr. George Engel as those of **shock and disbelief, developing awareness,** and **restitution and recovery.**[2]

Dr. Elisabeth Kübler-Ross describes stages of dying that are similar. They are the stages of **denial and isolation, anger, bargaining, depression,** and, finally, **acceptance.** These stages are distinct emotional states, but they invariably overlap and intertwine. Shock is usually the first stage, and resolution (acceptance) is usually the final stage, but in between the stages vary tremendously. (Table 28-1 summarizes the stages of grieving and dying.)

Shock and disbelief. At first, the person experiences shock and disbelief at the loss. The patient who is told he must undergo amputation of a leg or the person who is told of a death in the family usually reacts by denying the fact. This is one nurse's description of the denial exhibited by a mother whose son was dying of leukemia:

> Even though she [the mother] had been specifically told by her son's physician that his periodic episodes of rectal bleeding were due to leukemic infiltration of his gastrointestinal tract, she denounced this fact by attributing this bleeding to the "rupture of internal hemorrhoids."[3]

Occasionally, patients will deny that they are dying until the very moment of death. One woman dying of cancer, for example, believed (or pretended to believe) that she was only the victim of a slightly new strain of flu.[4]

[2] George L. Engel. 1964. Grief and grieving. *American Journal of Nursing* 64:94-96.
[3] Linda Goldfogel. 1970. Working with the parent of a dying child. *American Journal of Nursing* 70:1677.
[4] Thomas Powers. 1971. Learning to die. *Harper's Magazine* (June 1971):76.

Occasionally, patients will deny that they are dying until the very moment of death.

Stage	Kübler-Ross (Dying)	Engel (Grieving)
Initial	Denial and isolation	Shock and disbelief
Intermediate	Anger	Developing awareness
	Bargaining	
	Depression	
Final	Acceptance	Restitution and recovery

TABLE 28-1
Stages of Grieving and Dying

Developing awareness. Usually, the person soon acknowledges the reality of the loss. He alternates between denial and bewilderment. He is distressed, sorrowful, and regretful, and usually can think of nothing but his loss. He feels a painful yearning and longing for the lost person, social role, or bodily function, and in the early stages of grief, sexual desire and a capacity for even small pleasures are greatly diminished. He may feel "unreal."

The perceptions of the grieving person may be distorted. He may believe that he hears the voice of the lost person, or he may feel the presence of the deceased person, even though he recognizes that these experiences are illusions. Dreams and nightmares are common. Guilt also is not an uncommon reaction. The bereaved may recall the ways in which he mistreated the deceased, or he may feel guilty about his past functioning as a family member. The dying person may also feel a sense of guilt.

Crying is typical during the early stages of grief. The greatest degree of anguish or despair is experienced and expressed at this time. This may be expressed in a variety of ways, depending on the cultural expectations. Some cultures demand loud and public lamentation, whereas others expect restraint.[5] This is one situation in which even adults are allowed to cry and act somewhat "childish."

The stage of developing awareness in grieving is similar to Dr. Kübler-Ross's stages of anger, bargaining, and depression in dying. In her experience, dying patients often expressed anger toward hospital personnel. Anger is often vented on the doctors for doing nothing, and on relatives because they are going to live. Other patients are blamed for not being so ill, nurses for being young and healthy, and God for being unjust.[6] The dying and the chronically ill often resent the attributes of those around them—the vitality, freedom, and purpose that they no longer possess.

The bargaining stage in dying or other types of impending or recent loss is characterized by the patient's attempt to make a deal with God or with fate, promising some act in exchange for more time or for a full recovery. If the patient does live longer than is expected, the promise is usually not kept and bargaining begins anew.

After these stages, the patient progresses to the stage of depression.

[5]Engel, p. 95.
[6]Powers, p. 76.

This may be a **reactive depression,** which comes from a nonacceptance of one's condition. It may also be a preparatory depression, which comes from a grieving for future losses, and is a step toward acceptance.[7] The patient discourages visitors, rarely speaks, and is preparing himself to give up the things that are meaningful to him.

Restitution and recovery. For Engel, the third stage in grieving is one of restitution and recovery. This is made easier for the grieving by rituals such as the funeral. These types of rituals make clear the reality of the loss. Since the ceremony takes place within a group, feelings can be more readily expressed and supported. The grieving person attempts to deal with the painful awareness of loss, but he cannot yet think of a new love object to replace the lost person.

During the earlier stages, he may have felt numb, but now he begins to experience physical discomfort. This may include shortness of breath, weakness, exhaustion, loss of appetite, and insomnia. Many other physical manifestations are common.

For the patient who is dying, a final stage of acceptance (Kübler-Ross) is reached when he can truly say, "I am ready to go." Dying patients who remain fully conscious, or nearly so, say they are tired, feel a growing calm, are ready to go, and are perhaps even happy.[8] This stage can occur only if there is an extended period in which the person is dying, and only when there is proper support from others. For some people, the need to control is so strong that they must fight until the very end. Others are prevented from progressing through the stages of dying by other people.

According to Engel, idealization begins in the normal grieving process when the person develops a completely positive image of the deceased person. He idealizes that person, and represses all negative and hostile feelings toward him.

Many other acute depressive symptoms may occur, but they are usually not indicative of any pathology unless they persist. The acute stage should be over within a few months, but it may take a year for complete recovery.

Restitution and recovery are complete when the individual returns to his prior level of functioning. He is then able to establish new relationships and express interest in other people. He can enjoy the pleasures of life without shame or guilt. Grief is resolved when the bereaved person can remember realistically, and without discomfort, both the positive and the negative attributes of the lost relationship or function.

Types of grief

Anticipatory grief occurs before the loss actually takes place. Today, when the process of dying often takes place over an extended period of

[7]Lisa Roseman Shusterman. 1973. Death and dying: A critical review of the literature. *Nursing Outlook* 21:466.

[8]Powers, p. 80.

> For the patient who is dying, a final stage of acceptance is reached when he can truly say, "I am ready to go."

There are people who are unable to express feelings of grief in public, and grieve only when alone.

time, the family, or the patient himself, may begin to grieve for the expected future loss.

Absent, delayed, or **inhibited grief** occurs in a number of situations, and it may not be indicative of maladaptation. The relationship between the lost function, role, or person and the bereaved may have been an ambivalent one, or there may have been a separation with the development of new relationships prior to the death.

Delayed grief often occurs when many details must be attended to immediately, and the person may not feel the full impact of the loss until later.

There are people who are unable to express feelings of grief in public, and grieve only when alone. They are admired because they appear to be strong. However, this pattern limits the degree to which the person can express grief or receive support.

Other individuals are not aware of feeling deeply grieved. These persons may feel intensely ambivalent about the deceased person. They feel that a strong emotional reaction will reveal feelings of hostility as well as feelings of love. They feel guilty, and they react defensively, busying themselves with activity.

Chronic grief is really a denial of the grief process. The individual acts as if the tragic event had not occurred, almost as if a return of the deceased is expected. Parents who leave a deceased child's room at home untouched are exhibiting this reaction pattern.

Depression. Depression, although it may seem similar to the developing awareness stage of normal grief, is actually a qualitatively different state. It differs from a normal grief reaction in that after a reasonably short period of time, the normally grief-stricken person's mood will lift at times. He will be responsive to the support and reassurance of the people around him. The depressed person will not respond to these stimuli, and the ability to experience pleasure is virtually nonexistent. Also, the depressed person appears to be more concerned with himself than with the deceased person. He engages in self-deprecating behavior, and feels that he will never get better. He moves slowly, has a poor appetite, is unable to sleep well, and does not appear to be interested in the world outside his preoccupations.

Hypochondriasis. In **hypochondriasis** (a morbid anxiety about one's health), the person expresses concern about a physical problem rather than about the loss and its consequences. Symptoms of hypochondriasis may occur for a short period in grief, as symptoms of depression, or they may exist independently. The symptoms represent an expression of intense anxiety, hostility, or guilt after the loss of a loved one. This type of reaction also needs professional attention.

Acting-out. When the person handles his feelings of loss by compulsively seeking out new relationships or by immersing himself in work or other activities, his behavior is called acting-out. The person is actually denying that real feelings of loss exist, although it may appear that he is handling the situation adequately given the expectations of his culture.

These stages are general, and are to be used as guidelines. They are not hard and fast rules of behavior. Within these categories, there are many variations, and the nursing student should allow for maximum individualization of grieving from person to person.

Death in twentieth-century America

Death is inevitable. But one would not think so in modern American culture. We prolong, preserve, and restore life, and even attempt to develop ways of returning to life once death occurs. Television commercials reflect many of our society's values. We are told to stay beautiful, live forever, and, most of all, never grow old. Skin creams, hair implants, face-lifts, elixirs, and exercises—all guarantee, for a time at least, a "youthful" look. They also postpone the realization that aging must occur and that it inevitably leads to death.

Our ancestors thought much more about death. They had to. Survival to old age was the exception, and one could not count on living a complete life cycle. The occasion of death was not a surprise; people experienced deaths within their family from an early age. In most cases, nothing could be done to delay the dying process.

Today, however, our world is completely different. We expect to live to a "ripe old age"; in fact, the life expectancy for us is more than twice that of most of our ancestors. It is no longer natural to die at an early age—"natural" deaths occur only in the aged.

Another difference between our experiences and those of past generations is that the structure of our society shields us from the fact of death. Throughout the history of mankind, the sight of death was a common experience. Today, dying has become more and more separated from everyday life. Many young people grow up without ever seeing a dying person. Even those people who remind us of death, the aged, tend to be segregated from the rest of society.[9]

Death has become the province of specialists—medical, pastoral, and commercial. It is no longer the shared experience of many. The bereaved family seldom deals with many of the details of dying. The hospital cares for the person while he is dying, the physician "pronounces" the final moment of death, and the nurse prepares the body. After death, the funeral director arranges the burial ceremony, and a representative of the clergy eulogizes.

> Today, dying has become more and more separated from everyday life.

[9]Herman Feifel. 1963. Death. In Norman L. Farberow, ed., *Taboo topics,* p. 113. New York: Atherton.

Awareness contexts

The degree to which the probability of death is acknowledged by the patient and by the people around him is involved in what is called the **awareness context.** The awareness context is the total combination of what each person involved knows about the identity of the other and his own identity in the eyes of the other.[10] This awareness determines much of the interplay between the patient, his family, and the health care personnel. (The latter are the group of people who, because of the trend in care of the dying, are with the patient most during the process of dying.)

The various types of awareness contexts are **closed awareness, suspected awareness, mutual pretense awareness,** and **open awareness.**[11]

Closed awareness. A closed awareness context creates an atmosphere in which the patient has not been informed of his prognosis. It appears that most American physicians choose not to reveal the prognosis to their patients. Since many of the involved families and personnel follow the lead of the doctor, many consequences follow. Since the patient assumes that he will recover, he plans his future accordingly. He may not know that certain care could extend his life, and he may initiate plans that could shorten his life. The family members are unable to share their feelings of grief with the patient. The members of the health care team are also subject to a great deal of strain when the prognosis is withheld.

Suspected awareness. In the suspected awareness context, the patient suspects that he is dying, but he is unable to confirm the fact with the health care personnel. The patient may receive hints about his condition. These hints include transfer to an intensive care unit, treatment with radiotherapy, and uncomfortable and evasive reactions on the part of the health care staff. The reason for withholding the truth, some doctors say, is that the patient would find it too upsetting. These doctors feel that patients need hope in order to keep on fighting for life, that one never can be absolutely certain of a diagnosis, and that patients do not really want to know.[12]

Mutual pretense awareness. A mutual pretense awareness context is the pretense, on the part of the patient, the family, and the health staff, that the terminal prognosis is not a reality. Although both are fully aware of the prognosis, the staff will not mention the subject, and the patient refrains from bringing it up. Often, the patient is discouraged by the behavior of the staff from discussing anything even related to the topic.

[10] Anselm L. Strauss and Barney G. Glaser. 1964. Awareness contexts and social interaction. *American Sociological Review* 29:670.

[11] Anselm L. Strauss and Barney G. Glaser. 1970. Awareness of dying. In Schoenberg, ed., *Loss and grief,* p. 300.

[12] Powers, p. 74.

Pretense may provide some degree of dignity and privacy for the patient. On the other hand, an open awareness context allows for much more participation in the acceptance of death by both the patient and the people around him. Most of the research done with dying patients indicates that acceptance of death is more likely if the patient is allowed to speak openly about his feelings and to tie up the loose ends in his life.[13]

If the patient understands his prognosis, he can plan more appropriately for his remaining time. He can finish essential work, reconcile important relationships, settle plans for his family, or plan something that he has always wanted to do. He can even have some control over some of the aspects of his dying.

The patient is not, however, always ready to deal with the dying process. He may not be able to accept death, and may die with more anguish and with less dignity than he might have if he were unaware of the prognosis.

Some of the behaviors of the fully aware patient (for example, constant complaining, angry demands, withdrawal) may not be acceptable to the hospital staff. With the sharing of feelings among the patient and staff members, the personal involvement with the patient may become too charged with emotion. This may lead to a total avoidance of the patient.

Planning, implementation, and evaluation

The nurse and the dying patient

Death and the period of dying have moved, in many cases, out of the home and into the hospital. As a result, the dying patient has become more the responsibility of hospital personnel and less the responsibility of the family. It is therefore important that the nursing student become aware of the ways in which the present caretakers of the dying and the supporters of the grieving are responding to this relatively new facet of professional responsibility. Since most care of the dying patient and support of the bereaved are less than ideal, there are several factors involved in hospitalized care that must be considered.

First, hospitals are dedicated to restoring health, and health professionals are committed to assisting patients to recovery. Therefore, the dying patient represents an awkward contradiction for both the system and the professional. The equipment and technical skills of life-saving measures are emphasized to a great degree in the hospital. On the other hand, the care of the dying, those beyond expertise and mechanical restoration, is being relegated to a less significant place. "One often hears physicians praise the quick-thinking skill of the nurse in the intensive care unit, but does one hear much praise for those who care for the dying? Not often."[14]

> If the patient understands his prognosis, he can plan more appropriately for his remaining time.

[13] Shusterman, p. 467.

[14] Frances Mervyn. 1971. The plight of dying patients in hospitals. *American Journal of Nursing* 71:1988.

Second, the hospital is an organizationally based medical order, and the dying must fit into this organization.[15] A certain amount of work must be performed in a prescribed length of time. This work is usually made up of innumerable kinds of tasks to ensure that a large number of patients receive baths, medications, intravenous fluids, and treatments on time. Time spent with distressed patients does not "count" on the nurse's task-oriented daily agenda. Even if the nurse has some time after her responsibilities are completed, the patient may not at that moment be in need. (Some of this busyness is an attempt to avoid the very difficult confrontation with the questions and pleas of dying patients.)

If the nursing staff were to become genuinely involved with the needs of each dying patient, and with the responses of the grieving family, much more emotional support of the staff would be necessary than now exists. Patients going through angry, depressive, and hostile behaviors are considered "problem" patients to hospital staffs. These behaviors disrupt the attempts of often short-staffed units in completing the assigned work.

Because the nurse often does not know what to say in this situation, or is afraid that she will say the wrong thing, the patient is often ostracized and avoided. Health professionals apparently have accepted the notion that left to themselves, people die quietly and with few or no problems.

Defense mechanisms used by nurses. In order to protect themselves when the patient has not been adequately informed of his prognosis, nurses adopt certain defense mechanisms. They are used to maintain professional composure and to avoid involvement. Some of these mechanisms are:

1. *The nurse purposefully avoids the patient, or she may "expressively" avoid the patient.* This means that during the time she must confront the patient to give care, she ignores the "person" part of the patient and focuses on the treatment needs only. She ignores him, wears a bland professional expression, and exudes dignity and efficiency. She often refuses or evades conversation, or else does her chores quickly and attempts to leave before the patient can say anything.[16]

2. *"Role-switching" is another defensive measure.* The nurse counters any direct questioning from the patient by referring him to his doctor. She also does this with the family.

3. *When dying is particularly prolonged or painful, the nurse, although she wishes that the patient would expire, develops a "miracle rationale."* This is especially true if the patient is receiving experimental treatments. The nurse hopes that something miraculous will result from the research modality.

4. *The quality of conversation can be used to defend against patient distress.* The nurse refrains from asking questions such as "How are you?" to avoid the possibility that the patient may bring up the dangerous topic of his

[15]David Sudnow. 1967. *Passing on*, p. 84. Englewood Cliffs, N.J.: Prentice-Hall.
[16]Barney G. Glaser and Anselm L. Strauss. 1965. *Awareness of dying*, p. 237. Chicago: Aldine.

prognosis. The nurse may find it necessary to speak as little as possible to avoid the subject.

She may give the patient a "professional brush-off"—a silent, pleasant smile, a "We're doing all we can" or "We'll pull you through."[17] She restricts her conversation with the patient to the here and now, and avoids mention of any possible future plans that the patient might have.

5. *The family is isolated from the scene of medical care in order to avoid confrontation and communication.* This structural arrangement, aided by the use of doors as shields, separates the nurse from the family. It decreases her involvement, and prevents the family from disturbing her composure.

6. *The nurse may only "selectively hear" what the patient has to say about his fears and anxieties.* If a patient says, "I'm afraid, I'm afraid, I can't breathe, and I do a lot of coughing," the nurse will focus on the least threatening subject—the problem of coughing. She also may "not hear" any of the more detailed explanations about the patient by the family, about the indicators of social loss—his children, spouse, job, or talent.

7. *She may directly deny the possibility of death as an outcome of the illness, or she may treat his symptoms as unimportant.* In the beginning stages of a terminal illness, this response creates no suspicion on the part of the patient that his disease may be fatal.

8. *In some situations, the nurse perceives the patient as "unaware," and behaves openly about his prognosis.* She "discounts" the patient's awareness. With infants and premature infants, the nurse can openly show her feelings and devotion. She talks to the infant, and can talk to others in his presence.

When the nurse believes that the patient is permanently unconscious she can also talk freely and behave as if the patient were a "nonperson." The patient is considered socially dead.

Nurses often resort to cynical joking in the presence of these patients, or with patients who are considered senile. Since the patient is unaware, the nurse feels as though she can speak openly to him or speak with others about him in his presence. The staff members can converse together on many other topics during the time that care is being given, or, as nurses have said themselves, while "watering the vegetables."

9. *Even when there is nothing more the medical profession can do for the patient, the nurse must direct her activity toward the patient's comfort.* She feels negligent and guilty that nothing more can be done and works hard to make sure that the patient is comfortable and free of pain. Sometimes the nurse can only maintain her composure by making sure her patient is completely free of pain.

Helping the dying patient. How can dying patients be treated more humanely? The nurse must first start with herself. She must examine her own concept of death. When health workers become aware of their own

[17] Ibid., p. 233.

At times there is little or no need for words; a touch or silence may be enough. Stay with the patient; do not desert him.

reactions and how these reactions affect patients, they can more realistically approach the task of assisting patients and grieving families to accept death. To be able to discuss death with patients, the nurse must come to grips with her own feelings about pain, grief, loss, helplessness, hopelessness, life, and death.[18]

The nurse personalizes her care for the dying when she talks with the patient while taking care of his medical needs. She does so when she maintains eye contact with the patient and responds to what she senses he feels. She also does so when she exchanges her thoughts, feelings, and ideas with him.[19]

To assist nurses in their care of the dying, a nursing plan for the dying patient has been devised.[20] Its implementation will depend, of course, on the individual needs of each patient and the willingness of the nurse:

1. Recognize how you, as a person and as the nurse, feel about death, since each death reminds us of our own and we fear destruction.
2. Talk with the patient long before his death actually happens and when he indicates he wants to. Most dying patients know they are dying and when they are dying.
3. Help patients to live until they die; dying is a normal part of life.
4. Recognize and try to understand what the patient is experiencing. Identify the times when your feelings contradict those of the patient— for example, you want him to live, but he wants to rest and die in peace.
5. Make the patient feel like an important individual whether he can be helped or not; remember he has a right to decision making.
6. At times, there is little or no need for words; a touch or silence may be enough. Stay with the patient; do not desert him.

Emotional support of the dying

After the initial stages of dying, the patient's need for emotional reassurance is greater than his need for facts.

Some of the needs that can be met by the nurse are:[21]

1. *The dying patient needs relief of his loneliness, his fear, and his depression.* He needs someone to spend time with him and listen.

2. *The dying patient needs maintenance of security, self-confidence, and dignity.* He should not be isolated or abandoned. To ensure that these needs are met, the nurse should help the family in their support of the patient (see p. 498). The family will be comforted if they feel that they can trust the nurse, that she will be available, compassionate, and competent. They want

[18] Jeanne Quint Benoliel. 1970. Talking to patients about death. *Nursing Forum* 9:266.
[19] David E. Sobel. 1969. Personalization on the coronary care unit. *American Journal of Nursing* 69:1439–42.
[20] Barbara Allen Davis. 1972. . . . Until death ensues. *Nursing Clinics of North America* 7:308-9.
[21] V. Ruth Gray. 1973. Dealing with dying. *Nursing '73* 3:28–29.

to see that she is human and capable of grief. This will assist them in expressing their own feelings of grief.

3. *For the dying patient, everyday needs are heightened.* The patient should be provided with the basic necessities without strain on his part. Diversional activities that are relevant to the patient can provide a change in routine and a point of interest by focusing on the here and now and on short-term goals.

4. *The patient, even in the last stages of dying, tolerates the idea of death more readily if he still has some degree of hope.* Hope is compatible with an intellectual acceptance of the reality, because, in fact, no one really does know the future. In many cases, patients have had a remission when the prognosis was extremely poor, and patients who hope for a miracle drug are not all that unrealistic about this hope.

Physical needs of the dying patient

Some of the physical needs associated with dying patients include:[22]

1. Sensation and power of motion as well as reflex activity are lost first in the legs and then gradually in the arms. Pressure on the extremities seems to bother the patient. Sheets should not be snug, the patient should be turned frequently, and special attention should be given to the positioning of the legs.
2. As peripheral circulation fails, there is a "drenching sweat," and the body surface cools, regardless of the room temperature (see chapter 25). To compensate, body temperature begins to rise, and restlessness is often caused by a sensation of heat. Patients need lighter clothing and fresh, circulating air.
3. The dying patient always turns his head toward the light. As sight and hearing fail, the dying see only what is near and hear only what is distinctly spoken to them. Indirect lighting should be provided in the room, and a loved one should be seated near the patient at the head of his bed. Nurses and relatives should never draw the shades in the room, never talk in whispers, and never fail to answer honestly any of the patient's questions.
4. The dying patient's touch sensation is diminished, yet the dying can sense pressure. The nurse should find out if the patient likes to be touched, and should make sure that there are no points of pressure on his body.
5. The dying patient seems to be in pain throughout the dying process. If, however, all of his other needs are met and if he is at the stage of acceptance where he has said all he feels he needs to say, he may need minimal pain medication.
6. The dying patient is often conscious to the very end. And the nurse, to the very end, needs to give total care.

[22] Ibid., pp. 29–30.

The family will be comforted if they feel that they can trust the nurse, that she will be available, compassionate, and competent.

The nurse should recognize that she will witness many different kinds of grieving customs in her nursing career.

Support of grieving families

In order to assist the people close to the dying patient, the nurse needs to make sure that adequate information regarding the prognosis has been given. She must see to it that they are allowed to prepare for the patient's expiration before death is imminent. The people close to the patient may be the target of the patient's anger, and they will need to have this behavior explained to them. They should also realize that the patient's wish to limit the number of visitors is not a personal rejection of family members. They should be made aware that the person is psychologically removing himself from meaningful human contact in order to accept death.

Family members often feel much more relieved if they are allowed to assist in the care of the patient. This participation may help them in their grief. They will be able to reflect not only on the support their presence brought to their loved one but also on the comfort their ministrations of care gave him.[23]

The following are some guidelines to follow in situations that the nurse commonly finds herself in with grieving family members:[24]

1. The request to see the dead patient should not be denied family members or others close to the deceased person. This need to take leave, to ask forgiveness, to touch, to kiss, or to caress the dying or dead loved one is of overwhelming importance to some. It will not be requested by those for whom it will be disturbing.
2. Since the nurse knows that the first stage of grief is shock and disbelief, she should anticipate that visitors and family members may react in highly disturbed ways when informed of the death. She should take the relatives to a quiet place where they can grieve in private. She should understand that their denial, anger, or other uncontrollable behavior is to be expected.
3. The nurse should recognize that she will witness many different kinds of grieving customs in her nursing career. These cultural and religious rituals are often essential to enable the family to tolerate the initial period of distress.

Special considerations—fatally ill children and adolescents

Children. Because society places a high value on children, parents of fatally ill children often exhibit more intense emotional reactions than they would if the terminally ill patient were an older member of the family. And because of the societal taboo on the subject of death, children often are not told that they are dying.

Hospital personnel also have strong feelings about caring for fatally ill children. They often identify with the child (who is seen as a younger

[23] Engel, pp. 97–98.
[24] Fran C. Northrup. 1974. The dying child. *American Journal of Nursing* 74:1067.

brother or a son). They react with anger about the fact that he will not be able to develop normally. Finally, they feel it unfair that a child should die when he can hardly comprehend the meaning (that is, the adult meaning) of death. These are all normal grief reactions that occur with the staff, but such strong emotional responses may create problems of care for the patient himself.

Care must involve the parents. They should be informed of any changes and be included when the child receives explanations from medical personnel. Including parents decreases the child's fear because he sees he has his parents' support, and senses that they understand and agree with what is being done for him.[25]

Adolescents. For the fatally ill adolescent, terminal illness interrupts and compounds the developmental tasks of establishing values, choosing a vocation, adjusting to the opposite sex, and developing independence. Because a fatal illness limits his development in all of these areas, special considerations should be given to the adolescent patient and his parents.

Here are some of the areas of developmental difficulty, as described by a nurse, of one hospitalized adolescent boy with leukemia:

Adolescence is a time of joining groups and seeking acceptance. One of Tony's first concerns was that his friends would abandon him. It was difficult for Tony to continue identifying with his peer group because he felt very different. Nor was it possible to identify with adults; his life would probably not extend into adulthood.

How could Tony develop an occupational and vocational orientation for his adult life if there was to be no adult life?

How could he attain the goal of independence and emancipation from his parents when he was forced into increased dependence on his family?[26]

Moral and philosophical considerations

Today, the entire body of traditional thinking on the subject of death is being reevaluated. The right of the patient to determine his own fate is becoming a pressing issue. Some people have devised "living wills" to ensure that extraordinary measures to prolong their life are not carried out at some future point. A contemporary writer, Marya Mannes, claims that one of the inalienable rights of the dying is a claim to "the good death," free from pain and artificial life supports.[27]

What seems to be changing is the previously accepted notion of the "absolute sanctity of life"—the classical doctrine of medical idealism in

[25]Christine Mitchell Lacasse. 1975. A dying adolescent. *American Journal of Nursing* 74:1067.

[26]Gray, pp. 27–28.

[27]Christopher Lehmann-Haupt. 1974. Speaking of the unspeakable. *The New York Times* (January 11).

its prescientific phases.[28] Concern is directed today more toward the quality of life than toward the absolute value of life in any form. This thinking is reflected in the current legislation allowing abortion on demand without medical or psychiatric reasons.

Although the responsibility of the medical profession in making life or death decisions has become a controversial issue in recent years, some historical and theological precedents have established that responsibility. Pope Pius XII declared in 1957 that the duty to maintain life necessitates only treatment of the standard or conventional type, but that "extraordinary" efforts are not obligatory.[29] "Extraordinary" is a term that means that life is not necessarily to be maintained under conditions that involve great expense, inconvenience, or hardship, and which at the same time offer no reasonable expectation for recovery.

One of the difficulties in today's health care system is the imprecise definition of "death." **Clinical death** may mean the moment at which the brain is no longer functioning, spontaneous respiration has ceased, and the heart has stopped beating. **Biological death** is defined as death of the tissues. The patient may have an adequate cardiovascular system with no evidence of a functioning brain (as indicated by flat electroencephalograph readings for a specified period of time). This ambiguity as to the exact parameters of "death" leads to many legal and ethical questions.

SUMMARY

Loss is the state of being deprived of something that one has had. The loss may be of a significant loved or valued person, external objects, or an aspect of the self. Developmental changes are also considered a form of loss.

There are a number of reactions to loss. Normal grief is a temporary state of bereavement characterized by the stages of shock and disbelief, developing awareness, and restitution and recovery. The acute stages will subside within several months, although complete recovery may take as long as a year.

The stages of dying are similar. Dr. Kübler-Ross describes the stages of denial and isolation, anger, bargaining, depression, and acceptance in dying persons. While the initial reaction is usually denial and the last stage is acceptance, individual reactions in between vary tremendously. In addition, not all people are able to complete all of the stages.

Some of the conditions that are considered maladaptations to loss are hypochondriasis, acting-out, chronic grief, and depression. These states require professional attention. Unlike normal grief, they do not follow a smooth course to recovery.

Death is an inevitable consequence of living. However, at this particular point in time, the values of American society emphasize youth, vitality,

[28]Joseph Fletcher. 1973. Ethics and euthanasia. *American Journal of Nursing* 73:671.
[29]Nathan Hershey. 1968. Questions of life or death. *American Journal of Nursing* 68:1910.

and productivity. With an increase in the numbers of aged people in the United States, and with the technological advances in medical care, more and more people will not be able to conform to these values. Many elderly cannot sustain their lives economically. Chronic illness, limited mobility, and the psychological effects of being considered no longer valuable to the society increase as serious problems of living. When prepared to die, the elderly and others who are dying are not allowed even this; instead, they are brought back to some form of "life." Many have their physiological lives maintained with machinery against their wishes, when they are, in fact, socially dead.

Awareness contexts determine the kind of interaction that will develop between the dying patient, his family, and the medical personnel. Awareness contexts may be closed, suspected, mutual, or open.

The dying patient should be encouraged to maintain his basic functions, and should ambulate and exercise if able. Physical breakdown should be prevented, and he should be kept as comfortable as possible and free of pain.

The nurse, in order to personalize care for the dying, will encounter difficulties with the system that is structured to rehabilitate the moribund, not to care for the dying. She must recognize her own reactions to death and dying, and how these reactions are affecting patients. She can then more realistically approach the task of assisting dying patients and their families.

STUDY QUESTIONS

1. What is loss? Define the four major types of loss and give examples of each.
2. What are the major types of normal grief? How do they differ from one another? How does normal grief differ from depression, hypochondriasis, and acting-out?
3. Compare and contrast Kübler-Ross's stages of dying with Engel's stages of normal grief.
4. What is meant by the term "awareness contexts"? Define the four types of awareness contexts discussed in this chapter. How do these awareness contexts affect the nurse-patient relationship?
5. How can the nurse meet the physical needs of the dying patient?
6. Based on your own experience, analyze the defense mechanisms you have used when interacting with a person who is dying. Why did you use these defenses? How can they be overcome?

SELECTED BIBLIOGRAPHY

Engel, George L. 1964. Grief and grieving. *American Journal of Nursing* 64:93–98.
Glaser, Barney G., and Strauss, Anselm L. 1965. *Awareness of dying.* Chicago: Aldine.
Kavanaugh, Robert E. 1974. *Facing death.* Baltimore: Penguin.
Kübler-Ross, Elisabeth. 1969. *On death and dying.* New York: Macmillan.
Schoenberg, Bernard, et al., eds. 1970. *Loss and grief.* New York: Columbia University Press.

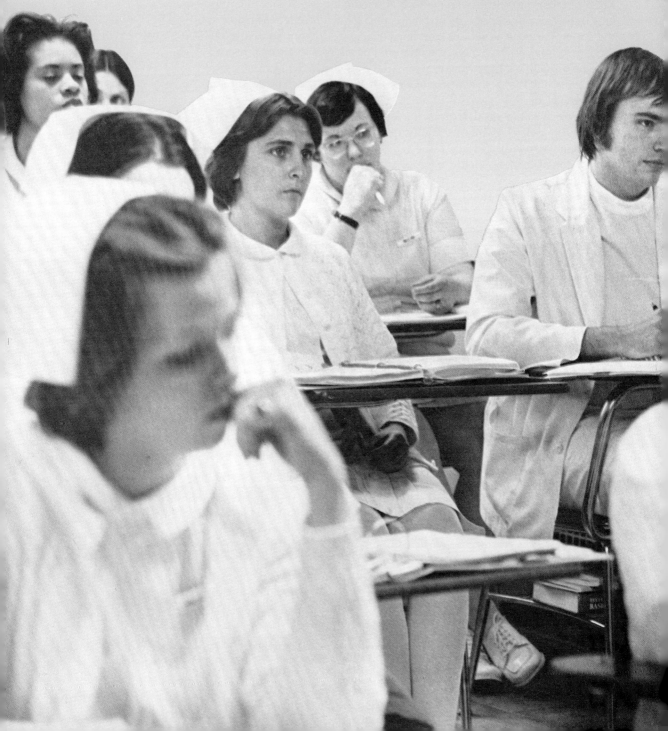

Part Seven

Conclusion

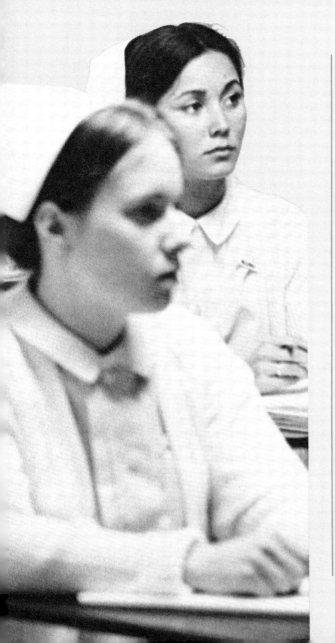

"Here's to health and happiness," the guests said as they toasted Anita on her fiftieth birthday. The Harrisons and some friends had gathered to celebrate the occasion. The family unit has changed over the past 10 years. Linda is married and has two children, and Paul has moved into his own apartment. Estelle Tanner, now 81, moved in with Richard and Anita 2 years ago, after it became evident that she could no longer live alone.

But perhaps the biggest changes in the family's life-style have been brought about by Richard Harrison's job-related illness and partial disability. About 5 years ago, Richard started developing a variety of physical problems that kept him out of work more and more. Finally, he was hospitalized for observation and tests at the local satellite health center. Surgery was recommended, and the operation took place at a centralized facility some 200 miles from the Harrisons' home.

Richard's postoperative convalescence had been lengthy, but eventually he was able to enroll in a vocational rehabilitation program sponsored by a nearby satellite hospital. Here, under the supervision of vocational therapists,

503

Richard learned how to repair and work with electronic calculators. With the help of a counselor, Richard was able to find a part-time job that allowed him to use his new skills.

During his hospitalization and convalescence, Richard noticed that more and more of his care was being planned as well as administered by nurses. He and Anita were also involved and consulted to a far greater extent than they had been during past contacts with the health care system. The team approach now characterized all aspects of Richard's care.

With Richard now able to resume most aspects of his own care, Anita has been able to find a job of her own. She works part-time as a teacher's assistant in the school attended by 10-year-old Kathy, their youngest. The job is satisfying to her, and the salary and employee benefits help supplement Richard's reduced income. Medicare and Medicaid have also helped to meet the expenses of Richard's lengthy recovery.

Both Richard and Anita now visit their local health maintenance organization for regular checkups. The examinations and interviews are carried on by nurse-practitioners. They also see a physician at the HMO for help with special problems. In addition, Richard is involved in a group counseling program sponsored by the vocational rehabilitation staff at the local hospital. The group meets twice a month to discuss and explore physical, social, and emotional problems its members may have encountered.

How has the family unit changed for the Harrisons?

How have these changes affected each member of the family?

How will nurses be involved in the ongoing health care of this family?

29 A look to the future in nursing

There is no question that the nurse of the next few decades will play a role considerably different from that of her forbears. First, rapid advances in biomedical knowledge have created much wider vistas for everyone involved in health care. Nurses will take on increasing responsibility and consequently will have access to greater professional opportunities.

Changes in nursing roles

Response to health needs

Major changes in nursing practice will result from changes in the types of illnesses being treated. In the last quarter century, for example, the incidence of acute febrile disease has dropped dramatically. Thanks to improved sanitation, the introduction of antibiotics, and new immunization procedures, former terrors such as scarlet fever, pneumonia, and typhoid fever are almost reduced to memories. As the incidence of communicable disease has diminished, chronic illness has assumed an ever-growing place in health care. Today, cardiovascular diseases are the greatest killers in the United States. Patients often suffer for years, requiring long-term nursing care, not just episodic treatment. People are living longer, and diseases such as arthritis and diabetes assume greater importance.

Thanks to prepaid hospital insurance, many people are seeking medical treatment who in the past might have stayed home to save money. As a result, demands on hospitals have swelled tremendously, and the types of care demanded have also grown in number.

The type of care expected of nurses has also changed as a result of the increasing mobility of the American people. In the past, a person who became ill often had the support of aunts, uncles, and grandparents in addition to the immediate family. Today, many people are isolated, especially older people. They may not be able to share their feelings of helplessness and inadequacy with the family as they can with the nurse.

Consumerism also has had an effect on nursing. One nurse has stated it this way:

Upon completing this chapter, the reader should be able to:

1. Trace the development of the roles and responsibilities of the individual within the profession of nursing.

2. Identify and discuss the changes that have taken place within nursing in response to such factors as changing health needs, consumerism, and the knowledge explosion.

3. Give examples of the role and function of the primary nurse, clinical specialist, and community-based nurse.

4. Discuss the role of research in advancing the concept of nursing as a learned profession.

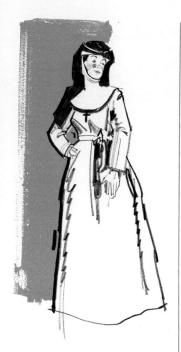

The nursing uniform worn in the year 1242.

We must, as a collective group, become social activists. By this, I mean the great need for nurses to become involved in all things going on in this society pertaining to the health, education and welfare of the people of this country, and in fact the world. I do not mean involvement only in things of a purely professional nature such as lobbying for a new nurse practice act. But I mean involvement, particularly political involvement, in all areas that concern life, liberty and the pursuit of happiness.[1]

Explosion of scientific and technical knowledge

The rapid strides in scientific knowledge and the proliferation of new diagnostic and treatment methods create a great challenge for the nurse of the future. Not only must the nurse know how to use special equipment but she must be able to recognize unfavorable responses, assess positive responses, and understand the appropriate nursing responsibilities related to each.

In what specific ways will the practice of nursing be affected by technology? In making hospital rounds, the nurse may be assisted by a computer programmed by health experts. While making a home visit to a convalescing cardiac patient, she might pick up the phone and describe distressing signs she has observed. The computer might tell her immediately what to do, or it might ask for more information.[2]

A nurse visiting a convalescent home might need the advice of a physician stationed at a nearby health center. He will be able to see the patient on the television telephone, and will also be able to ask the computer to display on the television screen the patient's family record and medical history. Once he has given the nurse a medical decision, she prepares the total care plan.

The nurse will still retain her traditional functions, but with a dramatic change in activities. "Computers, television, scanning, and other technological 'hardware' will extend her eyes, ears, and intellectual capacity," one author predicts.[3]

As the scientific basis for nursing continues to widen and deepen, so must the nurse be continually adding to her knowledge and skill. In order not to become obsolete, she must make a specific effort to keep informed of new developments in her areas of interest as well as in health-related fields in general.

Many nurses graduate from an educational program with relief; finally, their studying days are over. For the conscientious nurse, those days never end. Many agencies offer continuing education courses that nurses are

---

[1] Teresa E. Christy. 1973. New privileges . . . new challenges . . . new responsibilities. *Nursing '73* 3:11.

[2] Helen K. Mussalem. 1969. The changing role of the nurse. *American Journal of Nursing* 69. Reprinted in Joan P. Riehl and Joan W. McVay, eds., *The clinical nurse specialist: Interpretations*, pp. 495-96. New York: Appleton-Century Crofts, 1973.

[3] Ibid., p. 496.

encouraged to attend. Opportunities for continuing education are also available through community groups and national health organizations.

The learning process depends not on exposure but on motivation. Many nurses will find they can keep themselves abreast of new developments simply by spending time in the library on their own. In some institutions, self-instructional programs are available that the nurse can work into her own time schedule.

Clinical specialization

The concept of the clinical specialist originated some years ago, but only now is it being recognized as a major trend in nursing. The clinical specialist has been defined as a nurse who

provides a model of nursing activity appropriate to all nursing practitioners and works with the other nurses in a particular specialty area to achieve a high level of quality care for patients and a higher level of competence by all the nurses participating in their care. The clinical specialist is particularly prepared to assess the patient's responses to illness, to select the appropriate nursing intervention, and to assess the patient's response to that intervention.[4]

The term was coined in 1943 by Frances Reiter, chairman of the Committee on Education of the American Nurses' Association.[5] She felt that direct nursing care was the one area over which the nurse should have complete control. Clinical competence, she maintained, involves "range of function, depth of understanding, and breadth of services."

Under range of function she classified care, cure, and counseling. Personal care lies at the heart of nursing practice, whether it be palliative, protective, or rehabilitative.

By curative nursing, Reiter meant not just technical expertise but also a sound knowledge of the principles of rehabilitation. Curative nursing calls for an understanding of medical and therapeutic goals and for close cooperation with physicians.

Counseling, too, must be based on a deep level of understanding, not of physiology but of the dynamics of human behavior. "By counseling I refer to the kind of emotional, intellectual, and psychological support that sometimes borders on the realm of social work but is still a part of professional nursing practice," she commented. "Within this range, too, I see such nursing responsibilities as health promotion, preventive teaching, working with families, and the full therapeutic use of one's self in relationships with patients."[6]

Reiter found another set of "Cs" to define her concept of breadth of service: coordination, continuity, and collaboration. The nurse should be

[4]Dagmar E. Brodt. 1970. Excellence or obsolescence: The choice for nursing. *Nursing Forum* 9:24.
[5]Frances Reiter. 1966. The nurse-clinician. *American Journal of Nursing* 66:274.
[6]Ibid., p. 276.

> The concept of the clinical specialist originated some years ago, but only now is it being recognized as a major trend in nursing.

The nursing uniform worn in 1880.

responsible for coordinating all patient care activities, for making sure that care between hospital and home or between hospital specialists is continuous, and for collaborating with physicians.

Reiter's concept of the clinical specialist has been translated into programs across the country. Although the nurse practitioner or clinical specialist is essentially a nurse, she is often more independent than her colleagues because of additional education or training. She is comfortable performing duties that many nurses would shy away from. Also, the nurse practitioner is often based in a clinic or private office rather than a hospital.

It was in 1965 that the first of the formalized nurse practitioner programs was established. This was a program for pediatric specialists at the University of Colorado School of Nursing. Many other programs have sprung up since that time.

What motivates this new type of nurse? "I was getting tired of a lack of real patient contact," notes Shirley Carlin, a nurse-practitioner trainee at the University of California, San Francisco.

I want to do something more exciting than hospital nursing, where most of the "nursing" is done by nurses' aides. In our program, we take histories; do physical exams, including pelvics; take pap smears; GC (gonococcal) cultures, and hematology. We follow up on return appointments to determine the well being of patients and fetal development. If they want it, we teach breast feeding and do sexual counseling.[7]

[7] Alice M. Robinson. 1973. The nurse-practitioner: Expanding your limits. *RN* 36:29–30.

Primary care

The concept of primary care nursing originated at the University of Minnesota Hospital in 1958.[8] Today, several institutions are developing similar programs, which they call either primary care or total patient care. Essentially, these programs aim to return the nurse to the one-to-one patient relationship that was once her hallmark. Impetus for the Minnesota program came from the desire of staff nurses to get closer to the patient, to make decisions about his care, and to eliminate centralized nursing-service control.

Primary nurses are given complete responsibility for four or five patients round the clock, from admission to discharge. Other RNs, called associate nurses, provide care when the primary nurse is off duty, but they follow the primary nurse's treatment plan.

When the patient is admitted, the primary nurse talks with him and his family. She writes instructions for nursing care either on the interview sheet or on the Kardex. The primary nurse takes charge of physical care of the patient, although she may delegate duties such as bathing the patient or making his bed. She communicates daily with other health personnel and keeps the nursing care plan up to date. She initiates referrals when necessary, plans for the patient's discharge or transfer, and writes the summary.

The primary nurse's role is based not on additional training but on reorganization of duties. Assignments are patient-centered rather than task-oriented. Rather than perform an isolated technical procedure for a number of patients, such as taking temperature readings, the nurse carries out several care activities during one patient visit. She thus has time to talk to the patient and find out how he feels and what he needs.

And, as so often happens, the patient may have difficulty comprehending some medical language and terminology used by the physician. The nurse can help clarify a problem and thereby foster better understanding.[9]

Community-based nursing

As the delivery of medical care continues to expand beyond the hospital, the community nurse will play an increasingly crucial and varied role. A number of experts have called for a change in the health care delivery system that would take ambulatory care out of the hospitals.

A well-staffed ambulatory care center, located in areas of need, could provide preventive, diagnostic, and education and treatment services for an entire community, they point out. Some communities would be well

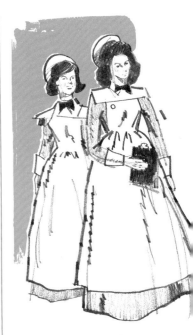

The uniform worn in the year 1900.

[8] Alice M. Robinson. 1974. Primary nurse: Specialist in total care. *RN* 37:31.

[9] Kathy Bakke. 1974. Primary nursing: Perceptions of a staff nurse. *American Journal of Nursing* 74:1434.

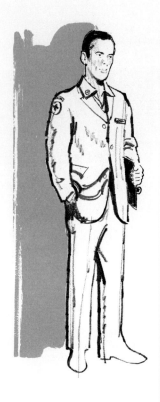

served with subcenters, with major centers being the focal point for community health manpower, including private physicians and group practitioners.

For the community nurse, such ambulatory care centers would become the base of operation. She could then communicate and plan more easily, and could work flexibly in a variety of community programs. These programs include drug addiction services, maternity training, abortion counseling, preschool care, and nutrition instruction.

"It is obvious that nurses must build into their present functioning maximum use of their present skills, and add some," a well-known public health nurse contends.

Public health nurses in many places have long assumed a wide range of responsibilities for patient care that generally are not formalized. Community nursing agencies must become more direct in defining an expanded role for nurses and provide the preparation and the policies to see it through.[10]

Research

What is involved in nursing research? One author says that research means to:

R   *eview the literature*
E   *volve a theoretical framework*
S   *tate the problem, purpose, and hypothesis*
E   *volve a methodology for data gathering*
A   *nalyze and interpret the data gathered*
R   *eport conclusions and recommendations*
C   *ommunicate results*
H   *elp to implement findings*[11]

Educators are in agreement on the importance of increasing research in both nursing practice and education. Twenty years ago nursing research centered on the questions of education and who was qualified to practice. Also of importance in research at that time were questions of how many people, and of what type were needed to organize and deliver nursing care. The attitude was that if there were enough professionals treating the patient, he would receive high-quality care.[12]

Today the shortage of trained personnel continues to perplex organizers of nursing care. However, manpower is not considered the only important factor in quality care. Cost and accessibility of service are also taken into consideration. Moreover, nursing researchers are now looking at how

[10]Eva M. Reese. 1970. To perpetuate the hospital-focused system seems illogical . . . . *American Journal of Nursing* 70:2125.
[11]Alberta R. Kovacs. 1972. What does it mean "to research"? *Nursing Forum* 11:395.
[12]Susan R. Gortner. 1973. Research in nursing: The federal interest and grant program. *American Journal of Nursing* 73:1052–53.

nursing education and practice affect the patient. They are trying to find ways to help the patient leave the hospital early and return to work, as well as ways to prevent complications, maintain health, and prevent future illness.

The government's interest in nursing research is channeled through the Division of Nursing, Bureau of Health Manpower Education, National Institutes of Health. The division provides financial aid for conferences on research in nursing, including such subjects as doctoral education, nursing theory, and quality of nursing care. The division also supports nursing research in academic settings and awards grants for improving nursing school curriculums, continuing education, and expanding existing clinical programs.

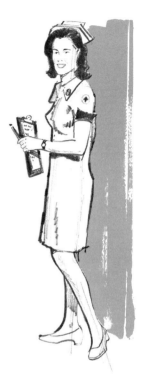

Educational nursing research includes studies of the characteristics and achievements of nursing students, as well as of effective means of teaching. Practice research focuses more directly on improved methods of delivering nursing care. More and more research projects are exploratory rather than descriptive in nature. An increasing number of studies are being conducted in the laboratory before being moved into a clinical setting. Recently, researchers examined the nature of explanations that can be given to patients who are about to undergo unpleasant procedures. Descriptive and exploratory work preceded actual clinical testing.

The purpose of nursing research, one author maintains, is not only to improve the status of the nurse or to develop nursing theory but also to improve service to patients.

Nursing, like other professions, exists only on the mandate of society. To fulfill that mandate, it must meet the societal needs that provide the reason for its existence. Chronic failures to meet these needs will inexorably lead to decline and loss of professional status and to the mushrooming of other groups to fill the void in service.[13]

SUMMARY

Where is nursing headed? Although analysts of this question differ in specifics, they agree on the fact that the nurse of the future will be answering to challenges far greater than those faced by nurses of the past.

One reason the role of the nurse must change is that health care itself is in the process of constant change. Diseases which in the past claimed many lives, such as tuberculosis and cholera, no longer pose a major threat to health. In their place, the chronic diseases have risen to a new magnitude. People are living longer, and the ailments that beset them, such as heart disease, hypertension, and diabetes, are matters for long-term care.

The public, with the help of insurance, is demanding more care and more value for its dollar. People are also demanding a voice in the planning and delivery of medical care.

[13]Katherine B. Nuckolls. 1972. Nursing research—good for what? *Nursing Forum* 11:376.

Technical advances will also change the practice of nursing. As a citizen of the electronic age, the nurse will adjust to the many ways in which computers are being utilized. The explosion of knowledge also means that she must constantly be learning new techniques and informing herself of new developments in health care.

One way that nurses have reacted to the increasingly heavy load of knowledge in each specialty is to become more specialized themselves. The clinical specialist is a nurse who focuses on a particular area of care, such as pediatrics. She undergoes special education, and often she offers her services from a clinic or private office base rather than a hospital. Many nurses have found that clinical specialization brings them closer to direct patient care.

The primary nurse is a relatively new phenomenon. In current programs, the primary nurse takes complete charge of four or five patients. She is able to develop a close relationship with each one and to communicate his needs to other staff members.

Thanks to the proliferation of health care in a nonhospital setting, the community nurse will also find increased opportunity for challenge and for varied responsibility. And all nurses will find that research becomes a more important part of their professional development. Funds for nursing research are available from several sources, offering the possibility for in-depth study of special areas of interest.

STUDY QUESTIONS

1. What effect has the increase in the average life span had on the health care field?
2. What factors have influenced the development of clinical specialties in nursing? How is this development related to the growth of community-based nursing?
3. What are some of the areas in which nursing research is being conducted? In what additional areas do you think research is needed?
4. How has modern technology influenced nursing as a profession?
5. In what ways do you think nursing will change in the next 10 years?

SELECTED BIBLIOGRAPHY

Alfano, Genrose, et al. 1970. Nursing in the decade ahead. *American Journal of Nursing* 70:2116–25.

Brodt, Dagmar E. 1970. Excellence or obsolescence: The choice for nursing. *Nursing Forum* 9:19–31.

Christy, Teresa E. 1973. New privileges . . . new challenges . . . new responsibilities. *Nursing '73* 3:8, 11.

National Commission for the Study of Nursing and Nursing Education. 1973. *From abstract to action*, pp. 187–222. New York: McGraw-Hill.

Secretary's Committee to Study Extended Roles for Nurses, U.S. Department of Health, Education and Welfare. 1972. Extending the scope of nursing practice. *Nursing Outlook* 20:46–52.

Glossary

Abscess A collection of pus formed in solid tissue.

Acceptance The second psychological stage of illness, characterized by adoption of the sick role and withdrawal from the normal world. Also, the fifth of Kübler-Ross's five stages of dying.

Acetone A colorless liquid found in urine which sometimes gives an ethereal odor to urine and breath.

Acid-citrate-dextrose (ACD) solution A solution used to preserve blood.

Acidity The amount of the chemical compound acid in a fluid.

Acting-out In the context of loss, the compulsive seeking out of new relationships or other activities which represent an attempt to deny feelings.

Active immunity Resistance to infection acquired naturally, through recovery from a communicable disease, or artificially, through immunization.

Active transport A mechanism whereby ions move from areas of lesser to areas of greater concentration.

Acute Sharp, active; the second phase of illness.

Adaptation The process by which an organism responds to its environment, both consciously and unconsciously.

Adenosine triphosphate (ATP) A nucleoside involved in the active transport process.

Adequately nourished Eating and digesting an appropriate amount and mixture of the vital nutrients.

Adipose tissue Fatty tissue.

Adolescence The time of life between puberty and adulthood, approximately 9 to 18 years of age.

Adrenal cortex Outer portion of the paired endocrine glands of the abdominal cavity.

Adrenal medulla Inner portion of the endocrine glands of the abdominal cavity.

Affective Emotional.

Agent In the infection process, the disease-producing organism.

Air bed A bed with an air-filled mattress which provides uniform support for the body and minimal pressure on the skin.

Alcoholism A disease condition characterized by addiction to alcoholic beverages.

Alert In full possession of one's senses; watchful.

Alkalinity The amount of a basic substance called alkali in a fluid.

Alpha rhythm A recurring, regular wave pattern characteristic of the first phase of sleep.

Alveolar Pertaining to the lungs.

Ambient Atmospheric.

Amino acids Organic compounds which form the structure of proteins.

Anabolism Assimilation of body matter.

Anal Pertaining to the anus; one of Freud's stages of psychosexual development.

Anaphylactic Showing great sensitivity to foreign material.

Anions Electrolytes which develop negative charges.

Anorexia The lack or loss of an appetite for food.

Anorexia nervosa A personality disorder characterized by a complete lack of interest in food.

Anoxia A total lack of oxygen.

Antibiotic A substance taken from a mold or bacteria which prevents the growth of other microorganisms.

Antidiuretic hormone (ADH) A hormone used to treat diabetes insipidus and to stimulate intestinal motility. Also called vasopressin.

Antihistamines Drugs used in treating allergy which are antagonistic to histamine, a depressor amine.

Antimicrobial Tending to prevent the growth of pathogens.

Antipyretic Fever-reducing.

Antisepsis The destruction of germs to prevent infection.

Anxiety Uneasiness, apprehension, nervousness.

Apical beat Measurement of rhythm, rate, and quality of the heartbeat.

Apnea Complete cessation of breathing.

Apothecary system A system of weights and measures used in pharmacy. The basic unit is the grain.

Appetite The desire for and anticipation of eating food.

Arrangement Modification of a message by choice of words.

Arterial pressure The tension within the arteries, usually 200 mm Hg.

Artificial circulation The use of external cardiac compression to get the blood moving.

513

Asepsis Freedom from pathogenic organisms.

Assessment The act of reviewing a situation in order to identify a problem and then communicate it to others.

Assisted ventilation The process of applying intermittent positive-pressure breathing.

Atrophy Wasting of part of the body.

Audit committees Groups of professionals who evaluate the performance of hospital staff members, using patient records.

Auditory system The sensory system which specifies the nature of vibratory occurrences.

Auscultation Listening to chest sounds by means of a stethoscope.

Autistic thinking The tendency to hear, see, and understand exclusively according to one's own desires.

Autonomic Involuntary.

Bacteria Microorganisms, some disease-producing.

Basal metabolic rate (BMR) The rate at which an awake individual produces body heat.

Base-line patient data Information about the patient gathered at the time of admission, including historical, physiological, and laboratory facts. Base-line patient data make up the first component of the problem-oriented record.

Basic orienting system The sensory system which specifies the direction of gravity and the movements of the body.

Bed cradle A device used to keep the weight of the bedclothes off the patient.

Bed rest Confinement to bed prescribed as part of therapy.

Biped A two-footed animal.

Blood pressure The tension of the blood within the arteries. There are two types: systolic and diastolic.

Body language Communication through movement and manner.

Bone matrix The formative portion of bone tissue, including inorganic bone salts, collagen, and ground substances.

Body mechanics The physical correlation of the various systems of the body.

Bradypnea Excessively slow breathing.

Brain waves Alternations in electrical charge in the brain.

Bronchogram The radiogram obtained after injection of radiopaque material into the tracheobronchial tree.

Bronchoscopy Examination of the inside of the tracheobronchial tree using an endoscope.

Buccal administration The giving of medication between tongue and teeth.

Bulk-former A class of laxative containing substances that actively increase the bulk in the stool.

Calcium deficiency A form of malnutrition resulting from a lack of calcium foods.

Calculi Stones.

Calisthenics Gymnastic exercises.

Carbohydrates Organic compounds composed of carbon, hydrogen, and oxygen. Carbohydrate foods include starches and sugars.

Carbonic acid A major component of the hydrogen ion concentration.

Cardiac apex The extremity of the heart; the point at which the apical beat is measured.

Cardiac arrest A cessation of cardiac function.

Cardiac output The quantity of blood circulated by the heart.

Carrier A person who provides a source of disease because of the pathogens he carries.

Catabolism Breakdown of body matter.

Cathartic Medication taken to stimulate the movement of fecal matter.

Cations Electrolytes which develop positive charges.

Center of gravity The point in any object or individual at which all mass is centered.

Chart A sheet of paper for the recording of data related to the patient's condition.

Cheyne-Stokes breathing A form of arrhythmic breathing caused by cardiac failure.

Cilia Short, hairlike growth found on many cells.

Circadian rhythm A 24-hour biological cycle.

Circuit A pathway in the homeostatic process for communicating responses to an effector mechanism.

Clinical nurse specialist A nurse who has undergone clinical training for a particular specialty, such as pediatrics. Also called a nurse practitioner.

Cognition The process of perceiving or obtaining knowledge.

Cold sore An eruption around the mouth. Also called fever blister (herpes simplex).

Colonic irrigation (Harris flush) A process in which the colon is alternately filled with and drained of fluid until there is no further release of gas.

Comatose In a state of profound unconsciousness.

Commensal An agent-host relationship where the microorganism is dependent on the host's body but neither harms nor helps it.

Communication Interchange of thoughts and feelings through words, actions, and gestures. Through communication, the nurse establishes rapport with her patients.

Compensation A conscious or unconscious attempt to make up for real or imagined handicaps by becoming successful in other areas.

Conduction The transmission of heat through direct contact between objects.

Conjunctiva The mucous membranes which cover the front of the eyeball and line the eyelid.

Conscious motivation A recognized rationale for behavior.

Constant Unchanging.

Constipation Infrequent or incomplete bowel movements.

Contracture Permanent muscle contractions resulting from prolonged immobilization of a joint.

Convalescence The third psychological stage of illness, characterized by a return of physical strength and reintegration of a healthy personality.

Convection The transmission of heat by the mass movement of heated particles, as in air, gas, or liquid currents.

Conversion The attempt to resolve conflicts and prevent anxiety by the development of physical symptoms in areas of the body controlled by the sensory-motor system.

Corticoid Hormone secreted by the adrenal cortex.

Cortisone A steroid isolated from the adrenal cortex used in treating rheumatoid arthritis, adrenal insufficiency, and other conditions.

Credé maneuver Exertion of manual pressure over the bladder to induce emptying of the bladder.

Crisis intervention Application of the problem-solving process to a traumatic event.

Critical thinking One of the intellectual components of the nursing process, involving the ability to extract meaning from an assemblage of facts.

Decision making One of the intellectual components of the nursing process, involving the ability to decide on a coures of action.

Decoding A step in the communication process in which the receiver relates a message to the picture in his mind.

Decubitus ulcer Pressure sore resulting from prolonged confinement to bed.

Deductive From the general to the particular. Deductive reasoning means drawing inferences from general conclusions.

Defense mechanisms Unconscious processes in which anxieties that result from inner conflicts are prevented from reaching consciousness or are relieved.

Delta waves Large, slow waves that appear on the encephalogram in the third stage of sleep.

Denial Complete disregard of a disturbing situation.

Dependence A need to rely on someone else.

Depressants Drugs which have a sedative effect by lowering nervous or functional activity.

Development The growth of personality functions.

Developmental tasks Points of accomplishment which accompany each phase of growth. Part of Erik Erikson's system of psychosocial development.

Diabetes mellitus A derangement of carbohydrate metabolism caused by a deficiency of insulin. The illness has many complications, often sustained for a lifetime.

Diagnosis The act of determining the nature of a disease or problem through examination and observation.

Diarrhea The passage of loose, watery stool and an increase in the frequency of bowel movements.

Diastolic pressure The minimum blood pressure, occurring at the end of flow after pressure has been applied.

Diffusion A process whereby molecules move from higher concentrations of solution to lower concentrations.

Digestion The conversion of ingested food into forms usable by the body.

Discharge notes The final phase of progress notes, focusing on plans for management and providing information for future analysis of the problem.

Displacement The transference of feelings from one idea, object, or situation to another, more acceptable one.

Dissociation The splitting off of one portion of consciousness from the rest; for example, the separation of feeling from memories.

Distension Enlargement of segments of the intestine and spasms in the muscle layers.

Diurnal variation Fluctuation according to the time of day.

Drop factor The number of drops in one ml of liquid in a needle.

Drowsiness Sleepiness.

Dyspnea Difficult breathing.

Effector mechanism The element which corrects disturbances in the homeostatic process through the process of output.

Effleurage A long, smooth stroke used in giving a massage. The hands move up the spine, then lightly down the sides.

Ego identity Recognition of the unconscious self.

Egocentric Self-centered.

Elderly Advanced beyond middle age. In Theodore Lidz's division of old age, the elderly period is first, corresponding with independence.

Electroencephalograph (EEG) An apparatus for recording the electric potentials of the brain using scalp leads.

Electrolytes Chemical substances which develop electrical charges when placed in water.

Emaciation Extreme thinness.

Emerging identities The second phase in the nurse-patient relationship, when the two begin to establish a bond.

Emotional immobilization Psychological block that results from excess stress.

Empathy The fourth phase in the nurse-patient relationship, when the nurse gains the ability to enter into the patient's psychological state and thus to understand him.

Employeeism The belief, held by employees, that the employer has the employees' best interests at heart and will therefore be just and fair in bestowing benefits.

Encoding Setting information or feeling into a form that can be transmitted. A step in the communication process.

Endotracheal intubation Insertion of a tube into the trachea.

Enema Fluid solution introduced via the anus into the rectum and colon.

Epigenetic principle The theory that humans develop through phases as a result of five primary circumstances.

Erythema Skin inflammation.

Etiologic agent The pathogen which produces infection.

Evaluation The act of appraising the effectiveness of a plan.

Excursion Movement from one point to another and back, as in the expansion and return to normal of the chest.

Expiration The act of exhaling.

Extracellular Outside the body cells.

Face tent A device applied to the face to increase oxygen concentration or to supply mist.

Facultative parasite A parasite which is able to live independently of the host as well as with it.

Fat An oily substance found in the bodies of animals. Fatty foods include butter and gristle.

Fear The emotion which arises in response to an observable external danger; a painful sense of dread.

Feedback A process which allows us to control our communication signals by incorporating information about their effects.

Fever A body temperature above 98.6° F (37° C).

Fever blister An eruption around the mouth. Also called cold sore or herpes simplex.

Fibrin A protein formed by blood coagulation.

Fight or flight Confrontation or avoidance of a threat, representing the body's reaction to stressful situations.

Filtration The process in which liquid is passed through a filter.

Fistula A hollow passage from one cavity or abscess to another.

Fixation Arrest at a point of development.

Flatus bag A bag attached to a rectal tube for the collection of any expulsion through the tube.

Flora Harmless microorganisms found in various parts of the body.

Flow chart Chronological listing of observations about the patient's progress, most often used in rapidly changing situations. Also called a flow sheet.

Flow sheet Chronological listing of observations about the patient's progress, most often used in rapidly changing situations. Also called a flow chart.

Fluoroscopy Examination of the internal organs using an apparatus which makes visible the shadows of X-rays.

Foley catheter A triple-lumen type of indwelling catheter which allows urinary drainage through one channel, inflation of the bag with water or air through a second channel, and a continuous irrigation of the bladder through the third channel.

Four-point gait A crutch-walking technique where the right crutch is advanced, then the left foot, then left crutch, then right foot.

Frontal Relating to the anterior.

Frostbite Destruction of tissue as a result of freezing.

Fulminating Characterized by unusually severe symptoms and the rapid approach of death.

Gait Pattern of walking.

Gastric suction Removal of fluids through the stomach.

Gastric tube A tube inserted into the stomach.

Gastrointestinal motility Movement within the stomach and intestines.

Gatch bed A bed with cranks and screws which allows for elevation of the patient's head and knees.

General adaptation syndrome Selye's theory of the entire process of stress and the body's reaction to it.

General malaise A feeling of being out of sorts, uncomfortable.

Generativity The desire to establish and guide a new generation. The seventh stage of Erik Erikson's system of psychosocial development.

Genital Pertaining to the sexual organs.

Gluconeogenesis The deposition of glycogen.

Glucose Blood sugar.

Gravity The mutual attraction between the earth and another object.

Gravity line An imaginary line which passes through the center of gravity downward to the base of support of the object or individual.

Haptic system The sensory system responsible for touch, with receptors located throughout the body.

Health maintenance organization A private, comprehensive, prepaid medical care program.

Heat stroke A severe illness resulting from exposure to extremely high temperatures and characterized by headache and temperature rise.

Hemoglobin A protein compound in the blood.

Herpes simplex A viral infection characterized by the eruption of vesicles at various sites.

Homeostasis A state of equilibrium or balance in physiological and psychological areas of functioning. The drive for homeostasis is both conscious and unconscious.

Hormones Chemical substances that are formed in a part of the body and can alter structural activity.

Host The organism which provides nourishment for a parasite.

Humidifier A device used to provide moisture when a patient is receiving high concentrations of oxygen.

Hunger A strong desire to eat after prolonged food deprivation.

Hydraulic lift A device used to transfer a totally dependent patient to and fro. Also called a patient lifter.

Hydrostatic pressure The pressure of water or other liquids produced by the pumping action of the heart.

Hyperalimentation Administration of essential nutrients through a venous catheter.

Hyperbaric oxygen treatment The administration of oxygen in a compression chamber.

Hyperthermia A condition in which body temperature is abnormally high as a result of disturbance of the heat-regulatory mechanism.

Hypertonic solution A solution that has a higher osmotic pressure than another.

Hyperventilation Excessive elimination of carbon dioxide leading to respiratory alkalosis.

Hypodermic Beneath the skin.

Hypodermoclysis The injection of fluids into the subcutaneous tissues.

Hypothalamus A group of nuclei at the base of the brain which send out signals in alarm reaction.

Hypotonic solution A solution that has a lower osmotic pressure than another.

Hypoventilation Reduced exchange of air in the lungs which causes short, shallow breathing.

Hypoxia A condition resulting from inadequate oxygen supply.

ICU-itis A state of disorientation which often affects patients in an intensive care unit.

Idealization The overestimation and exaggeration of valuable attributes or qualities.

Identification The unconscious modeling or patterning of the self after another person.

Idiopathic insomnia Sleeplessness without apparent cause.

Ileostomy The creation of a fistula into the ileum.

Immobilization Prescribed or unavoidable restriction of movement in any area of a person's life.

Impaction Situation which occurs when the rectum and the sigmoid colon become filled with feces material.

Implementation The translation of a plan into action; also, the third phase of the nursing process.

Incontinence A condition in which the bladder is unable to retain urine.

Independence Ability to govern oneself.

Inductive From the particular to the general. Inductive reasoning means drawing general conclusions from specific instances.

Infancy The earliest stage of life.

Infectious diseases Illnesses resulting from the action of a microorganism, capable of being transmitted.

Ingestion Eating and drinking.

Inhalation therapist A specialist in the administration of oxygen.

Initial encounter The first phase in the nurse-patient relationship, when both nurse and patient form ideas about each other.

Input The stimulus that affects the receptor in a homeostatic mechanism.

Insomnia Inability to sleep at normal sleeping times.

Inspiration The act of inhaling.

Instinct An aptitude or action that comes naturally, without reflecting.

Intellectual immobilization Inability to acquire knowledge, such as occurs in mental retardation.

Interferon A virus-killing protein produced in cell cultures or host tissues.

Intermittent Alternating between periods of quiet and periods of activity.

Intermittent positive pressure-breathing apparatus (IPPB) An airway-applied respirator.

Interpretation The part of the perception process in which the receiver decodes the message being sent him.

Interstitial fluid The liquid outside the blood vessels and between the body cells.

Interviewing A goal-directed method of questioning which involves effective interaction between two people.

Intestinal suction The aspiration of fluids from the intestines.

Intracatheter A long, plastic tube inserted through a metal needle.

Intracellular Within the body cells.

Intradermal Into the skin.

Intramuscular Into the muscle.

Intravenous Into the vein.

Intubation The insertion of a tube into part of the body, for example, the stomach.

Invert sugar A mixture of levulose and dextrose sugar.

Ionize To develop an electrical charge.

Ischemia Local anemia caused by obstruction.

Isometric Involving a muscular contraction occurring when the ends of muscles are fixed so that tension increases without change in muscle length.

Isotonic Involving a muscle contraction accompanied by a change in muscle length.

Kardex A system for recording patient data, used for quick reference. Individual cards are stored in a portable index file.

Ketones Chemical substances, one of which is acetone, found in the blood.

Kinestheses Receptors for the sense of movement, located in the muscles, the joints, and the inner ear.

Korotkoff's sounds Noise of the blood flow heard over the artery when pressure changes.

Latency Arrested development.

Laxative Medication taken to stimulate bowel activity.

Learning The discovery of meaning by acquiring and interpreting new information or experience.

Lesion An injury, wound, or individual point in a multifocal disease.

Litmus paper Paper which, when dipped into urine, indicates pH through color change.

Macrominerals Those minerals of which the body needs more than 100 mg per day, including calcium and potassium.

Malabsorption Gastric imbalance in the digestive tract.

Malpractice Misconduct or unreasonable lack of skill in treating a disease or injury.

Maturation The growth of bodily functions.

Maturity The stage of life where a person is fully developed.

Medicaid An amendment to the Social Security Act, passed in 1965, which provides a program of grants to states for medical assistance. Also called Title XIX.

Medical diagnosis The physician's evaluation of a patient's problem based on assessment of data about his condition.

Medicare An amendment to the Social Security Act, passed in 1965, which provides for a federally administered program of health insurance for the aged. Also called Title XVIII.

Menarche The first menstruation.

Metabolic alkalosis A fluid imbalance characterized by shallow respiration, muscle hypertonicity, and personality changes.

Metabolism The chemical changes taking place in the cells of the body.

Metric system A system of weights and measures used in pharmacy. The basic unit is the gram.

Microbiology The study of microorganisms.

Microminerals Those minerals of which the body needs only small amounts, such as cobalt and copper. Also called trace minerals.

Microorganism A plant or animal of microscopic size, such as a bacterium.

Micturition The process by which the body rids itself of urine in the bladder; voiding.

Minerals Inorganic substances occurring in the earth and in certain foods. Iron is a mineral vital to health.

Minimal daily allowances (MDA) Amounts of various nutrients that have been determined as minimal for adequate nutrition.

Modification The act of redesigning a plan based on an evaluation of its effectiveness.

Morphology Form and structure.

Motor activity Use of the nerve capabilities; part of physical development.

Muscle strength The maximal tension which muscles can exert.

Narcolepsy The tendency to fall asleep quickly and at inappropriate times.

Narcotics Drugs which induce sleep or lethargy.

Narrative notes Records of the patient's progress, containing entires by all members of the health care team.

Nasal cannula A tube connected to an oxygen source and inserted into the nostrils. Also called a nasoinhaler.

Nasal catheter A hollow tube passed through the nostrils and used when high concentrations of oxygen are needed.

Nasoinhaler A tube connected to an oxygen source and inserted into the nostrils. Also called a nasal cannula.

Nausea The desire to vomit; stomach sickness.

Need What an individual must have in order to survive or function within the limits of what is considered normal.

Negative feedback Change in one direction which triggers change in the opposite direction. Most homeostatic mechanisms are regulated by negative feedback.

Neighborhood health centers Treatment facilities located in rural or inner-city areas short on traditional health manpower. These centers, authorized by Congress in 1966, provide a wide scope of services.

Neurotic anxiety A painful sense of uneasiness provoked by an unrealistic threat.

Nightingalism Selfless idealism that precludes concern with economic and job conditions.

Nocturia (bed wetting) An inability to control the release of urine when asleep.

Nocturnal myoclonus Jerking of the leg muscles at night.

Nosocomial Hospital-related.

Nurse practice acts State laws regulating the functions and responsibilities of the nurse.

Nurse practitioner A nurse who has undergone clinical training for a particular specialty, such as pediatrics. Also called a clinical nurse specialist.

Nursing care plan An outline of nursing actions based on assessment of the patient's problems.

Nursing diagnosis The process of evaluating observable data about a patient and finding a pattern in those data that will determine the nursing care plan.

Nursing history Data which the nurse collects about the patient from him and others.

Nursing order A direction based on both medical and nursing diagnoses and communicated to the staff.

Nursing process A system, derived from the scientific method, of organizing the delivery of nursing care. It provides guidelines for the intellectual and physical activities needed to analyze the patient's problems, determine their solution, carry out a plan of action, and assess the plan's effectiveness.

Obligatory A relationship in which a microorganism depends completely on the host for survival and propagation.

Oedipal Characterized by erotic attachment to the parent of the opposite sex.

Oncotic pressure The pressure exerted by substances with high molecular weights, such as protein. Also called colloid osmotic pressure.

Oral Pertaining to the mouth.

Orientation The first phase of the nurse-patient relationship, during which the patient reveals—directly or indirectly—where he needs help.

Orthostatic hypotension A sudden drop in blood pressure that occurs when a person stands up.

Osmosis A process by which water passes through a semipermeable membrane from a high concentration of water to a lower concentration.

Osmotic diuresis Excessive excretion of urine due to a high concentration of osmotically active substances.

Osmotic pressure The pressure necessary to prevent the passage of solvent into a solution.

Osteoporosis Bone shrinkage.

Output The action taken by the effector mechanism in the homeostatic process.

Overweight Weighing more than what is considered the acceptable range for height, age, and sex.

Oxidation Conversion of oxygen into energy and other elements.

Oxygen poisoning Physical disturbances caused by breathing high partial pressures of oxygen.

Oxygen tension The relationship between the amount of oxygen and the pressure under which it is contained.

Oxygen tent A device used to provide oxygen for patients too disoriented or uncooperative for other methods.

Panic Complete preoccupation with a state of anxious distress, usually accompanied by physical symptoms such as shaking or sweating.

Paranoid schizophrenia A psychosis in which the victim thinks he is being persecuted and has delusions of grandeur.

Parasite An animal or plant which lives on or in another and draws its nourishment from the other.

Parasitic An agent-host relationship where the agent feeds off the host, but the host derives no benefit from the agent.

Parenteral By means other than through the intestinal canal.

Passive immunity Resistance to infection acquired through transfer of protective substances, either from mother to fetus or from serum taken from a person who has recovered from the disease to another person.

Pasteurization Destruction of bacteria through heating of milk, wine, and other liquids.

Patency Freedom from obstruction.

Pathogen Disease-causing microorganism.

Patients' rights What is owed to the patient ethically, legally, morally, and medically.

Pearls Single, fragile containers used for inhaled drugs such as amyl nitrite.

Pediculosis capitis Head lice or scabies.

Perception The process by which particular signals, verbal or nonverbal, strike the receiver's sensory end organs.

Percussion Tapping with the finger in order to determine the density of a part of the body; also, repeated blows or taps to remove secretions.

Pétrissage A stroke used in giving a massage. The masseur takes large pinches of skin between his fingers, moving up the sides of the vertebral column, then over the back.

pH level A urine measurement that indicates the balance between acidity and alkalinity.

518

Phagocytes Cells capable of ingesting bacteria, foreign particles, and other cells.

Phagocytosis The process by which foreign particles are engulfed or digested by specialized cells.

Phallic Pertaining to the penis.

Phenylketonuria A congenital deficiency of the enzyme phenylalanine hydroxylase which can lead to brain damage.

Piggyback Tubing and a needle attached to a medication bottle and inserted into a rubber stopper.

Pinocytosis The process by which cell membrane folds inward to incorporate substances of high molecular weight.

Pituitary gland A small organ attached to the floor of the brain which produces several hormones and is considered to be the "master" gland of the endocrine system.

Planning The weighing of priorities and design of methods for the resolution of problems.

Plantar flexion A downward turning of the foot or toes.

Plasma The liquid portion of the blood.

Plastic needle A small, plastic tube mounted on a metal needle.

Pledget A ball of lint, cotton, or wool.

Pleural friction rubs Loud, grating sounds heard upon ausculation of the chest.

Popliteal space The back surface of the knee.

Positive feedback A self-perpetuating system where one change causes more of the same.

Posture The alignment of the parts of the body with each other, and of the body as a whole.

Primary care The first contact which a patient has with the health system.

Problem A barrier to a goal; an obstruction of some kind that prevents a need from being met.

Problem list Itemization of areas requiring further observation, diagnosis, management, or education. The second component of the problem-oriented patient record.

Problem-oriented Organized according to a patient's needs. Problem-oriented hospital records emphasize not who gives the care, but the problem for which the care is given.

Problem solving A combination of inductive and deductive reasoning which provides the rationale for nursing action. One of the intellectual components of the nursing process.

Prodromal Initial, early. The first phase of illness.

Professional collectivism The feeling held by nurses that the profession's high standards of service are the individual responsibility of each practitioner.

Progress notes Data about the patient's response to treatment, contributed by everyone involved in his care. The fourth component of the problem-oriented record.

Projection The attribution of one's own ideas and impulses to another, freeing one from association with the action.

Properdin A chemical found in the blood which provides protection against bacteria.

Protein An amino acid substance found in all animal and vegetable matter. Meat and eggs are among protein foods.

Protein deficiency A form of malnutrition resulting from a lack of protein foods.

Psychological homeostasis State of emotional balance.

Psychosexual Including both psychological and sexual aspects.

Psychosocial Including both psychological and social dimensions.

Puberty The age of attainment of sexual maturity.

Pulmonary unit An area including the respiratory bronchiole, alveolar duct, atria, and alveolar sac.

Pulse rate Measurement of the rhythmical dilation of an artery.

Purification The freeing of a substance from impurities.

Pus A yellow-white, creamy substance produced by inflammation.

Radiation The process whereby heat is transferred from one object to another without direct contact.

Rales A fizzing sound heard on auscultation of the chest and caused by lung or bronchial disease.

Range of motion The maximum amount of movement possible at a joint in one direction.

Rapid eye movements (REM) A phenomenon noticeable in a person who is in the dreaming stage of sleep.

Rapport The final phase of the nurse-patient relationship, when the two share harmonious feelings.

Rationalization A way of justifying behavior by stating motives (usually with an element of truth) other than the genuine ones.

Reaction formation A denial of real feelings resulting in behavior as if the exact opposite were true.

Receptor A sensing device that detects disturbances in the internal and external environments.

Recommended daily allowances (RDA) Amounts of various nutrients that have been recommended for good nutrition.

Rectal suppositories Medicated pellets that melt on insertion in the rectum, to relieve pain or irritation.

Rectal tube Device inserted in the anus which allows gas to be expelled without the patient straining to open the anal sphincter.

Regression Reversion to earlier ways of behaving.

Rehabilitation Restoration of a sick or disabled person to as normal functioning as possible, using medical and vocational techniques.

Remittent Characterized by periods when symptoms diminish temporarily, although never disappear completely.

Repression The unconscious exclusion from awareness of unacceptable, inappropriate thoughts, memories, or impulses.

Reservoir The environment in which a pathogen lives and multiplies and which provides the source of infection.

Respiration Movement of air through the bronchi and lungs, heard on auscultation.

Respiratory arrest Cessation of breathing.

Rest A state of tranquility and freedom from anxiety; relaxation.

Restless leg syndrome Tingling and pain in the legs, causing restlessness at night.

Retention A condition in which the bladder is unable to empty itself of urine.

Rhonchi Loud, whistling sounds heard on auscultation of the chest.

Role confusion Failure to achieve recognition of the unconscious self.

Roughage High-fiber foods.

Sagittal In an anteroposterior direction, i.e., left and right.

Satiety Fullness.

Second childhood A return to childish ways that characterizes the senile adult.

Self-image The way a person perceives himself or believes himself to be.

Senescence Old age.

Senile Aging. In Theodore Lidz's division of old age, the senile period is the last, and is also termed second childhood.

Sensation The part of the perception process in which stimuli strike the sensory end organ of the receiver.

Sensory alteration A state of changed perception that occurs when an individual is exposed to an environment very different from what he is used to.

Sensory deprivation A decrease in the amount or intensity of the stimuli available to the senory organs.

Sensory distortion A state where sensory stimuli are presented out of the usual time or spatial sequence.

Sensory integrity Awareness of stimuli.

Sensory system A system based on the ability to receive mental impressions through the sense organs and to organize the stimuli received.

Sensory underload A state where sensory stimuli are inadequate or monotonous.

Shivering Trembling from excessive cold.

Side effects Consequences other than the intended therapeutic effects for which a drug is prescribed.

Side-lying Lying on one's side; the lateral position.

Sigmoid colon Lower area of the large intestine which temporarily stores the residual waste products of the body as feces.

Sitz bath A therapeutic soak where the patient sits in a small tub with his legs outside.

Sleep A natural, periodically recurring physiological state of rest.

Sleep apnea Periods of cessation of breathing during sleep.

SOAP Acronym for Subjective data, Objective data, Assessment, and Plan. SOAP represents a systematic format for writing progress notes used in the problem-oriented record.

Social immobilization Restraint of normal human interaction caused by physical confinement.

Somatic Physical, bodily.

Somatization The attempt to resolve conflicts and prevent anxiety by the development of physical symptoms in areas of the body controlled by the autonomic nervous system, such as the internal organs.

Somatotropic hormone A hormone which regulates growth, influences fracture healing, lowers blood cholesterol, and stimulates tissue healing. Also called growth hormone.

Stryker frame A device, consisting of two frames with a pivot device at each end, which allows for the turning of the patient.

Stupor A state of seemingly total loss of consciousness.

Subcutaneous Under the skin.

Sublimation The channeling of strong urges such as hunger or aggression into constructive purposes.

Somnambulism Sleepwalking.

Source-oriented Divided according to origin. Source-oriented hospital records separate the patient's history and treatment according to the doctor's observations, nurses' observations, lab reports, etc., with no attempt to integrate.

Specific gravity An indicator of the kidney's ability to concentrate and dilute urine.

Sphygmomanometer A device which measures blood pressure.

Splint A device which prevents joint movement or fixes a movable part in position.

Splinting The application of a device to prevent movement of a joint or to fix a movable part.

Spores Small structures which protect the microorganism from outside elements and also permit it to reproduce.

Stages of sleep A repeating pattern of four phases of intensity of sleep, detectable by EEG tracings.

Staphylococcus A genus of bacteria found on the skin, in skin glands, on the nasal and mucous membranes, and in a variety of foods.

Sterilization The destruction of microorganisms by one of several means, such as steam.

Steroids Chemical substances, both natural and man-made, including many hormones, vitamins, and body constituents.

Stethoscope An instrument for listening to sounds within the body.

Stool softener Medication which serves to lubricate the fecal mass and prevent the loss of water.

Streptococcus A genus of bacteria found in the mouth and intestines, in dairy and other food products, and in fermenting plant juices.

Stress Any internal or external influence which interferes with satisfaction of basic needs or with homeostasis; "wear and tear" on the body.

Stress incontinence A form of incontinence that occasionally occurs when intra-abdominal pressure increases.

Stressors The agents of stress that bring about structural and chemical changes.

Stroke volume Amount of blood ejected per heartbeat.

Sublingual administration The giving of medication under the tongue.

Suctioning The process of aspirating fluids.

Superego The operating conscience.

Superficial Located on or near the surface.

Supine Lying on the back.

Suppression The conscious exclusion from awareness of unacceptable, inappropriate thoughts, memories, or impulses.

Symbiotic An agent-host relationship where both the agent (the microorganism) and the host (the body) benefit.

Symbolization A representation of an object, idea, or act.

Sympathy The third phase in the nurse-patient relationship, when the nurse is concerned about the patient's distress.
Synergistic effects The consequences of taking two or more drugs at the same time.

Tachypnea Excessively fast breathing.
Tapotement A technique used in giving a massage. The edge of the hand is used in a hacking motion over the back.
Taste-smell system The sensory system involved in eating, including receptors of the nose and mouth.
Temperature Degree of heat intensity.
Termination The fourth phase of the nurse-patient relationship, when the patient prepares to leave the nurse's care.
Therapeutic Curative.
Therapeutic effects The desired results for which a drug is prescribed.
Therapeutic hypothermia Deliberate lowering of body temperature for a therapeutic purpose.
Thermometer Temperature-measuring device.
Thoracentesis Removal of chest fluid using a trocar and cannula.
Thorax The closed cavity in which the lungs are contained.
Three-point gait A crutch-walking technique where the weight is shifted to the uninvolved extremity while the crutches are advanced.
Thrombus Clot in a blood vessel or in one of the cavities of the heart.
Tidal volume The amount of air inhaled and exhaled in normal breathing.
Topical medications Ointments, lotions, and solutions applied to the skin surface.
Torsion Twisting, rotation.
Toxin Poisonous substance within a cell or tissue.
Trace minerals Those minerals of which the body needs only small amounts, such as cobalt and copper. Also called microminerals.
Tracheostomy The formation of a slit in the trachea.
Traction A pulling force created by various means.
Transactional Interpersonal, involving common experience and mutual influence.
Transition The first psychological stage of illness, characterized by the onset of noticeable signs and symptoms.
Transverse Crosswise; upper and lower.
Trendelenburg's position A supine position where the pelvis is higher than the head.
Treponema pallidum A parasite which causes syphilis.
Two-point gait A crutch-walking technique where the left crutch and right foot are advanced together.

Unconscious motivation An unrecognized rationale for behavior.
Underweight Weighing less than what is considered the acceptable range for height, age, and sex.
Undoing An attempt to negate previous behavior and cancel a painful feeling.
Urticaria An eruption of itching hives.

Venous spasm An involuntary contraction of the veins resulting from administration of cold or irritating solution.
Ventilation The exchange between ambient and alveolar air that takes place in the lungs.
Vertical planning The timing of nursing activities to coordinate with the patient's biological rhythms as well as the activities of other staff members.
Vibration A technique for removing lung secretions in which the nurse presses the patient's thorax downward, then releases the pressure after the patient exhales.
Visual system The sensory system which functions in accommodation, pupillary adjustment, fixation, convergence, and exploration.
Vital signs Bodily functions that are basic indicators of a person's physical status.
Vitamin Any of many complex organic substances found in foods and vital to health. Fruits and vegetables contain many vitamins.
Vitamin A The vitamin needed for growth, normal vision, and healthy skin. Found in dark green and deep yellow fruits and vegetables.
Vitamin B The vitamin group important for maintenance of mucous membranes and other body surfaces. Includes thiamine, riboflavin, pyridoxine, and cyanocobalamin.
Vitamin C The vitamin needed for healthy gums and body tissues, found in citrus fruits and green leafy vegetables.
Vitamin D The vitamin necessary for proper bone growth and structure, obtained from sunshine and from enriched milk.
Voice action Modification of a message by tone of voice.
Vomiting Regurgitation of matter from the stomach through the mouth.

Water A liquid composed of hydrogen and oxygen.
Water bed A bed featuring a nylon mattress filled with water, which allows for minimal pressure on the patient's skin.
Wheezes High-pitched, continuous sounds heard on chest auscultation.
Working The second phase of the nurse-patient relationship, when the patient begins to come to grips with his experience.

Young adult A person between the ages of approximately 18 and 30.

Index